Clinical Doppler Ultrasound

Content Strategist: Michael Houston
Content Development Specialist: Poppy Garraway
Content Coordinator: Trinity Hutton
Project Manager: Umarani Natarajan
Design: Miles Hitchen
Illustration Manager: Jennifer Rose
Illustrator: Hardlines/Antbits
Marketing Manager: Abigail Swartz

3rd Edition

Clinical Doppler Ultrasound

Myron A. Pozniak, MD, FACR, FSRU, FARS
Professor of Radiology
Department of Radiology
University of Wisconsin School of Medicine and Public Health
Madison, WI
USA

Paul L. Allan, BSc, DMRD, FRCR, FRCPE
Consultant Radiologist and Director of Imaging Services
Department of Radiology
Royal Infirmary of Edinburgh
Edinburgh
UK

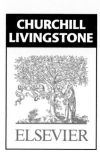

CHURCHILL
LIVINGSTONE

ELSEVIER

Edinburgh   London   New York   Oxford   Philadelphia   St Louis   Sydney   Toronto   2014

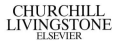

CHURCHILL
LIVINGSTONE
ELSEVIER

Second edition 2006
First edition 2000

The right of Myron A. Pozniak and Paul L. Allan to be identified as authors of this work has been asserted by them in accordance with the Copyright, Designs and Patents Act 1988.

Notices
Knowledge and best practice in this field are constantly changing. As new research and experience broaden our understanding, changes in research methods, professional practices, or medical treatment may become necessary.

Practitioners and researchers must always rely on their own experience and knowledge in evaluating and using any information, methods, compounds, or experiments described herein. In using such information or methods they should be mindful of their own safety and the safety of others, including parties for whom they have a professional responsibility.

With respect to any drug or pharmaceutical products identified, readers are advised to check the most current information provided (i) on procedures featured or (ii) by the manufacturer of each product to be administered, to verify the recommended dose or formula, the method and duration of administration, and contraindications. It is the responsibility of practitioners, relying on their own experience and knowledge of their patients, to make diagnoses, to determine dosages and the best treatment for each individual patient, and to take all appropriate safety precautions.

To the fullest extent of the law, neither the Publisher nor the authors, contributors, or editors, assume any liability for any injury and/or damage to persons or property as a matter of products liability, negligence or otherwise, or from any use or operation of any methods, products, instructions, or ideas contained in the material herein.

ISBN: 9780702050152
e-book ISBN: 9780702055379

Printed in China
Last digit is the print number: 9 8 7 6 5 4 3 2 1

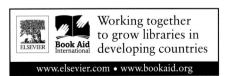

Working together
to grow libraries in
developing countries

www.elsevier.com • www.bookaid.org

Contents

Video Table of Contents

Access all videos online at expertconsult.com. See inside front cover for activation code.

Preface

It has been almost 20 years since the original proposal for a book dealing with Clinical Doppler Ultrasound evolved into reality. It was designed as a practical introduction to the principles and practice of Doppler ultrasound in the clinical setting. Progressive advances in the science and technology of ultrasound and Doppler require continuing revision of the original text, now entering its third edition.

In this edition we have remained true to our initial philosophy – to provide practical information and guidelines on the applications and limitations of Doppler ultrasound. Our contributors all have significant experience in diagnostic ultrasound and all of the chapters have been re-written to incorporate more recent knowledge and developments. This edition features a new chapter on intraoperative and interventional applications of Doppler. The Doppler evaluation of dialysis grafts has so evolved that it now appears as a separate chapter. The images have been updated and expanded; the references brought up to date.

Computed tomographic angiography and magnetic resonance angiography continue their evolution, but the authors remain convinced of the importance of Doppler ultrasound in the investigation of vascular disorders. With the continuing miniaturisation and decreasing cost of ultrasound technology, its distribution into the hands of the clinicians now gives the patient benefit of a more timely diagnosis, provided the practitioner is properly trained in the use of their new device. It is important that those performing Doppler ultrasound examinations have a clear understanding of the underlying principles of this powerful tool, and that continues to be our motivation in creating this book.

We dedicate this book to our families who endured our disappearing from them as we worked incessantly on this new edition. We thank our sonographers and technologists, together with our colleagues, for providing support, tolerating our demanding pursuit of quality and providing the occasional image and advice. We encourage you, the reader, to be a persistent practitioner of Doppler and to understand the underlying principles. It is only with constant use that you will evolve comfort and expertise with the modality. Eventually, these waveforms will sing to you (your ears are the most sensitive spectrum analyser available) and your patients will be the ultimate beneficiaries.

Myron Pozniak
Paul Allan

List of Contributors

Paul L. Allan, BSc, DMRD, FRCR, FRCPE
Consultant Radiologist and Director of Imaging Services, Department of Radiology, Royal Infirmary of Edinburgh, Edinburgh, UK

Lauren F. Alexander, MD
Assistant Professor, Department of Radiology, University of Alabama at Birmingham, Birmingham, AL, USA

Jonathan D. Berry, BSc, FRCR
Consultant Radiologist, Department of Radiology, North Cumbria University Hospitals Cumberland Infirmary, Newtown Road, Carlisle, UK

Peter N. Burns, PhD
Professor of Medical Biophysics and Imaging University of Toronto, Sunnybrook Health Sciences Centre, Toronto, ON, Canada

Michael T. Corwin, MD
Director of Body MRI, University of California, Davis Medical Center, Department of Radiology, CA, USA

Peter R. Hoskins, PGCert, BA, MSc, PhD, DSc
Professor of Medical Physics and Biomechanics, Centre for Cardiovascular Science, University of Edinburgh, Edinburgh, UK
Adjunct Professor of Medical Imaging, Department of Mechanical, Aeronautical and Biomedical Engineering, University of Limerick, Limerick, Ireland

Mark E. Lockhart, MD, MPH
Professor, Department of Radiology, University of Alabama at Birmingham, Birmingham, AL, USA

W. Norman McDicken, PhD, FIPEM
Emeritus Professor Medical Physics and Medical Engineering, Medical Physics, The University of Edinburgh, Edinburgh, UK

John P. McGahan, MD
Vice Chair and Director of Abdominal Imaging, University of California, Davis Medical Center, Department of Radiology, Sacramento, CA, USA

Imogen Montague, MB ChB, FRCOG, DOU
Fetal-Maternal Medicine Consultant, Obstetrics and Gynaecology, Plymouth University Hospitals NHS Trust, Plymouth, UK

Fred T. Lee, Jr, MD
Professor of Radiology, Department of Radiology, University of Wisconsin School of Medicine and Public Health, Madison, WI, USA

Fred Lee, Sr
Rochester Urology, PC, Rochester Hills, MI and Crittenton Hospital, Rochester Hills, MI, USA

Myron A. Pozniak, MD, FACR
Professor of Radiology, Chief of Body CT, Department of Radiology, University of Wisconsin School of Medicine and Public Health, Madison, WI, USA

Michelle L. Robbin, MD
Professor Department of Radiology, University of Alabama at Birmingham, Birmingham, AL, USA

Paul S. Sidhu, BSc, MRCP, FRCR
Professor of Imaging Sciences, King's College London, Department of Radiology, King's College Hospital, Denmark Hill, London, UK

Therese M. Weber, MD, FACR
Professor, Department of Radiology, University of
Alabama at Birmingham, Birmingham, AL, USA

Michael J. Weston, MB ChB, FRCR, MRCP
Consultant Radiologist, Ultrasound Department,
St James's University Hospital, Leeds, UK

Heidi R. Umphrey, MD
Assistant Professor, Department of Radiology,
University of Alabama at Birmingham,
Birmingham, AL, USA

Chapter 1

Physics: Principles, Practice and Artefacts

W. Norman McDicken and Peter R. Hoskins

A number of techniques have been developed which exploit the shift in frequency of ultrasound when it is reflected from moving blood. This frequency shift is known as the 'Doppler effect'.[1] Five types of diagnostic Doppler instrument are usually distinguished:

1. Continuous wave (CW) Doppler
2. Pulsed wave (PW) Doppler
3. Duplex Doppler
4. Colour Doppler imaging (CDI; colour velocity imaging, colour flow imaging)
5. Power Doppler imaging.

The characteristics of an ultrasound beam, the propagation of ultrasound in tissue and the design of transducers as found in B-mode imaging are all relevant for Doppler techniques.[2-6]

The Doppler Effect and Its Application

For all waves such as sound or light the Doppler effect is a change in the observed frequency of the wave because of motion of the source or observer. This is due either to the source stretching or compressing the wave or the observer meeting the wave more quickly or slowly as a result of their motion. In basic medical usage of the Doppler effect, the source and observer (receiver) are a transmitting and a receiving element usually positioned next to each other in a hand-held transducer (Fig. 1-1A). A continuous cyclic electrical signal is applied to the transmitting element and therefore a corresponding CW ultrasound beam is generated. When the ultrasound is scattered or reflected at a moving structure within the body, it experiences a Doppler shift in its frequency and returns to the receiving (detecting) element. Reflected ultrasound is also detected from static surfaces within the body but it has not suffered a Doppler shift in frequency. After the reflected ultrasound is received, the Doppler instrument separates the signals from static and moving structures by exploiting their different frequency.

Motion of the reflector towards the transducer produces an increase in the reflected ultrasonic frequency, whereas motion away gives a reduction. The system electronics note whether the detected ultrasound has a higher or lower frequency than that transmitted and hence extract information on the direction of motion relative to the transducer.

When the line of movement of the reflector is at an angle θ to the transducer beam, then the Doppler shift, f_D, is given by:

$$f_D = f_t - f_r = f_t . \frac{2.u.}{c} \cos\theta$$

where f_t is the transmitted frequency, f_r is the received frequency, c is the speed of ultrasound and $u.\cos\theta$ (i.e. $u \times \text{cosine}\theta$) is the component of the velocity of the reflecting agent along the ultrasonic beam direction. For a typical case of blood flow in a superficial vessel:

Transmitted frequency, $f_t = 5$ MHz $= 5 \times 10^6$ Hz
Velocity of sound in soft tissue, $c = 1540$ m/s
Velocity of blood movement, $u = 30$ cm/s
Angle between ultrasonic beam and direction of flow, $\theta = 45°$

The Doppler shift is therefore:

$$f_D = (5 \times 10^6 \times 2 \times 30 \times \cos 45)/154\,000$$
$$= 1372\text{Hz}$$

The shift in frequency is small and within the audible range. In an ultrasonic Doppler instrument, the

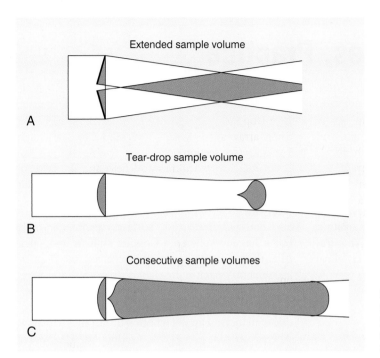

FIGURE 1-1 Sample volumes in Doppler techniques. (A) For dual crystal continuous wave Doppler unit. (B) For pulsed wave Doppler unit. (C) Neighbouring sample volumes along a beam for imaging Doppler units.

electronics are designed to extract the difference in frequency, $f_D = f_t - f_r$ (the Doppler shift frequency). The instrument can therefore feed a signal of frequency f_D to some output device such as a loudspeaker or frequency analyser.

So far we have considered an ultrasound beam being reflected from a structure moving at a fixed speed and hence generating a Doppler shift of one particular frequency. In practice, there are many reflecting blood cells and their speeds are different. The ultrasound signals returned to the detector from the different cells therefore have suffered different Doppler shifts and add together to give a complex signal containing a range of frequencies. The Doppler shift frequencies are extracted from the detected complex signal and can be fed to a loudspeaker where they can be interpreted by listening. High-frequency (high-pitch) components in the audible sound are related to high speeds, whereas low-frequency components correspond to low speeds. Strong signals, namely those of loud audible volume, correspond to strong echoes that have received a Doppler shift. Strong signals could be due to the detection of many blood cells, say in a large vessel, or to echoes from

tissue. An output display called a spectral display or spectrogram is often used to portray the frequency content of Doppler signals.

In the PW Doppler technique, the electrical excitation signal is applied to the transmitter element at regular intervals as pulses, each containing typically 10 cycles, and therefore a corresponding train of pulses of ultrasound are transmitted, separated by non-transmission intervals of duration around 20 times that of each pulse. Regularly spaced echoes are then received back from a reflector and they can be regarded as samples of the signal which would be received if a continuous wave had been transmitted. If the reflector is moving the system electronics can extract a Doppler shift signal from the samples. The Doppler equation again applies to this Doppler shift and can be used to calculate the speed of the reflector.[7]

A bonus of PW Doppler is that since pulsed ultrasound is employed, the range of the moving target may be measured from the echo-return time, as well as its speed from the Doppler shift. The range can be measured from one echo signal; however, the calculation of the Doppler shifts and hence speed of the reflector, typically requires 50–100 echoes. As in the CW case, a group of blood cells moving with different velocities produces a range of Doppler shift frequency components in the output signal.

It was noted above that the frequency of reflected ultrasound is shifted upward or downward depending on whether the motion of the reflector is toward or away from the transducer. A numerical example illustrates this point and emphasises the small changes in frequency that the instrument must distinguish. When 2 MHz ultrasound is reflected from an object travelling at 30 cm^{-1} toward the transducer, it returns to the receiver with a frequency of 2.00078 MHz, a shift of +0.00078 MHz. If the object moves at 30 cm^{-1} away from the transducer, the ultrasound returns with a frequency of 1.99922 MHz, a shift of −0.00078 MHz. Virtually all Doppler instruments which measure velocity preserve this direction information.

Continuous and Pulsed Wave Doppler Instruments

Doppler blood flow instruments are required to be extremely sensitive and to be capable of detecting weak signals from moving blood in the presence of much stronger signals from static or moving tissues; the latter give rise to low-frequency Doppler shift 'clutter' signals. The magnitude of the scattered signal from blood is typically 40 dB below that received from soft tissues, i.e. the blood echo amplitude is typically one hundredth of the soft tissue echo amplitude. The dB (decibel) unit is a measure of the size of a signal relative to another signal; the second signal is often a reference signal or perhaps the input signal to an amplifier to which the output is compared. Blood flow signals may be detected even though the vessel is not clearly depicted, for instance in the fetal brain, or the renal artery of the neonate.

The transducer of a basic CW Doppler unit has two independent piezoelectric elements. Since the transmitting element is continually driven to generate a continuous wave of ultrasound, a second element is used to detect the reflected ultrasound. When a CW Doppler mode is implemented as part of an ultrasound system which uses array transducers, separate groups of array elements are used for transmission and reception. On extraction of the Doppler shift frequency a

filter, the 'wall thump' filter, is often used to remove large, low-frequency components from the signal, such as those from slowly moving vessel walls. Typically in a Doppler unit operating at 5 MHz, Doppler shift frequencies below 100 Hz are removed by filtering. Basic CW Doppler instruments are small and inexpensive; CW Doppler mode facilities are incorporated into some array systems to allow them to detect high velocities (see section on Aliasing artefact, below).

The transmitted ultrasound field and the zone of maximum receiving sensitivity overlap for a particular range in front of the transducer (Fig. 1-1A). Any moving structure within this region of overlap will contribute a component frequency to the total Doppler signal. The shape of the region of overlap (the beam shape) can be considered as having a crude focus which depends on the field and zone shapes and on their angle of orientation to each other. In practice, the beam shapes are rarely well known for CW Doppler transducers. A 5 MHz blood flow instrument might be focused at a distance of 2 or 3 cm from the transducer and a 10 MHz device at a distance of 0.5–1 cm. CW Doppler instruments normally have ultrasonic output intensities (I_{spta}) of less than 10 mW cm^{-2} although they may be significantly higher when used in conjunction with duplex systems to measure high velocities.

A PW Doppler instrument, operating with 5 MHz ultrasonic pulses, may have a pulse repetition frequency (PRF) of 10 000 per second, i.e. 10 kHz. The highest velocity that the instrument can measure is directly proportional to its PRF (see Aliasing artefact, below); therefore the PRF is made as high as possible while still avoiding overlap between successive echo trains. A train of echoes is produced as a transmitted pulse passes through reflecting interfaces and regions of scattering targets. After amplification, successive echo signals from a specific depth are selected by electronic gating and the Doppler shift frequency is extracted as described above.

Pulsed Doppler devices can be used on their own by altering slowly the beam direction or the gated range depth while listening to the output, for example in transcranial blood flow studies. Identification of vessels is made easier by combining the PW Doppler mode with a real-time B-scan mode to form a duplex system; however, this obviously adds to the cost and complexity.

Since the ultrasound is pulsed and the excitation time is short, a stand-alone PW unit uses a single crystal transducer for transmission and reception (Fig. 1-1B). On setting the electronic gate to select a signal from a specific range, reflectors within a volume, known as the sample volume, contribute to the signal. The shape and size of the sample volume are determined by a number of factors: the transmitted pulse length, the beam width, the gated range length, and the characteristics of the electronics and transducer. The sample volume is often described as a tear drop in shape (Fig. 1-1B). Sample volume lengths are usually altered by changing the gated range length. In a blood flow unit for superficial vessels, the sample volume length may be as short as 1 mm, whereas in a transcranial device it can be 1 or 2 cm; however, the precise lengths are rarely known.

The ultrasonic output intensity of pulsed Doppler instruments varies considerably from unit to unit. The intensity (see Safety section, below) may typically be a few hundred $mW\ cm^{-2}$ but can be as high as $1000\ mW\ cm^{-2}$, particularly when they are required to penetrate bone, as in transcranial Doppler. At present the most common use of stand-alone PW units is in transcranial examinations of cerebral vessels.

A summary of technical factors relating to the use of continuous wave and pulsed wave Doppler instruments is given in Box 1-1.

Imaging and Doppler

There are three types of imaging used with Doppler techniques. The first, known as 'duplex Doppler', uses a real-time B-scanner to locate the site at which blood flow is to be examined then a Doppler beam interrogates that site. The second type creates an image from Doppler information, i.e. an image of velocities in regions of blood flow.[8] Known as 'colour Doppler', 'colour flow imaging' or 'colour velocity imaging', it is normally combined with a conventional real-time B-scan so that both tissue structure and areas of flow are displayed. The third type of Doppler imaging is similar to colour Doppler, but generates an image of the power of the Doppler signal from pixel locations throughout the field of view and is known as 'power Doppler imaging' (power Doppler).[9] A power Doppler image depicts the amount of blood moving in each region, i.e. an image of the detected blood pool.

BOX 1-1 TECHNICAL FACTORS IN THE USE OF CW AND PW DOPPLER

1. Doppler beams are subject to the same physical processes in tissue as B-mode beams, i.e. attenuation, refraction, speed of sound variation, defocusing, etc.

2. Since stand-alone CW and PW units are used blind, the beam direction and also the sample volume in the PW case must be systematically moved through the region of interest to maximise both the volume and pitch of the audible Doppler signal.

3. PW Doppler is subject to the aliasing artefact in the measurement of high velocities, CW Doppler is not.

4. The sensitivity (gain, transmit power) of the Doppler unit should not be so high that noise detracts from the signal quality.

5. The instrument should be assessed on normal vessels where the blood flow pattern is known and the expected Doppler signal well understood.

6. The wall-thump filter should just be high enough to remove the strong low-frequency signal from vessel walls and any other moving tissue.

7. The final result in many cases should be a distinct display, called a 'spectrogram' or 'sonogram' (see section on the Spectrum analyser, below), with a clearly defined maximum-velocity trace.

8. Since the beam–vessel angle is unlikely to be known, the sonogram cannot be calibrated in velocity and the vertical axis remains as Doppler shift frequency.

9. Care should be taken to ensure good acoustic coupling between the transducer and the patient. Since there is no associated image it is not always apparent that a weak signal may be due to a lack of coupling agent.

10. If possible, information should be obtained on the shape of the sample volume for both CW and PW beams. The sample volume size can then be related to the size of the vessel under study. With CW Doppler there is very little depth discrimination. With PW Doppler the sample volume depth and size are set by the user.

DUPLEX INSTRUMENTS

Duplex systems link CW or PW Doppler features and real-time B-scanners so that the Doppler beam can interrogate specific locations in the B-scan image (Fig. 1-2). CW duplex is normally only used where very high velocities have to be measured without the aliasing artefact, for example in the estimation of the velocity of a jet through stenosed heart valves. The direction of the CW beam is shown as a line across the B-scan image.

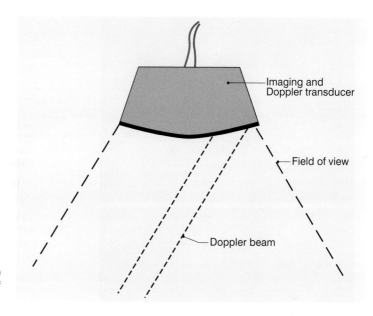

FIGURE 1-2 Duplex system combining real-time B-mode (– – – –) and a Doppler beam (----) of variable position across the B-mode field of view.

In the case of PW Doppler, markers on the beam line show the position of the sample volume. The Doppler beam is often directed across the field of view so that it does not intersect the blood flow at 90°.

In duplex systems, the transmitted ultrasound frequency in the Doppler mode is often lower than that for the B-mode. The low Doppler beam frequency is to enable higher velocities to be handled before aliasing occurs, while the high B-scan frequency is to optimise resolution in the image. An example could be 5 MHz for Doppler and 7 MHz for B-mode when studies of superficial vessels are undertaken.

A summary of technical factors relating the use of duplex Doppler instruments is given in Box 1-2.

COLOUR DOPPLER IMAGING

Pulsed Doppler techniques require between 50 and 100 ultrasonic pulses to be transmitted in each beam direction for the determination of velocities of blood in a sample volume. It is therefore not possible to move the beam rapidly through the scan plane to build up real-time Doppler images of velocity of flow. Such imaging became possible when signal processing was developed which could quickly produce a measure of mean blood velocity at each sample volume from a small number of ultrasonic echo pulses. A technique called 'autocorrelation processing' of the signals

from blood quickly gives the mean velocity in each small sample volume along the beam (Fig. 1-1C). This real-time colour Doppler imaging processes between 2 and 16 echo signals from each sample volume. In addition, the direction of flow is obtained by examining the signals for the direction of the shift as for CW and PW Doppler devices. Each image pixel is then

BOX 1-2 TECHNICAL FACTORS IN THE USE OF DUPLEX DOPPLER

1. The factors quoted above for CW and PW Doppler may also be relevant.

2. A spectrogram can be obtained from a known vessel and a known location within the vessel.

3. The Doppler beam may be refracted and not pass along the line shown in the B-mode image.

4. The beam–vessel angle may be measured manually, allowing blood velocity to be estimated.

5. Simple estimates of blood flow rate may be obtained from the measured diameter and mean velocity.

6. Spectral broadening due to the use of wide aperture transducers to give good focusing can cause large errors in the measurement of maximum velocity.

7. Since the Doppler beam is held fixed and the PRF is high, particular attention should be paid to the outputs of PW units in relation to safety.

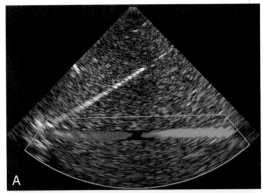

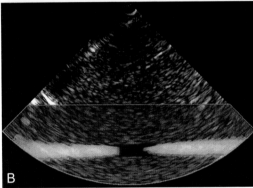

FIGURE 1-3 (A) Colour flow image of flow from left to right in a straight tube. When the flow velocity component is along the beam towards the transducer it is colour-coded red, when the component along the beam is away from the transducer it is coded blue. (B) Power Doppler image of flow in a straight tube. Direction of flow is not measured so it is not colour-coded.

colour-coded for direction in relation to the transducer and mean Doppler shift (Fig. 1-3A).

B-scanning and Doppler imaging are carried out with the common types of real-time transducer. Echo signals from the blood and tissues are processed along two signal paths in the system electronics (Fig. 1-4). Going along one path, the signals produce the real-time B-scan image; going along the other path, autocorrelation function processing and direction flow sensing are employed to give a colour flow image. An important exclusion circuit in the autocorrelation path separates large-amplitude signals which arise from tissue and excludes them from the blood velocity processing. The B-mode and mean velocity images are then superimposed in the final display. Strictly speaking, the flow image is of the mean Doppler shift frequency and not

the mean velocity, since the beam–vessel angles throughout the field of view are not measured. Colour shades in the image can indicate the magnitude of the velocity, for example light red for high velocity and dark red for low velocity. Turbulence, related to the range of velocities in each sample volume, may be presented as a different colour or as a mosaic of colours.

Doppler images typically contain about 64 genuine lines of information and 128 consecutive sample volumes along each line. The frame rate varies from 5 to 40 frames per second, depending on the depth of penetration and the width of the field of view. As in B-scanning, the appearance of the image is usually improved by inserting additional lines or frames whose data are calculated from the genuine lines, a process known as interpolation. Alteration in flow can occur rapidly over the cardiac cycle, therefore a

BOX 1-3 TECHNICAL FACTORS IN THE USE OF COLOUR DOPPLER IMAGING

1. The mean Doppler frequency shift is the quantity which is presented in a colour-coded form in each pixel. When the colour bar is labelled in velocity the beam–vessel angle has been assumed to be zero throughout the image.

2. The velocity component along the Doppler beam is heavily dependent on the angle between the direction of flow and the beam direction (the cosine θ dependence). The colours depicted in the image are therefore heavily angle dependent.

3. The flow pattern on the colour Doppler display can be related to the structures shown in the B-mode image.

4. Colour Doppler imaging is a pulsed technique so aliasing is a problem.

5. A good colour Doppler machine is one which discriminates well between signals from tissue and those from blood.

6. The colour Doppler field of view box should be adjusted to cover only the region of interest and therefore maximise the frame rate.

7. The velocity range covered by the colour scale should be carefully matched to the velocities expected in the study.

8. A cine-loop is useful for the review of fast-changing blood flow patterns.

9. A change in the colour registered in a vessel from, say, blue to red may not mean a change in the direction of flow along a vessel. It may merely mean the beam–flow angle has changed from less than 90° to more than 90°.

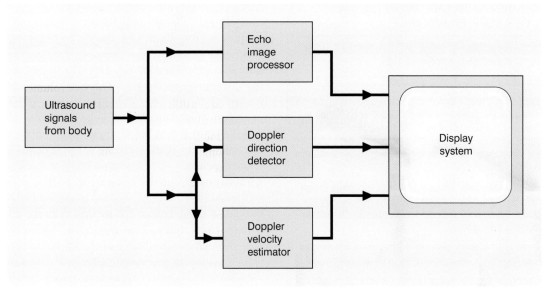

FIGURE 1-4 B-mode and Doppler imaging signal processing paths in a scanning machine.

cine-loop store of say the last 128 frames is of value for review purposes. Doppler spectrograms can be made by selecting the appropriate beam direction and sample volume location in the image and then switching to the PW or CW mode. PW and CW Doppler techniques provide more detailed information on blood velocities than colour Doppler, so spectral information is still of value.

A summary of technical factors relating to the use of colour Doppler imaging is given in Box 1-3.

POWER DOPPLER IMAGING

The power of the Doppler signal from each small sample volume in the field of view may be displayed rather than the mean frequency shift (Fig. 1-3B). The power of the signal from each point relates to the number of moving blood cells in that sample volume. The power Doppler image may be considered to be an image of the blood pool. The power mode does not measure velocity or direction and therefore the image shows little angle dependence, nor does it suffer from aliasing; however, it obviously presents less information about blood flow. The attraction of power Doppler images is that they suffer less from noise than velocity images, as the power of the background noise for any sample volume with no blood flow signal is less than the power of the background noise plus Doppler signal when blood flow is present. The background noise may be used to set a threshold above which signals are accepted for Doppler flow. Noise from sample volume regions lacking blood flow is therefore reduced in the power image by a threshold detector. However, when the same signal is used in the velocity imaging mode, the noise will produce a mean velocity value which the machine will treat as a genuine blood velocity and which will therefore appear in the image. The power Doppler mode is therefore less prone to noise and hence more sensitive and can be used to detect small vessels. Further sensitivity can be obtained by averaging power images over several frames to reduce spuriously distributed noise even more. In velocity imaging there is interest in showing quick changes in blood flow and hence less averaging is used.

Power Doppler imaging often provides a more complete image of the vasculature than velocity imaging. This has made it popular in clinical use and it is commonly used initially to locate regions of interest prior to investigation by colour Doppler or duplex methods. It is also possible to use the direction

BOX 1-4 TECHNICAL FACTORS IN THE USE OF POWER DOPPLER IMAGING

1. In the power Doppler image, the power of the Doppler signal at each pixel is colour-coded.

2. No velocity information is displayed.

3. The power Doppler signal is direction insensitive; so the display is the same regardless of whether the blood is flowing toward or away from the transducer. However, some systems do display different colours depending on the direction of blood flow by including some directional Doppler information.

4. The power Doppler image is insensitive to angle except near 90° where the Doppler signal may fall below the clutter filter, which cuts out low Doppler shifts, and no signal is displayed.

5. There is no aliasing, because the frequency information (i.e. velocity) is not estimated from the Doppler signal.

6. The power Doppler image is very sensitive to movement of the tissue or probe (the flash artefact). Some machines incorporate a flash filter to try to reduce this effect.

information in the signal to colour-code the corresponding power image.

A summary of technical factors relating to the use of power Doppler imaging is given in Box 1-4.

Ultrasonic Microbubble Contrast Agents

A number of agents have been considered which can enhance the scattering of ultrasound from blood and hence could be employed as echo-enhancing or contrast agents. Ophir and Parker[10] have reviewed contrast agents. From this review and more recent experience it has become obvious that agents in the form of encapsulated microbubbles are by far the most likely to be successful echo-enhancing agents in the immediate future. This is due to the large difference in acoustic impedance between the gas in the bubbles and the surrounding blood. In addition, bubbles of a few microns in diameter have a fundamental resonance frequency of a few megahertz. For example, 4 μm diameter bubbles resonate at 4 MHz, which is well within the range of medical ultrasound systems. Bubbles of these dimensions are important since, even with only very thin wall encapsulation, they are able to pass through the capillaries of the lung into the systemic circulation. An investigation by a committee of the American Society of Echocardiography concluded that contrast echocardiography carried a minimal risk for patients and that there were few residual or complicating side-effects.[11] Other studies have confirmed these conclusions; however, more work is required on new agents as they become available.[12]

The development around 1990 of contrast agent microbubbles that can be used by percutaneous venous injection was the breakthrough which gave rise to the current high level of activity in this field. Table 1-1 gives examples of agents which are currently under commercial development. Large gas molecules are encapsulated in some agents to reduce the rate of diffusion and so increase the lifetime of the bubbles.

TABLE 1-1	**Properties of Some Commercially Available Ultrasound Contrast Agents**					
Agent	**Manufacturer**	**Type of Agent**	**Capsule**	**Gas**	**Bubble Size**	**Concentration**
DEFINITY/ LUMINITY	Lantheus Medical Imaging	Microsphere	Lipid	Octafluoropropane	Mean diameter 1.1–3.3 μm (98% <10 μm)	10×10^8 μ bubbles/mL
OPTISON	GE Healthcare	Microsphere	Albumin	Octafluoropropane	Mean diameter range 3.3–4.5 μm (95% <10 μm)	5–8×10^8 μ bubbles/mL
SONOVUE™	Bracco	Stabilised microbubble	Phospholipids	SF_6	Mean diameter 2.5 μm (90% <6 μm)	2–5×10^8 μ bubbles/mL

By courtesy of CM Moran, University of Edinburgh.

Typically the lifetime in blood ranges from 2–3 min up to 20–30 min. An attraction of contrast agents is the ability to increase the signal obtained from small blood vessels which are difficult to detect by conventional Doppler methods, such as cerebral or renal vessels. There is also interest in perfusion studies, for example to observe and measure the wash-in and wash-out of agent in the myocardium in a manner analogous to nuclear medicine studies.

Enhanced scattering is obtained if a bubble is insonated with ultrasound of a frequency equal to that of the fundamental resonance frequency of the bubble. At low power (that is low ultrasonic wave pressure amplitudes) the oscillations of the bubble are about its centre and are directly in proportion to the size of the pressure fluctuations in the ultrasound wave. However, at higher powers the oscillations become distorted and ultrasound at frequencies different from that of the incident wave is generated by the bubbles. These frequencies are known as harmonics and are simply related to the fundamental resonance frequency of the bubble, so that the second harmonic frequency is twice the fundamental frequency. There is considerable interest in detecting and using the second harmonic, since tissue does not produce this effect to any great extent and the second harmonic signal comes predominantly from the echo-enhancing agent in the blood vessels. Both pulse–echo and Doppler systems have been designed to pick out the second harmonic component in the ultrasound returned to the transducer and use it to enhance the signal from the agent in blood, possibly by as much as 20–30 dB. These systems are being evaluated in clinical practice.[13]

The scattering from contrast agents can also be enhanced if the acoustic pressure fluctuations in the beam are large enough to damage the microbubbles, causing them to leak. An unencapsulated gas bubble then forms next to the original one; however, since it has no outer shell, the scattering from it is undamped and can be around 1000 times higher than that from the encapsulated bubble. This effect has been exploited in a technique known as 'intermittent' or 'transient' imaging, which allows time for the damaged bubbles to be replaced between sweeps of the ultrasound beam.[14]

A summary of technical factors relating to the use of microbubble contrast agents is given in Box 1-5.

Information from Doppler Signals

When the Doppler signal with the information on blood velocities has been obtained, it has to be interpreted. It is essential to obtain good-quality signals in order to be able to detect disease.

THE SPECTRUM ANALYSER

A Doppler signal may be analysed into its frequency components in order to give a display of the velocities of the blood cells at each instant (Fig. 1-5).[2] Short time intervals of the Doppler signal are analysed, for example a segment of 5 ms duration. This produces an instantaneous spectrum of the frequencies in the sample volume for that time period. If an angle correction is then applied, this spectrum will represent the range of velocities in the sample volume. The frequencies in each spectrum are displayed along a vertical line on which the power of each frequency component is presented as a shade of grey. The consecutive velocity spectra are then displayed as side-by-side grey-shade vertical lines. In this way a spectral display, or spectrogram, is built up (Fig. 1-6). Note the difference between the instantaneous velocity spectrum which

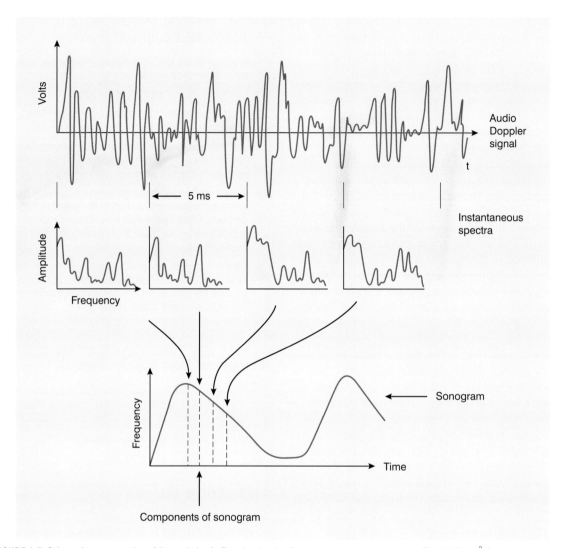

FIGURE 1-5 Schematic representation of the analysis of a Doppler signal to form a sonogram (spectrogram). (From McDicken[2], Copyright Elsevier 1991)

tells us about the pattern of velocities in the sample volume at that instant and the spectral display, or spectrogram, which shows how the velocity pattern varies with time. Spectrograms are generated in real time during the clinical examination and it is usually possible to store a few seconds of the trace in an analyser for subsequent review.

The temporal resolution in a spectrogram, that is the smallest discernible time interval, equals the length of the portion of Doppler signal used to produce each instantaneous spectrum and is typically 5–10 ms. The frequency (or velocity) axis of the spectrogram usually

has about 100 scale intervals each of 100 Hz. The Doppler signal is therefore resolved into frequency components separated by 100 Hz, the frequency resolution of the spectrogram.

It is often desirable to make measurements on a spectrogram, for example an estimate of the time between two events or of the maximum velocity during systole or diastole. Measurement is performed by placing a cursor on the relevant points of interest then a variety of calculations can be performed by the system computer. Indices related to the spectrogram shape and hence to normality or abnormality of flow

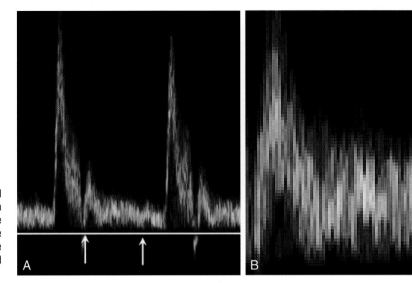

FIGURE 1-6 A normal sonogram (A); (B) a magnified view of the segment between the arrows illustrating the pixel structure and speckle pattern.

velocities can be calculated within the analyser and displayed on its screen. These are discussed later in this chapter. The oscillatory shape of a spectrum or a trace derived from it is often referred to as a waveform.

A summary of technical factors relating to spectral analysis is given in Box 1-6.

Spectrograms (Sonograms) and Indices

A good-quality audible Doppler signal will result in a good-quality sonogram. Degradation of a sonogram is due to electronic and acoustic noise which should only be a problem when the gain of the Doppler unit or analyser is very high for the detection of weak signals. Noise in sonograms creates considerable difficulties for the automatic calculation of quantities and they should therefore be used with caution. If the automatic mode cannot deal with the noise, then the traces should be drawn manually making use of the eye's ability to distinguish the true signal from the noise. It should also be remembered that the vertical axis of a sonogram can only be labelled as velocity after the beam–vessel angle has been measured.

BOX 1-6 TECHNICAL FACTORS IN RELATION TO SPECTRAL ANALYSIS

1. Arrange the frequency and time scales to best display the detailed information in the sonogram by adjusting velocity scale, baseline and sweep speed.

2. Arrange the grey tones, or colours, of the spectral display to give the best 'image' quality by adjusting the Doppler gain.

3. Treat with caution information from weak signals in a noisy background.

4. A clear spectrogram is required before the maximum frequency can be traced.

5. It is usually best to make measurements over at least five heart cycles. However, if this is not possible, perhaps due to respiratory movement, useful information can be obtained from one or two cardiac cycles.

6. Make use of the total storage capacity of the analyser and use the scroll facility to select the most suitable part of the spectrogram to make relevant measurements.

7. Check thoroughly the reliability and accuracy of automatic tracing techniques and calculations derived by the ultrasound system.

8. Note whether the vertical axis has been calibrated in velocity by allowing for the beam–vessel angle.

9. To obtain reproducible results, try to use the same beam–vessel angle for all examinations, e.g. 60°.

WAVEFORM INDICES

Waveform indices are derived from a combination of a few dominant features of the waveform.[3] Indices that have the same or similar names in the literature are occasionally defined differently, so a first step is to check the definition of any index to be used. In practice only two classes of index are used to any great extent, those related to the degree of diastolic flow and others related to spectral broadening. The variation in time of the maximum velocity displayed in a spectrogram is commonly used as a source of data for the derivation of an index (Fig. 1-7). Since the maximum velocity is not always clearly apparent in a spectrogram, some analysers produce a trace which is closely related to the maximum velocity trace. One example is a trace showing the upper velocity boundary below which the velocity components contain seven-eighths of the power of the Doppler signal.

The mean velocity waveform (average velocity waveform) is also employed (Fig. 1-7). To calculate the mean velocity at each instant, the values of velocity and the intensities of the signal for each velocity component in the instantaneous spectrum are used. The mean velocity is used together with the vessel cross-sectional area to calculate blood flow rate. However, it is difficult to measure mean velocity accurately and there are several other problems associated with calculating flow rates; these are discussed further in Chapter 2.

Since the beam–vessel angle may not always be known, the waveforms or spectrograms will not be corrected for angle. Indices are therefore defined involving ratios of velocities. In such a ratio, the angle factors appear on both the top and bottom and hence cancel each other out, so that the index is independent of beam angle. Errors are also reduced by averaging the calculated indices over several heart cycles.

A number of the most commonly encountered indices are briefly discussed below:

A/B Ratio

The A/B ratio is defined as the ratio of two specified velocities, e.g. maximum velocities, at two points in the cardiac cycle (Fig. 1-8). It is usually employed where there is no reverse flow in the waveform.

Resistance Index (RI)

In Fig. 1-8:

$$RI = \frac{S - D}{S}$$

High resistance in the distal vessels produces low diastolic flow in the supplying artery and results in a high value for this index; a low resistance results in a low value as there is higher diastolic flow. It is also known as the Pourcelot index.

Pulsatility Index (PI)

The pulsatility index (PI) is defined as:

$$PI = \frac{\text{maximum velocity excursion}}{\text{mean of the velocity}}$$

This ratio is used in vessels where reverse flow may occur, for example in the lower limbs (Fig. 1-8). The PI may typically have a value of 10 for the normal common femoral artery but be around 2 when proximal disease severely dampens the waveform.

As defined above, the PI index is heart rate dependent. To avoid this, PI can be calculated over a specified time from the start of systole, e.g. for the first 500 ms. The pulsatility index is then labelled 'PI(500)'.

Damping Factor

The damping factor is defined as the ratio of pulsatility indices at two sites along an artery. It quantifies the damping of the waveform downstream along a diseased vessel.

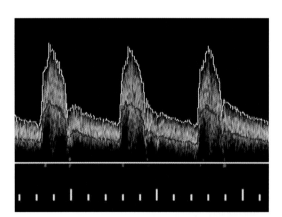

FIGURE 1-7 A spectral waveform showing maximum velocity trace (white) and mean velocity trace (blue).

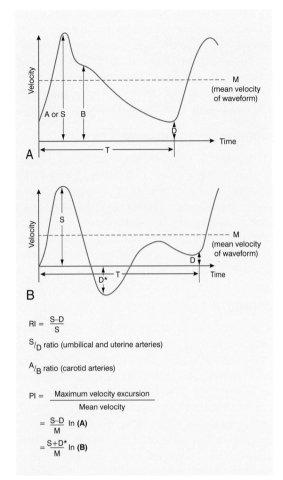

$$\text{Spectral broadening index (at systole)}$$
$$= \frac{\text{maximum velocity}}{\text{mean velocity}}$$

Conclusions with regard to the presence of turbulence should be made with caution and only after familiarity has been gained with the patterns for laminar and plug flow for the particular instrument being used. Other technical factors can cause spectral broadening: for example 'geometrical spectral broadening', which results from the range of Doppler angles which any given blood corpuscle subtends to different points on the face of the transducer.

Transit Time

The time for the pulse pressure wave to travel along a length of artery can be measured by placing a Doppler probe at either end of it. From this time and knowing the length, the pulse wave velocity (PWV) is calculated. Alternatively, using the electrocardiogram (ECG) and one Doppler unit the transit time can also be measured, the QRS of the ECG giving the time when the pressure pulse leaves the heart. The time is first measured for the pulse to travel from the heart to the proximal artery site; a second time is then measured for the pulse to go from the heart to the distal site. Subtracting these two times gives the transit time and, if the length of the artery is known, the PWV can be calculated. Any error associated with the assumption that the QRS represents the time at which the pulse leaves the heart is removed by the subtraction.

A normal aorta has a PWV of around 10 m/s. The transit time along 0.5 m is then 50 ms. Pulse wave velocity depends on disease states of the artery wall and blood pressure. This index is also mentioned for completeness, it is not widely used.

A summary of technical factors relating to waveform analysis is given in Box 1-7.

FIGURE 1-8 Waveform indices, normally calculated from a maximum velocity waveform, but the mean velocity waveform can also be used. (From McDicken[2], Copyright Elsevier 1991)

$$\text{Damping factor} = \frac{\text{PI (proximal site)}}{\text{PI (distal site)}}$$

The numerical value of this index increases as disease becomes more severe, a value of 2 being typical of a high degree of damping. This index is mentioned for completeness, it is not widely used.

Spectral Broadening

Turbulence increases the range of blood cell velocities in a vessel. One index to quantify this broadening of the spectrum of velocities is:

Artefacts in Doppler Techniques

The most important artefacts are mentioned here and methods of dealing with them are suggested. Further details can be found in other texts.[2,5] Artefacts are usually dealt with by explaining their origin or by recognising that they occur fairly frequently and are not of significance.

ATTENUATION

The reduction in echo signal size due to attenuation of the beam in tissue will be familiar from B-mode imaging and the same attenuation processes occur for Doppler techniques, so that stronger signals are detected from superficial vessels than from deep ones. With CW Doppler units this imbalance cannot be compensated. With PW stand-alone and duplex Doppler devices, the signals are from a sample volume at a selected depth and the gain can therefore be adjusted to optimise the signal. In colour Doppler and power Doppler imaging, time gain compensation (TGC) could help to compensate for attenuation but it is more usual just to process all signals that are above the noise level; obviously those from deep vessels will be closer to the noise level and hence will be more likely to be affected by noise.

REFRACTION

Refraction deviates a beam as it crosses at an angle the interface between two tissues in which the speed of sound is different. The direction of the transducer axis may not, therefore, coincide with the actual beam path. With duplex systems a weaker signal than expected from a well-imaged vessel is probably due to refraction of the Doppler beam. This is less of a problem with colour or power Doppler imaging instruments, since the presence of a signal is noted first in the image before any spectral analysis is attempted.

SHADOWING AND ENHANCEMENT

Attenuation of a Doppler beam at a structure may be so large that blood flow behind it cannot be detected, for example at a calcified plaque on a vessel wall. Microbubble contrast agents can also give rise to shadowing problems behind them. Signal enhancement occurs where the beam passes through a medium of low attenuation to reach the vessel, such as a collection of amniotic fluid, or the full bladder.

BEAM WIDTH

A wide beam can cause contributions to the Doppler signal from moving structures well off the central axis. This is most likely to be due to a strong reflector such as a heart valve leaflet, but it could also be due to a large blood vessel. A narrow beam may result in only partial insonation of a vessel with the related errors in the Doppler signal; for example, over-emphasis of the high-velocity flow at the centre of a vessel occurs when a narrow beam is directed into a vessel but does not encompass the slower-moving blood at the side.

SPECTRAL BROADENING

Spectral broadening is another artefact resulting from beam shape. As noted in the discussion on the spectral broadening index, this arises due to the ultrasound beam insonating a sample volume over a range of angles from different points on the transducer face.

OVERESTIMATION OF MAXIMUM VELOCITY

The maximum blood velocity is often of clinical interest since it is of physiological significance and often easy to identify on a spectrogram. However large errors can occur in its measurement if steps are not taken to avoid them. If maximum velocity is measured in the laboratory using a string phantom, which simulates a line of blood cells passing through a sample volume, it is found that the velocity is overestimated (Fig. 1-9A) and the error increases markedly as the angle approaches 90°. As an active array segment has a finite length, typically 20–40% of the full array, so different elements will register different beam–vessel angles and therefore Doppler shifts, as shown in Fig. 1-9B; the elements with the

higher angles will also be more affected by the angle error shown in Fig. 1-9A. The highest Doppler shift and hence the highest measured velocity will be registered by the elements with the smallest beam–vessel angles. Strictly speaking a correction should be applied to allow for the fact that the maximum velocity is not measured by ultrasound travelling along the central axis of the beam, as assumed in the basic Doppler equation, but manufacturers have not adopted this approach. The errors in maximum velocity estimation shown in Fig. 1-9 are typical of modern linear arrays. The errors for phased arrays, which are used in cardiology, are smaller due to their smaller Doppler apertures. In clinical practice with linear arrays, errors are reduced by the use of small angles (typically 45–60°) and by the use of indices employing velocity ratios as described in Fig. 1-8.[15,16]

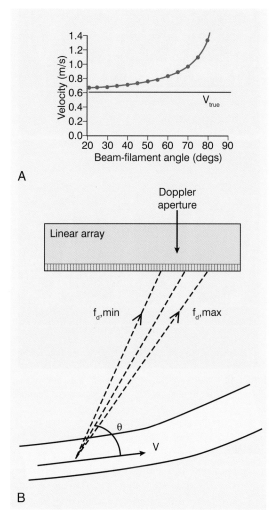

FIGURE 1-9 Overestimation of maximum velocity: (A) Velocity errors measured using a string phantom. The true string velocity is 0.61 m/s but the velocity measured using Doppler ultrasound is overestimated, with the degree of overestimation increasing as the beam-filament angle approaches 90°. (B) Geometrical spectral broadening due to the finite size of the active area of an array. Higher Doppler shifts are received at one end of the Doppler aperture, smaller shifts at the other end. The Doppler system will usually perform angle correction with respect to the centre of the aperture.

SPECKLE AND THE SPECTRAL DISPLAY

The speckled appearance of a sonogram results from fluctuations in the power levels of the velocity components in neighbouring pixels (Fig. 1-6). These fluctuations are due to variations in the ultrasonic signal received from the random distribution of blood cells. Due to this speckle noise, the power level in a pixel cannot be directly related to the number of cells moving with a particular velocity. Averaging the power levels in neighbouring pixels gives a more accurate measure of the number of cells moving with each velocity.

INADEQUATE COUPLING

Weak Doppler signals can be attributed to a lack of coupling medium between the transducer and the skin. In CW and PW Doppler applications this artefact is not as evident as in imaging techniques, where poor penetration is readily seen.

ELECTRICAL PICK-UP

Doppler devices are required to be highly sensitive and are therefore prone to electrical pick-up of stray signals. Some such signals can be recognised by their pattern in the sonogram. The spectrum analyser unit may allow the operator to attempt to clean up the sonogram by deleting spurious signals.

COMPRESSION OF THE SPECTRAL DISPLAY

Information is lost when a sonogram is compressed, either in its grey shades, or in its scale of presentation. A sonogram should be treated as a type of image and therefore presented with optimum grey-shade contrast and spatial detail. The latter means that the velocity and time axis scales should be selected to show detailed structure in the sonogram. The accuracy of measurements from the sonogram will also be affected by poor presentation.

ERRONEOUS DIRECTION SENSING

The direction-sensing circuitry does not always function correctly since its design and implementation are difficult. Flow will then be presented in the wrong direction, either in a sonogram or in a colour Doppler image; if this is suspected then the set-up of the system can be checked by examining a normal artery in which the direction of flow is known.

FILTERING

Filters are used to reduce low frequencies, such as those obtained from arterial walls. Filters also remove information on slow-moving blood but this is not usually a serious problem unless it is desired to measure mean velocity accurately or slow flow specifically (Fig. 1-10).

HARMONIC GENERATION BY LARGE SIGNAL DISTORTION

The harmonics of a frequency are higher multiples of that frequency; for example, harmonics of 100 Hz are 200 Hz, 300 Hz, etc. If a signal is too large to be handled by the electronics it becomes distorted and then contains additional harmonic frequency components. When such a distorted signal is analysed, the harmonics appear at regular frequency intervals in the spectral display. Strong blood flow signals exhibit harmonic components as a higher frequency part of the sonogram above that which would probably be obtained if the gain were reduced (Fig. 1-11).

HIGH OR LOW SENSITIVITY

In colour Doppler and power Doppler imaging, setting up the system with too low a sensitivity causes blood flow signal to be lost. Too high a sensitivity causes spurious echoes to be colour-coded as blood (Fig. 1-12).

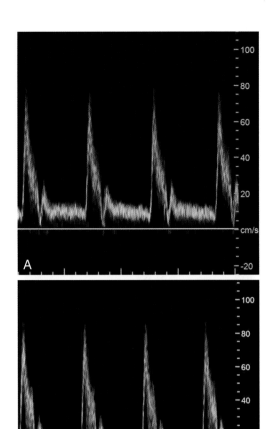

FIGURE 1-10 Filtering. (A) Standard sonogram. Raising the high pass (wall thump) filter (B) removes low-velocity signals and information.

ALIASING

Pulsed Doppler and colour Doppler units have to reconstruct the Doppler shift signal from regularly timed samples of information, rather than the complete signal as used in CW units. The sampling rate is equal to the PRF (pulse repetition frequency) of the Doppler unit. If the sampling rate is too low, less than half the Doppler shift frequency, then the frequency of the reconstructed Doppler signal is in error and the direction of flow is presented wrongly. In a spectral display or flow image, this is known as an 'aliasing' artefact (Figs 1-13 and 1-14).

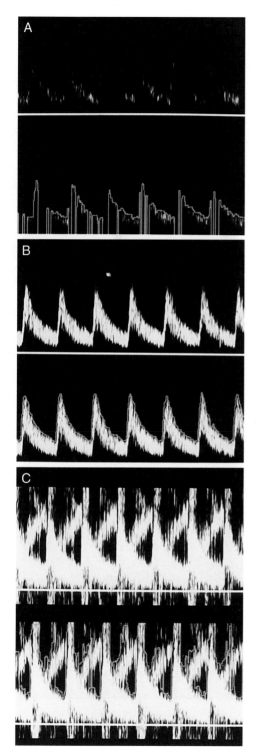

FIGURE 1-11 Increasing gain from (A) to (C). Very high gain distorts the signal and introduces harmonic frequencies.

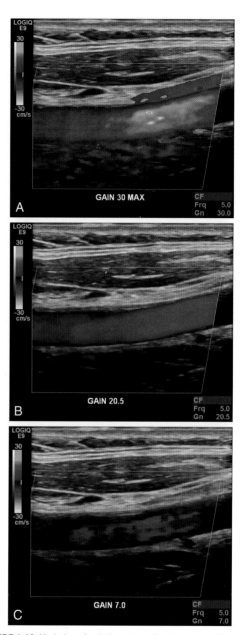

FIGURE 1-12 Variation of gain in a colour Doppler image. The image content is very sensitive to gain setting: (A) shows too much gain; (B) shows a satisfactory gain; (C) shows too little gain.

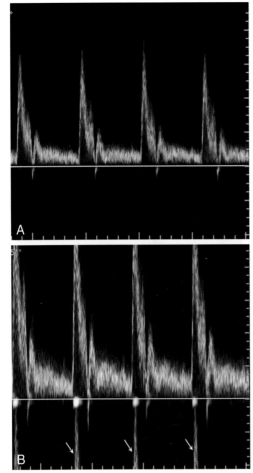

FIGURE 1-13 Aliasing in a sonogram. (A) Satisfactory PRF and spectral display. (B) PRF is too low and the highest velocity signals appear in the reverse channel (arrows).

The aliasing artefact is encountered when high-frequency Doppler shift signals are produced, usually by high-velocity flow. It also occurs when sampling deeper vessels, as the PRF is reduced to allow time for the echoes from a pulse to return before the next pulse is transmitted. If the PRF is too low for the Doppler shift frequencies from the blood in the vessel, aliasing will occur. An approach to raising the velocity level at which aliasing becomes a problem is to use a high PRF (the high-PRF mode), even although the echoes from deep structures have not died out before the next pulse is transmitted. If the deep echoes are strong enough, Doppler signals from deep vessels may then be super-imposed on those from a more superficial site. This uncertainty with regard to the source of the signal is

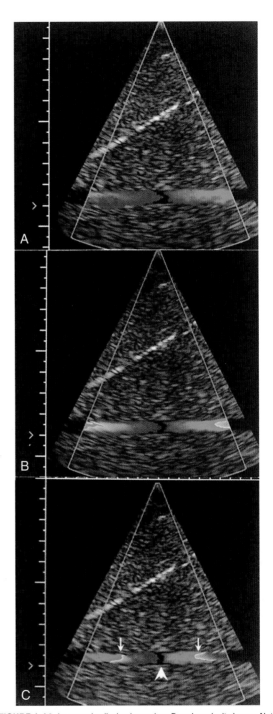

FIGURE 1-14 Increase in aliasing in a colour Doppler velocity image. Note that there is no black space between the red and blue pixels in the lateral colour displays (arrows), indicating that the pixel colour-coding has gone off the top of the red colours and wrapped round to the blue colours. However, there is a black space between the colour displays centrally (arrowhead), indicating reversal of flow direction in relation to the transducer.

referred to as 'range ambiguity'. The ultrasound display will show two or more sample volumes from which data are being analysed and the examination is best performed if only one sample volume is positioned in the vessel, with the others overlying non-vascular structures so that any Doppler shift detected is most likely to come from the vessel. Although this mode can be useful, it also increases the intensity of the beam, which is another reason for using it only when necessary. Aliasing can be of value in colour Doppler imaging since it allows high-velocity jets to be identified. Power Doppler does not suffer from aliasing.

EFFECT OF BEAM ANGLE TO FLOW DIRECTION

The quality of a Doppler signal depends on beam–vessel angle and above 70° it degrades quite rapidly (Fig. 1-15). If the direction of an ultrasound beam is at 90° to the direction of the flowing blood, no Doppler signal is expected since, in the Doppler equation, $\cos 90° = 0$. However, a poor-quality Doppler signal is usually obtained for two reasons. First, the ultrasound beam may converge or diverge slightly from the beam axis, so all of it is never at 90° to the flow. Second, there may be some turbulence in the flow, in which case the blood cells are not all travelling in parallel paths at 90° to the beam.

Colour Doppler images obtained at 90° to the direction of flow appear dark or noisy, corresponding to an absent or small Doppler shift (Fig. 1-3). Power Doppler images are relatively insensitive to angle, except near 90°, where the low Doppler frequencies may fall below the clutter filter and no power signal is displayed (Fig. 1-3).

In a vessel in which the direction of flow alters with respect to the ultrasound beam, different regions of the vessel will be colour-coded differently. Note that this may be due to a genuine change in flow direction as seen in the normal carotid bulb, or merely due to the changing beam angle (see Fig. 4-7) which is particularly common in sector scan imaging.

EFFECT OF VELOCITY SCALE

The choice of velocity scale can dramatically change the appearance of a colour Doppler image (Fig. 1-16). The scale should be chosen to accommodate the range of velocities thought to be present. Too low a scale will cause aliasing and too high a scale results in the flow being depicted as a few dark colours in colour Doppler imaging.

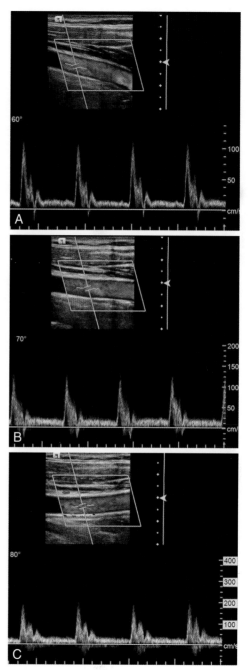

FIGURE 1-15 Variation of quality of signal with beam–vessel angle: (A) at 60°; (B) at 70°; (C) at 80°.

UNEXPECTED MACHINE ARTEFACTS

Doppler technology is developing rapidly and can still have gremlins in it. The operator must therefore check

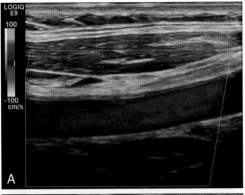

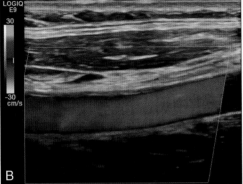

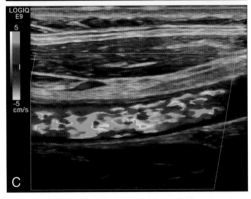

FIGURE 1-16 Effect of changing velocity scale (PRF): (A) scale set too high for flow velocity; (B) satisfactory setting; (C) scale set too low for flow velocity, resulting in aliasing.

artefact in which the maximum velocity measured varies with the beam position in the field of view. This has arisen because the transducer aperture used by the system is a different size in the different positions, resulting in a different amount of spectral broadening.

INTERFERENCE FROM NEIGHBOURING VESSELS

If part or all of a neighbouring vessel in addition to the vessel of interest is within the sample volume of a CW or PW instrument, the Doppler signal will contain a contribution from the extra vessel. Moving the sample volume or redirecting the ultrasound beam to try to interrogate only the vessel of interest may reduce this artefact.

VESSEL COMPRESSION

It is easy to compress superficial vessels by transducer pressure. Increased velocity of flow through the restriction in the compressed vessel results in a higher-pitched Doppler sound or a colour change in an image.

FACTORS AFFECTING THE PATIENT

It is necessary to have as complete a knowledge as possible of the patient's physiological status when undertaking blood flow studies, since many factors affect the cardiovascular system. Examples of these factors are exercise, heart rate, temperature, anxiety, posture, food, smoking and other drugs.

PATIENT OR VESSEL MOVEMENT

If movement causes the sample volume of a CW or PW beam to interrogate a different region, the blood flow signal will obviously be altered. It can be difficult to eliminate this factor, especially in abdominal examinations, and it is not always clear whether respiration has actually affected the flow or just moved the vessel.

FLASH ARTEFACT

Movement of the patient, an organ, or the transducer during Doppler imaging gives tissues a velocity relative

the performance and calibration of the instrument. This is most readily done in a situation where the flow pattern is considered to be well understood, such as in a clearly seen normal blood vessel or a flow test-object. Figure 1-17 shows an unexpected

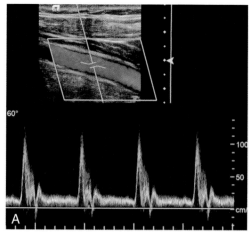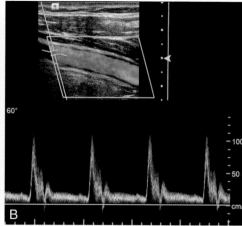

FIGURE 1-17 Variation of sonogram for different beam points of origin. A wider aperture is used towards the centre of an array for better focusing. This increases the range of angles of insonation, producing more spectral broadening (A) compared to a beam from the edge of the array (B).

to the transducer and hence scattered ultrasound is Doppler shifted; a large area of the image is therefore colour-coded for the duration of the movement. This artefact is more severe with power Doppler imaging due to its increased sensitivity.

TWINKLE ARTEFACT

This artefact is seen as an intense, rapidly changing mixture of colour signals behind strongly reflective stationary structures such as renal calculi (see Figs 9-7, 9-8 and 13-24). This artefact is thought to be produced by factors relating to the irregularity of the reflecting media, multiple reflections and tiny random variations in the clock that synchronises pulse transmissions (clock jitter). These factors result in fluctuating returned signals which the electronics present on the display as similar to colour-coded Doppler signals. The effect is highly machine and control setting dependent.[17,18]

BEAM POSITION WITHIN THE VESSEL LUMEN

The Doppler signal obtained from a vessel depends on how the beam insonates the vessel. The effect is less marked if the beam is wider than the vessel. A narrow beam through the centre of a vessel, however, overemphasises the high velocities while a beam through the side of the vessel detects lower velocities.

ONE-DIMENSIONAL SCAN

Blood flow often occurs in an unknown direction in space in relation to the transducer, for example in the heart or at a vessel bifurcation. Detecting the flow from one direction only measures the velocity component along that beam direction. Measurement of the actual velocity in these situations requires components to be measured in three directions not in the same plane. However, when laminar flow occurs in a vessel lying in an imaging scan plane, measurement of one velocity component and the beam–vessel angle permits measurement of the actual velocity.

Safety and Prudent Use of Doppler Instruments

Ultrasound beams transmit energy into tissue so the possibility of hazard has to be considered. The most likely mechanisms for harmful effects are thought to be tissue heating as the ultrasound energy is absorbed, or cavitation in which gas bubbles in the tissue react violently under the influence of the pressure fluctuations of the ultrasound field. The most sensitive structures are considered to be the developing fetus, the brain, the eye, the lung and bone–tissue interfaces.

There is a considerable amount of literature on bioeffects and safety of diagnostic ultrasound.[19] The literature is scrutinised by several national and international bodies who produce statements on safety and the prudent use of ultrasound. Organisations actively monitoring the safety of ultrasound are the World Federation for Ultrasound in Medicine and Biology (WFUMB),[20] the European Federation of Societies for Ultrasound in Medicine and Biology (EFSUMB),[21] the British Medical Ultrasound Society[22] and the American Institute of Ultrasound in Medicine (AIUM). It is still true to say that there are no confirmed harmful effects of diagnostic ultrasound. Often the possibility of an effect is reported but it is not confirmed by further work. There is a need for well-controlled studies but these are increasingly difficult to conduct since unscanned control populations are almost non-existent in the developed world. Although no harmful effects have been confirmed, there is some concern that the outputs of machines have been increasing by factors of as much as 3 or 5 since 1991, as manufacturers seek to produce better B-mode images and more sensitive Doppler units.[23] The situation is summed up in a commentary by ter Haar.[24]

Until the early 1990s, attempts were made to specify the maximum intensities permissible for different clinical applications. This proved to be both limiting and impractical, so the approach now is to use the ALARA principle (As Low As Reasonably Achievable) borrowed from the field of ionising radiations. The user is now informed of the output of the machine and has the responsibility to keep the exposure to a low value which will still give a diagnosis. Many systems now display the output on the screen in terms of a thermal index (TI), related to tissue heating, and a mechanical index (MI), related to the possibility of producing cavitation. These indices are defined in the Output Display Standard (ODS) developed jointly by the AIUM and the National Electrical Manufacturers Association (NEMA) in the USA.[25] The Food and Drug Administration (FDA) in the USA requires adherence to this standard and this is followed by many countries throughout the world. MI is also used to provide a measure of output during contrast agent studies and hence helps to describe the technique. When a new technique is to be implemented clinically, attention should be paid to the TI and MI values used by its developers. Transducer heating was a problem with some devices in the past due to inefficient conversion of electrical energy into acoustic energy. It is worth checking that the transducer face is not hot.

EFSUMB puts out regular statements on safety and currently it says that the use of B-mode is not contraindicated in routine scanning during pregnancy. However, it is more cautious with regard to pulsed Doppler, saying 'routine examination of the developing embryo during the particularly sensitive period of organogenesis using pulsed Doppler devices is considered to be inadvisable at present'.

A summary of technical factors relating the prudent use and safety of ultrasound is given in Box 1-8.

Future Instrumentation

The technical performance of Doppler ultrasound systems is regularly improved by the introduction of new transducers and computer processing algorithms for ultrasonic echo signals. Clinical performance is also improved by increased operator experience and the identification of new applications. The introduction of completely new technology typically occurs at the rate of one or two new instruments per decade.

The production of colour Doppler images by sweeping a single pulsed beam across a scan plane has already been discussed. With this technique the frame rate might typically be 5 to 40 frames s^{-1}. New techniques are being explored to increase frame rates and to overcome angle dependence in the measurement of velocity.

BOX 1-8 TECHNICAL FACTORS AFFECTING PRUDENT USE AND SAFETY

1. Use the lowest transmit power which will give a diagnostic result. This involves keeping the MI and TI less than 1 if possible.

2. Use high receiver gain rather than high output power to achieve high sensitivity.

3. Use the minimum scan time possible.

4. Check that the transducer ceases to transmit when the imaging mode is frozen.

5. Take particular care when a fixed beam direction PW Doppler mode is being used near sensitive tissues.

6. Compare the maximum output values (intensity, power, pressure amplitudes) for your machine to those quoted in the published data from equipment surveys.

7. Safety considerations related to contrast agents need to be studied at frequent intervals during their developmental stage.

Computer control of the excitation of the individual transducer elements and the reception of individual echo signals introduces great flexibility in the production of images. These new techniques allow the generation of frame rates in excess of 100 s^{-1} making it possible to image rapidly changing flow patterns in 2D and to have more useful volume scan rates in 3D.

At an interrogated blood flow site, techniques are being developed to measure velocity components in more than one direction (Fig. 1-18). Beam direction and interrogation sites can be altered very rapidly so that it is possible to interrogate flow sites across the scan plane and measure velocity components in quick succession. From these components the speed and true direction of flow at sites in the scan plane can be calculated, i.e. the velocity vector in the scan plane is obtained for each site. A quantity is called a vector in mathematics when its magnitude (speed in the present case) and direction are known. The velocity vector at each site in a blood vessel is then presented on the display as an arrow whose length is the magnitude of the velocity and whose direction is the direction of flow (Fig. 1-18). High frame rate vector Doppler images are possible because of the speed with which modern electronics can excite transducer elements and computers can process received echoes. High frame rates are very desirable in situations where flow patterns change quickly throughout the cardiac cycle, indeed low frame rates can be very misleading in such situations.

Advanced prototypes have been produced for both high frame rate colour Doppler flow and vector Doppler in blood vessels and the heart. The signal processing is more complex than that usually encountered in ultrasonic imaging and a number of different approaches have still to be evaluated.[26]

THREE-DIMENSIONAL DOPPLER FLOW IMAGING

Just as 2D colour Doppler flow imaging can be performed by scanning an ultrasound beam through a 2D plane, a 3D colour flow image can be produced by scanning a beam through a 3D volume. At present 3D images are often produced by stacking 2D images next to each other, i.e. a series of parallel scans. These images are proving useful for example in the study of flow through a cardiac valve or complex vascular bed (Fig. 1-19).

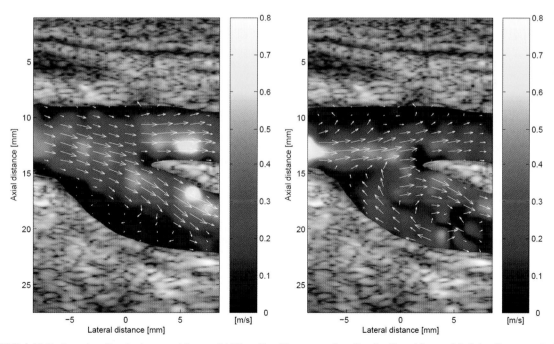

FIGURE 1-18 Vector colour Doppler images of the carotid bifurcation. The arrows show the direction of flow and their length represents the velocity at that point. (By courtesy of J Jensen, DTU Electro, Lyngby, Denmark.)

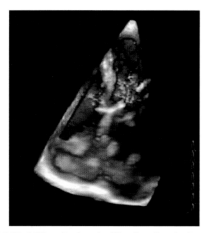

FIGURE 1-19 A 2D projection of a 3D colour Doppler image onto a display screen. The image can be rotated to provide a 3D impression of the flow in the 3D volume scanned. (Courtesy of Philips Medical.)

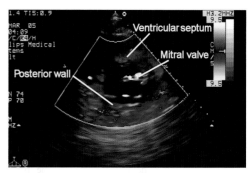

FIGURE 1-20 A longitudinal Doppler tissue image of a section through the left ventricle of the heart.

However true 3D flow imaging would involve measurement of the three velocity components of flow at each sample volume, i.e. at each voxel in the scanned volume. True 3D flow imaging is still at the laboratory development phase and quite far from clinical application.

TISSUE DOPPLER IMAGING

All Doppler instruments can be adapted to study tissue motion rather than blood flow. The echo signals from tissue are larger than from blood and the velocities do not reach the high values encountered in blood flow. Nevertheless the signal processing techniques remain valid for Doppler tissue motion.[27,28] Most commonly it is the myocardium that is studied by both PW Doppler and colour Doppler imaging (Fig. 1-20). The velocity information in 2D tissue Doppler images can be further analysed to give images of strain and strain rate in the myocardium.[29] Doppler tissue techniques have been incorporated in most cardiac imaging instruments.

CATHETER DOPPLER

High-frequency transducers can be miniaturised to dimensions of less than 1 mm making them suitable for insertion into arteries. PW Doppler catheters operating at 20 to 40 MHz have been commercially available for a number of years. The small transducer crystal is designed to transmit ultrasound along the artery in the direction of the axis of the catheter wire.[30]

In practice it can be difficult to know exactly how the ultrasound beam is interrogating the blood flow but high-quality low-noise signals may be obtained due to the catheter being immersed in the blood. Experimental systems have been made which combine Doppler imaging and grey shade B-mode imaging.

REFERENCES

1. White DN. Johann Christian Doppler and his effect – a brief history. *Ultrasound Med Biol* 1982;**8**:583–91.
2. McDicken WN. *Diagnostic Ultrasonics: Principles and Use of Instruments.* London: Churchill Livingstone; 1991.
3. Evans DH, McDicken WN. *Doppler Ultrasound: Physics, Instrumentation and Clinical Applications.* Chichester: Wiley; 2000.
4. Hoskins PR. Measurement of arterial blood flow by Doppler ultrasound. *Clin Phys Physiol Measure* 1990;**11**:1–26.
5. Taylor KJW, Burns PN, Wells PNT. *Clinical Applications of Doppler Ultrasound.* New York: Raven Press; 1988.
6. Fish P. *Physics and Instrumentation of Diagnostic Medical Ultrasound.* Chichester: Wiley; 1990.
7. Wells PNT. A range-gated ultrasonic Doppler system. *Med Biol Eng* 1969;**7**:641–52.
8. Kasai C, Namekawa K, Koyano A, et al. Real-time two-dimensional blood flow imaging using an autocorrelation technique. *Institute of Electrical and Electronics Engineers Trans Sonogr Ultrasonogr* 1985;**32**:458–64.
9. Rubin JM, Bude RO, Carson PL, et al. Power Doppler US: a potentially useful alternative to mean-frequency based colour Doppler US. *Radiology* 1994;**190**:853–6.
10. Ophir J, Parker KJ. Contrast agents in diagnostic ultrasound. *Ultrasound Med Biol* 1989;**15**:319–33.
11. Bommer WJ, Shah P, Allen H, et al. The safety of contrast echocardiography – report of the Committee on Contrast Echocardiography for the American Society of Echocardiography. *J Am Coll Cardiol* 1984;**3**:6–13.
12. Williams AR, Kubowicz G, Cramer E, et al. The effects of the microbubble suspension SHU 454 (Echovist) on ultrasound-induced cell lysis in a rotating tube exposure system. *Echocardiography* 1991;**8**:423–33.

13. Burns PN, Powers JE, Fritzsch T. Harmonic imaging; new imaging and Doppler method for contrast-enhanced ultrasound. *Radiology* 1992;**182**:142.
14. Porter TA, Xie F. Transient myocardial contrast after initial exposure to diagnostic ultrasound pressures with minute doses of intravenously injected microbubbles. *Circulation* 1995;**92**: 2391–5.
15. Hoskins PR. Measurement of blood velocity, volumetric flow and wall shear rate. *Ultrasound* 2011;**19**:120–9.
16. Oates CP, Naylor AR, Hartshone T, et al. Joint recommendations for reporting carotid ultrasound investigations in the United Kingdom. *Eur J Vasc Endovasc Surg* 2009;**37**:251–61.
17. Kamaya A, Tuthill T, Rubin JM. Twinkling artefact on color Doppler sonography: dependence on machine parameters and underlying cause. *Am J Roentgenol* 2003;**180**:215–22.
18. Rahmouni A, Bargoin R, Herment A, et al. Color Doppler twinkling artefact in hyperechoic regions. *Radiology* 1996;**199**: 269–71.
19. Starritt H, Duck FA. *Safety. Clinical Ultrasound*, vol. 1, 3rd ed. Edinburgh: Churchill Livingstone; 2011 [chapter 4].
20. Barnett SB, Ter Haar GR, Ziskin MC, et al. International recommendations and guidelines for the safe use of diagnostic ultrasound in medicine. *Ulltrasound Med Biol* 2000;**26**: 355–66.
21. Piscaglia F, Nolsøe C, Dietrich CF, et al. The EFSUMB Guidelines and Recommendations on the Clinical Practice of Contrast Enhanced Ultrasound (CEUS): Update 2011 on non-hepatic applications. *Ultraschall Med* 2012;**33**:33–59.
22. http://www.bmus.org/policies-guides/BMUS-Safety-Guide lines-2009-revision-FINAL-Nov-2009.pdf.
23. Henderson J, Willson K, Jago JR, et al. A survey of the acoustic outputs of diagnostic ultrasound equipment in current clinical use. *Ultrasound Med Biol* 1995;**21**:669–705.
24. ter Haar G. Commentary: safety of diagnostic ultrasound. *Br J Radiol* 1996;**69**:1083–5.
25. American Institute of Ultrasound in Medicine/National Electrical Manufacturers Association. *Standard for real-time display of thermal and mechanical acoustic output indices on diagnostic ultrasound equipment.* Rockville, MD: Am Institute of Ultrasound in Medicine; 1992.
26. Hansen KL, Udesen J, Oddershede N, et al. In vivo comparison of three ultrasound vector velocity techniques to MR phase contrast angiography. *Ultrasonics* 2009;**49**:659–67.
27. Anderson T, McDicken WN. Measurement of tissue motion. *Proc Instn Mech Engrs* 1999;**213**(Part H):181–91.
28. McDicken WN, Sutherland GR, Moran CM, et al. Colour Doppler velocity imaging of the myocardium. *Ultrasound Med Biol* 1992;**18**:651–4.
29. Heimdal A, Stoylen A, Torp H, et al. Real-time strain rate imaging of the left ventricle by ultrasound. *J Am Soc Echocardiogr* 1998;**11**:1013–19.
30. Doucette JW, Corl PD, Payne HM, et al. Validation of Doppler guide wire for intravascular measurement of coronary artery flow velocity. *Circulation* 1992;**85**:1899–911.

Chapter 2

Haemodynamics and Blood Flow

Peter R. Hoskins, W. Norman McDicken and Paul L. Allan

Principles of Blood Flow

This section describes the simple principles of blood flow which are of value in understanding the role of Doppler and for performing vascular ultrasound examinations. The underlying principles of fluid mechanics applied to the flow of blood are complex, and discussed in detail in a number of texts including those by McDonald,[1] Caro et al.,[2] Strackee & Westerhof[3] and chapters in the Doppler ultrasound books by Evans et al.[4] and Taylor et al.[5]

The blood vessels carry blood from the heart through the pulmonary and systemic arterial circulations and back to the heart through the venous network. Atheroma develops in the arteries and impedes the flow of blood to a greater, or lesser, extent depending on the degree of obstruction that results from its presence.

TYPES OF FLOW

The two essential flow states are laminar and turbulent. At low velocity, fluid flow is laminar (Fig. 2-1A). This is characterised by the motion of fluid along well-defined paths called streamlines. At very high velocities, fluid flow is turbulent (Fig. 2-1B); particular elements of the fluid no longer travel along well-defined paths, and there is a random component to the motion of the fluid.

Concepts of laminar and turbulent flow first arose from consideration of flow in long straight tubes. It was found that a dimensionless number called the Reynolds number (Re) was useful in characterising the fluid flow. The Reynolds number is defined as:

$$Re = \frac{\rho L V}{\mu}$$

where ρ is the fluid density, L is the vessel diameter, V is the mean velocity and μ is the fluid viscosity. For a wide variety of fluids the transition to turbulence takes place at a value of Re of about 2000. For flow in which Re is about 2000 the fluid flow will alternate between turbulent and laminar. When velocity is increased so that the Re is above the critical value, turbulence will take a small amount of time to develop. During pulsatile flow it is therefore possible for the flow to be laminar at values of Re higher than the critical value, because turbulence does not have time to develop before the blood velocity has decreased.

There is also a third flow state called disturbed flow, which refers to variations in velocity magnitude and direction which occur at low values of Re. The most important example of this is seen with the phenomenon of vortices, which are regions of circulating flow often produced when there is some obvious change in vessel geometry such as a stenosis, or the normal carotid bulb. The pattern of vortex production will change as the degree of stenosis and blood velocity increase. During steady flow at low Re values the vortex will be stable and limited to the region immediately behind the stenosis. At low velocity the fluid flow within the vortex is actually laminar. At higher Re values there will be vortex shedding at regular time intervals. Again this is not strictly turbulence, as the velocity magnitude and direction at any location is not random, but follows a regular pattern. At even higher Re values, the vortex shedding will be combined with the random flow patterns of true turbulence. Vortices which are shed travel a few diameters downstream and eventually die out as their energy is absorbed through viscous losses. During pulsatile flow, vortex shedding may occur for only a portion of the cardiac cycle.

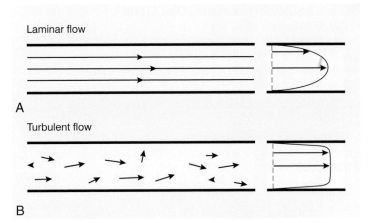

FIGURE 2-1 (A) Laminar flow consists of flow along well-defined streamlines; the velocity profile in a long straight tube under conditions of steady flow is parabolic. (B) The velocity vector magnitude and direction in turbulent flow have random components; the time-averaged profile is blunt.

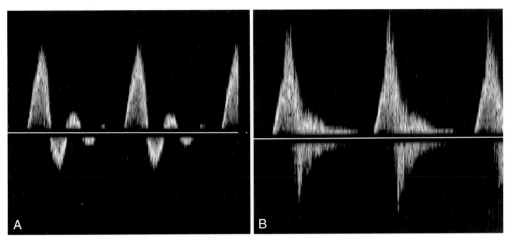

FIGURE 2-2 Femoral artery Doppler waveforms. (A) From a normal segment; the waveform has a smooth outline and the spectral width is low. (B) From the poststenotic region; in the early systolic phase the waveform has a clearly defined outline associated with the passage of blood which was at rest in the poststenotic region during diastole through the insonation site. In the later part of the waveform, blood which has passed through the stenosis has developed turbulent, disturbed flow with increased velocity. This appears as a region in which there is spectral broadening, with Doppler shifts above and below the baseline and high-frequency spikes.

The effect of the flow state on the Doppler waveform is illustrated in Figure 2-2. Doppler spectra are shown from the normal femoral artery in Figure 2-2A; in this case flow is laminar. Within the sample volume the blood velocity magnitude and direction are similar for all of the red cells, hence the spectral width is low and the waveform outline is smooth. In the post-stenotic region of a diseased artery the Doppler waveform is more complex (Fig. 2-2B). The blood which was at rest in the poststenotic region during diastole is accelerated through the sample volume. For this blood, flow is laminar and the initial up-slope of the waveform has a smooth outline with low spectral width, whereas blood which was in the prestenotic region during diastole has to pass through the stenosis, producing disturbed and turbulent flow within the sample volume. The variation in velocity magnitude and direction which this produces results in an increase in the spectral width (Fig. 2-2B), and the waveform outline is no longer smooth.

In the normal circulation, flow is mostly laminar; however, disturbed flow may occur in particular vessels such as the carotid arteries. Flow recirculation is

BOX 2.1 A SUMMARY OF POINTS CONCERNING FLOW STATE

1. In the normal circulation, flow is mostly laminar.
2. Disturbed flow may occur in particular vessels, e.g. in the region of the carotid bulb.
3. Disturbed and turbulent flow occur in the poststenotic region.
4. Disturbed and turbulent flow both give rise to spectral broadening.

BOX 2.2 PRESSURE AND ENERGY

1. The pressure drop across a stenosis is high as a result of energy loss in the poststenotic region.
2. For the estimation of the pressure drop across a cardiac valve stenosis, Bernoulli's equation may be simplified to $P = 4V^2$.

commonly seen in the region of the bulb and there may be disturbed flow in the distal region. For the purposes of clinical Doppler ultrasound, very little practical distinction is made between disturbed and turbulent flow. The presence of spectral broadening is often indicative of pathological change in the vessel.

A summary of points concerning flow state is given in Box 2.1.

PRESSURE AND ENERGY

In the circulation the essential principle is that a pressure gradient must be created in order for blood to flow; this is produced by the contraction of the heart and the resultant ejection of blood into the aorta and systemic vessels.

Energy is a useful concept in fluid mechanics. When there is steady flow of an incompressible frictionless fluid, the principles of conservation of energy can be used to give Bernoulli's equation.

Energy associated with blood pressure
+ Kinetic energy of moving blood
+ Potential energy associated with the height of the fluid above ground
= Constant

This is a simple expression which dem + onstrates that there will be an interchange between the different types of energy within the circulation. In the human body, however, the flow is not steady and the above equation must be modified slightly to account for the energy required to accelerate the fluid.[4] Energy is conserved in this simple ideal lossless system. In the circulation, energy is lost in the form of heat through viscous effects, manifested through friction of the blood at the vessel wall and between adjacent

layers of blood. Energy losses are highest in the region of a stenosis, as there is considerable friction during turbulent flow and vortex motion.

Within a stenosis there will be an increase in blood kinetic energy associated with increase in blood velocity, and according to Bernoulli's equation there is a corresponding fall in blood pressure. If there was no energy loss within the system then the decrease in velocity (and hence kinetic energy) in the poststenotic region would be compensated by a return of the pressure to the prestenotic level. In practice the loss of energy through turbulence and vortex shedding gives rise to a pressure drop across the stenosis whose magnitude is dependent on the degree of stenosis.

The most common application of Bernoulli's equation is in the prediction of pressure drop across a stenosed cardiac valve.[6] The equation may be simplified to:

$$P = 4V^2$$

where V is the measured velocity in m/s, and P is the pressure drop in mmHg. Points concerning pressure and energy are summarised in Box 2.2.

VELOCITY PROFILES

The Doppler ultrasound spectrum is critically related to the detailed variation of velocity within the vessel of interest. The velocity of the blood will vary as a function of its position within the vessel; this is called the velocity profile. The most commonly mentioned velocity profile is the parabolic velocity profile.

Strictly speaking, a parabolic velocity profile only applies to steady laminar flow in a long straight tube, when there is maximum velocity in the centre of the vessel and zero velocity at the edge of the vessel (Fig. 2-1A). The profile is radially symmetric, which means that it is the same regardless of which diameter is considered. The shape of the profile is an exact mathematical equation, that of a parabola.

Velocity profiles in vessels in the body are generally more complex; they may not be even approximately radially symmetric and they vary with time during the cardiac cycle. It is worth exploring the various effects that will influence true velocity profiles in the circulation.

Entrance Effect

The velocity profile in a vessel is strongly influenced by the distance of the region of interest from the entrance to the vessel. For a long straight vessel, when there is steady flow, the profile is initially flat at the entrance to the vessel. With increasing distance from the entrance the profile will change, becoming parabolic at a distance called the inlet length (Fig. 2-3).

Vessel Narrowing

For steady flow, a gradual narrowing taper will tend to sharpen the velocity profile.

Vessel Expansion

At regions where the cross-sectional area of the vessel increases, an adverse pressure gradient in the direction of flow is created; that is, there is a pressure decrease in the direction of flow, which tends to retard the flow. For the central high-velocity region, the high momentum opposes this, but at the edge of the vessel the velocities are low and the direction of motion near the wall will reverse if there is a sufficiently rapid increase in vessel cross-sectional area with distance. The phrase 'flow separation' is often used to describe this phenomenon; that is, the high-velocity central jet is located next to a region in which the flow is of low velocity and recirculating. The production of vortices in these circumstances was noted above; both the central jet and vortices die out after a length equivalent to a few diameters and laminar flow is re-established. Figure 2-4 shows the velocity profiles in the region of a small stenosis. When the expansion is less severe, such as a gradually widening taper, the velocity profile simply becomes more blunted.

Curved Vessels

Figure 2-5 shows that the velocity profile for steady flow in a curved vessel is skewed towards the outer wall when the entrance profile is parabolic, and skewed towards the inner wall when the entrance profile is flat.

Y-Shaped Junction

Figure 2-6 shows the velocity profiles from a Y-shaped junction and it can be seen that the profiles are skewed within the two branches, so that the higher velocities occur on the inner aspects of the two branches.

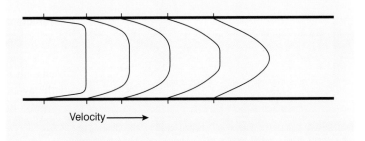

Velocity ⟶

FIGURE 2-3 Velocity profiles during steady flow at different distances from the entrance to a long straight tube from a reservoir. The parabolic velocity profile is restored at a distance from the entrance, the 'inlet length'. (After Caro et al.[2], with permission.)

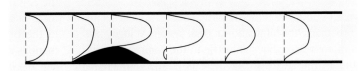

FIGURE 2-4 Velocity profiles from a stenosis model; the region of recirculation in the poststenotic region can be seen on the lower aspect.

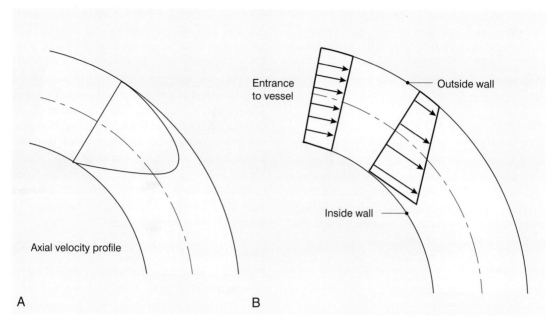

FIGURE 2-5 Velocity profiles within a curved vessel during steady flow. (A) A parabolic velocity profile at the entrance results in higher velocities on the outer aspect of the curve. (B) A blunt velocity profile at the entrance results in the higher velocities occurring on the inner aspect. (From Caro et al.[2], with permission.)

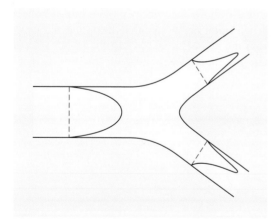

FIGURE 2-6 Velocity profiles in a Y-shaped junction with skewing of the velocity profile and higher velocities on the inner aspects of the two branches.

Figure 2-7 shows 2D velocity profiles taken in a realistic carotid bifurcation model with a moderate stenosis just proximal to the bifurcation at peak systole. Velocity profiles are reasonably symmetric in the common carotid and in the stenosis, but there is clear asymmetry at the entrance to the internal carotid artery.

Pulsatile Flow

During pulsatile flow the velocity profile will vary throughout the cardiac cycle. Figure 2-8 shows the profiles from a long straight tube with a velocity waveform similar to that found in the femoral artery.

Turbulence

As discussed above, the velocities during turbulence have a random component, so that it is necessary to take an average value over time. If this is done, then the averaged velocity profile during steady turbulent flow is found to be blunted, with high-velocity gradients near to the vessel wall (Fig. 2-1B).

Secondary Flow Motions

In many of the geometrical situations described above the components of flow are three-dimensional, which means that there will be some secondary flow motion in the plane perpendicular to the vessel axis. These motions may easily be demonstrated using flow models and dye-injection techniques, and there are a few in vivo studies which claim to have demonstrated this.[7,8]

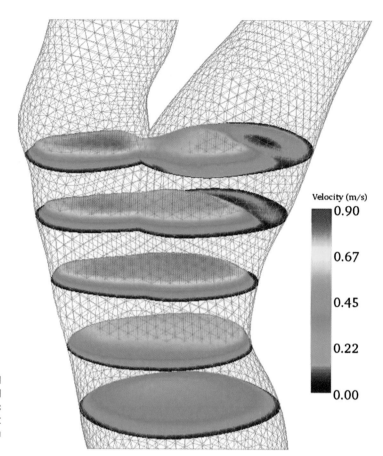

Velocity (m/s)

0.90

0.67

0.45

0.22

0.00

FIGURE 2-7 Velocity profiles in a realistic carotid bifurcation model with moderate stenosis proximal to the bifurcation, showing reasonably symmetric profiles in the common carotid and asymmetry at the entrance to the internal carotid artery. (From Hammer et al.[19], reprinted with permission.)

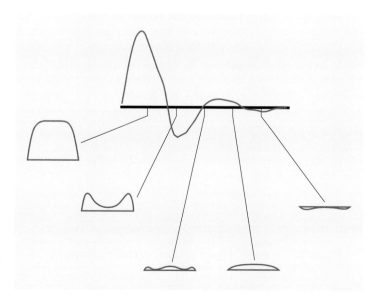

FIGURE 2-8 Changes in the velocity profiles across the vessel at various moments during pulsatile flow for a velocity waveform similar to that found in the femoral artery. (From Evans et al.[4], with permission.)

A summary of points concerning velocity profiles is given in Box 2.3.

A SIMPLE FLOW MODEL

The creation of a pressure gradient within the arterial system is performed by ejection of blood into the arterial tree by the heart. The resistance R to flow of a vessel segment may be defined as:

$$R = \frac{(P_1 - P_2)}{Q}$$

where Q is the flow through the vessel, and P_1 and P_2 are the pressures at the entrance and exit points of the vessel. One way of expressing this equation is to say that in order to maintain flow at a constant level, the pressure difference must be greater when the resistance to flow increases. Strictly speaking this formula only applies for steady flow conditions; it is therefore useful mainly as an aid in understanding general concepts of flow in arteries, and a more complex version of this equation must be used for pulsatile flow. For a long straight vessel the resistance to flow depends on the fourth power of the diameter. A segment of vessel 2 mm in diameter will therefore have a resistance 16 times that of a similar segment of 4 mm diameter.

A simple model of the flow to an organ is shown in Figure 2-9. The net flow is controlled by a combination of the small vessel (arteriolar) resistance and the large vessel (arterial) resistance. In the non-diseased circulation, the main arteries have relatively large diameters and their resistance to flow is small; the main resistance vessels are the arterioles. The essential clinical manifestations of atherosclerosis may be understood with the aid of this model; an increase in resistance in a large distributing artery because of atheroma must be compensated by a decrease in the resistance of the small arteries and arterioles in order to preserve flow to the capillary bed. As the disease progresses, flow is maintained by arteriolar dilatation until the point is reached where the arteriolar network is fully dilated. Further progression of the proximal disease results in a reduction in flow to the organ and the development of ischaemia because no further compensatory dilatation is achievable. In patients with lower limb claudication, the presence of severe proximal disease results in the distal arteriolar network being fully dilated at rest in order to maintain flow to the lower limb muscles. Whilst this is sufficient in the resting limb, the combination of the proximal stenosis and the maximum arteriolar dilatation means that no further increase in flow can be obtained to cope with the increased metabolic demands of limb exercise.

The concept of a critical stenosis follows from the above model. As the degree of narrowing at a single, isolated stenosis increases, a point is reached at which the distal arteriolar dilatation is at maximum. Consequently, any increase in the degree of stenosis beyond this point leads to a reduction in flow. Experiments performed on animals suggest that this point of critical stenosis is reached with an area reduction of about 90%, which corresponds to a diameter reduction of approximately 70%. Two quantities of interest in Doppler ultrasound are the volume flow rate and the velocity of the blood; the relationship between these two parameters, according to the model developed above, is shown in Figure 2-10.[9] As the calibre of the vessel is reduced, the volume of blood flowing along the vessel is maintained by increasing the velocity. However, above the point of critical stenosis (70% diameter stenosis), the volume

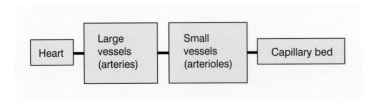

FIGURE 2-9 A simple model of flow from the heart to an organ through a large vessel (arterial) and small vessels (arterioles) to the capillary bed.

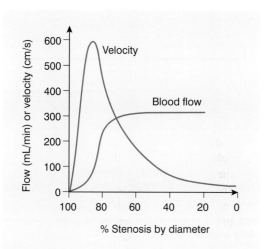

FIGURE 2-10 Flow rate and velocity based upon a single arterial stenosis inserted into an otherwise normal artery. (After Spencer and Reid[9], with permission)

of blood starts to reduce. It should also be noted that the velocity peaks at about 85% diameter stenosis, subsequently tailing off, so that in very tight stenoses the velocity is relatively low.

Two stenoses in series have a larger overall resistance compared with either stenosis considered individually. In practice the combined resistance of stenoses in series is dominated by the one with the smallest luminal diameter.

The concept of a critical stenosis is useful but its application to atherosclerosis should not be taken too far. As atherosclerosis develops, various other compensatory mechanisms come into play in an attempt to preserve perfusion. These include the development of a collateral circulation and a degree of local dilatation of the affected arterial segment. In addition, there is an increase in the extraction efficiency of oxygen from blood. A summary for this section is given in Box 2.4.

BOX 2.4 FINDINGS FROM SIMPLE FLOW MODELS

1. The degree of constriction of the distal arteriolar bed is one factor used to control the flow rate to the organ.

2. As the resistance to flow of diseased arteries increases, flow rate is maintained within normal levels as a result of distal arteriolar dilatation.

3. Very high degrees of stenosis are accompanied by a low flow rate and low velocities.

PULSATILE FLOW AND DISTAL RESISTANCE

Doppler ultrasound is commonly used to assess distal resistance to flow. The origin of pulsatile waveforms and their relation to distal resistance are considered here.

For a particular element of blood it is the pressure gradient, not the actual pressure, which accelerates the blood. The pressure gradient is related to the difference between the pressures on either side of the element of blood (Fig. 2-11). When the pressure gradient is positive the blood will be accelerated along the vessel; when the gradient is negative the blood will be decelerated. The corresponding flow waveform is found by detailed calculation of the pressure gradient at the site of interest.

Blood ejected by the heart in systole passes into the aorta, where it causes local expansion of the aorta and distal arteries due to the local high pressure. The expanded region passes down the arterial tree in the form of a pressure wave (Fig. 2-12). If the artery were long and straight then, at a particular location along the vessel, the pressure would reach a maximum and then decline to the baseline value (Fig. 2-13A), resulting in a flow waveform with forward flow only (Fig. 2-13B).[10] In practice it is known that flow waveforms in arteries can exhibit periods of reverse flow and this section is concerned with understanding the origin of this reverse flow.

FIGURE 2-11 The force acting on an element of blood is related to the difference in pressures on either side of that element.

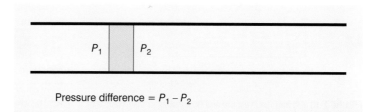

Pressure difference = $P_1 - P_2$

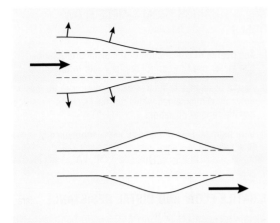

FIGURE 2-12 The blood ejected by the heart causes expansion of the elastic arteries. This expansion passes down the arteries in the form of pressure and flow waves.

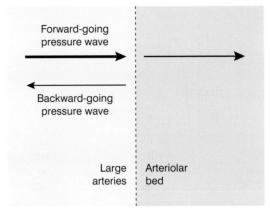

FIGURE 2-14 Reflected pressure and flow waves are produced from the distal arteriolar bed.

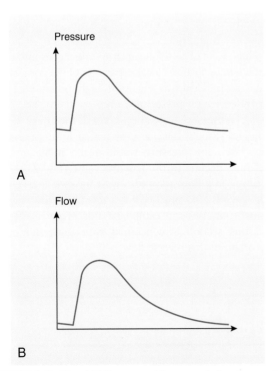

FIGURE 2-13 (A) and (B) Pressure and flow waves in the absence of distal reflection. (From Murgo et al.[10], with permission.)

Periods of reverse flow typically occur in arteries which supply muscle at rest, for example the brachial artery or the femoral arteries. However, on exercise, or during periods of reactive hyperaemia, the reverse flow disappears, and there is forward flow throughout the cardiac cycle. This difference in flow waveform is due to differences in the amplitude of reflected pressure and flow waves. As noted above in a long straight pipe there are no reflected waves. However the arterial system is a branching network and the site of the branches will cause a portion of the pressure wave to be reflected and travel back upstream. The major source of reflected waves occurs at the arteriolar junctions, which are the major resistance vessels in the body (Fig. 2-14). When the arterioles are tightly constricted as in the case in resting muscle the amplitude of reflected waves is high, leading to reverse flow. On the other hand, during exercise or reactive hyperaemia the arterioles are dilated, the amplitude of reflected waves is low and the reverse flow component is lost. This relationship between the degree of diastolic flow and the downstream resistance is used as a diagnostic tool, for example in obstetrics where umbilical artery Doppler waveforms are used to provide an indicator of placental resistance to flow. The normal placenta has a low resistance to flow and umbilical waveforms show flow throughout the cardiac cycle. Absent end-diastolic flow is associated with increased resistance to flow and abnormal placental development with an increased incidence of fetal compromise. Studies in sheep have provided good evidence for the basis for this work.[11]

Before considering the detail of how reflected waves give rise to reverse flow, it is worth considering the simple phenomenon of water waves to illustrate some of the concepts. If a buoy is placed in the ocean it will move up and down with the waves, but the height of the buoy does not provide any information on the direction of travel of the wave. If two waves are travelling towards each other from opposite directions and cross each other at the location of the buoy, then the height of the buoy will double as the waves cross due to the additive effect arising from two waves. Returning to the arterial system, there will be a reflected (reverse-going) pressure wave which will travel back up the arterial tree and combine with the forward-going pressure wave in an additive manner, hence the combined pressure will be greater (Fig. 2-15). There is also a reflected (reverse-going) flow wave which will also travel back up the arterial

tree. However in the case of the flow wave the direction of motion is important. Because the reverse-going flow wave is travelling in the opposite direction to the forward-going flow wave, the result will be a subtraction of the reverse-going from the forward-going wave, which then results in reverse flow (Fig. 2-16).

A summary of this section is given in Box 2.5.

BOX 2.5 PULSATILE FLOW AND DISTAL RESISTANCE

1. Reflected pressure waves from the distal arteriolar bed interact with the forward-going waves to produce the waveform causing increases in pulsatility of the flow waveform.

2. For some arteries the waveform pulsatility as measured using Doppler ultrasound may be a clinically useful indicator of disease.

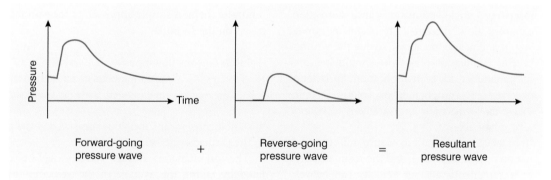

FIGURE 2-15 The resultant pressure wave is a combination of the forward-going wave and the reverse-going wave.

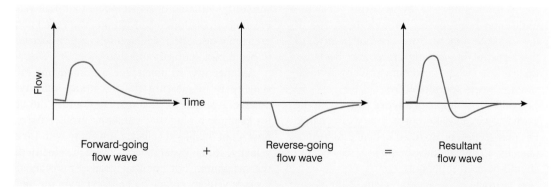

FIGURE 2-16 The resultant flow wave can be considered to be a combination of a forward-going flow wave and a reverse-going flow wave.

Quantitative Flow Measurement

Whilst it is possible to measure blood flow quantitatively, the error is usually rather large, probably between 20% and 100%.[12,13] In some applications such errors may be tolerable, for instance when a large change in flow in the order of 300% from normal to abnormal flow exists. However, one factor which mitigates against blood flow being a sensitive indicator of disease affecting an organ or limb is that circulatory regulatory mechanisms can often maintain the level of blood supply until the disease is quite advanced.

A variety of factors must be borne in mind when considering volume flow calculations in relation to the circulation of blood:

1. Flow is pulsatile, therefore the velocity varies over the cardiac cycle. The velocity also varies across the vessel lumen. In addition, turbulence and disturbed flow will result in vectors of flow off the central axis of the vessel, leading to inaccurate angle estimation and correction. Complex flow patterns can occur in curved vessels and near bifurcations, so that the assumption of laminar or plug flow should be carefully examined for each application. Turbulence observed in a sonogram or colour Doppler image makes accurate measurement of volume flow impossible.

2. In practice it is difficult to ensure uniform insonation of a blood vessel, and the resultant error in instantaneous average velocity can be very large, perhaps greater than 50%. Maximum velocity, for use in the calculation of instantaneous average velocity (see below), can be measured to around 5% by ensuring that the ultrasound beam passes through the centre of the vessel. It should always be borne in mind that spectral broadening errors can be large, up to 50%, when maximum velocity is measured by wide-aperture arrays.[14]

3. The calibre of compliant arteries varies with the cardiac cycle. Pulsation of an artery can change its cross-section by up to 20%, hence an instantaneous diameter measurement (see below) should be used if possible.

4. The accuracy of the measurement of the vessel diameter, or cross-sectional area, is inversely related to the size of the vessel and measurement errors are usually quite large, up to 20% for a 10 mm diameter vessel, rendering the technique of doubtful value for small vessels. The cross-sectional area and the velocity should be measured at the same site; in addition, errors will occur if the scan plane is not exactly at right angles to the axis of the vessel. Special efforts should be made to reduce the error in diameter measurement, since diameter is squared in the formula for cross-section (area $= \pi r^2$) and this increases the error.

5. For laminar flow in a straight vessel the beam–vessel angle can be determined to within 2° or 3°. However, even with this accuracy, if the beam–vessel angle is made greater than 60°, the error in the calculated velocity rapidly rises above 10%, so that the calculated velocities will have significant errors associated with them in this situation.

Knowing the sources of error, steps may be taken to minimise them. A simple approach to measurement is based on the formula:

$$\text{Instantaneous flow rate} = \text{instantaneous cross-section} \times \text{instantaneous average velocity}$$

'Instantaneous' means the value measured at the point in the cardiac cycle being considered.

The instantaneous average velocity may be calculated by taking the average of the velocities in the spectral display. Both the power level of each velocity in the spectrum and the velocity itself are used in this calculation. The power level for each velocity is a measure of the number of cells moving with that velocity. For this calculation to be accurate, the vessel must be uniformly insonated, which is not easy to achieve due to beam misalignment and distortion.

Another way to obtain the instantaneous average velocity is to measure the maximum velocity and assume a profile for the velocities across the vessel, for example a plug or a parabolic profile. With plug flow all of the blood cells are travelling with the same velocity, so the instantaneous average velocity equals the maximum. For parabolic flow the instantaneous average velocity equals half of the maximum velocity. The maximum velocity is readily measured from a spectral display, provided that part of the beam passes through the centre of the vessel.

The instantaneous cross-section is most easily calculated from the instantaneous diameter measured from an M-scan generated simultaneously with the sonogram; the assumption of a circular cross-section for a given diameter appears to be reasonable for arteries and introduces little error. The diameter can also be obtained from a B-scan provided that it is recorded at the same time and the same location as the spectrum being used from the sonogram.

Averaging the instantaneous flow rate over the cardiac cycle gives the average flow rate.

In practice, these measurements may not be easily achieved on some systems and the following is a more practical formula to use for volume flow rate, in mL/min.

$$\text{Flow rate (mL/min)} = \text{TAV}_{\text{mean}} \text{ (cm/s)} \times \text{area (cm}^2) \times 60$$

In these cases the time-averaged maximum velocity (TAV_{max}) can be calculated over several cardiac cycles and, assuming parabolic flow, divided by two to give a calculated time-averaged mean velocity (TAV_{mean}). Some systems will calculate the time-averaged mean velocity directly from the spectral display. Similarly, only a few systems will provide a time-averaged diameter measurement and therefore an instantaneous diameter measurement must be used to calculate area, usually from an image frozen in systole. Alternatively, the area of the vessel can be measured directly from a transverse image of the vessel, providing care is taken to ensure that the section is a true cross-section of the vessel made at systole.

Measurement of volumetric flow is difficult and not generally attempted, as it is easy to produce errors of 100%,[12] but there is little in the literature that gives accurate data on errors in practice. In general terms it should be considered as a research tool and the results treated with suitable caution with regard to the potential errors.

Arterial Motion

In the section on pressure and energy above, it was described how the blood ejected from the heart travels down the elastic arteries causing them to distend.

It is possible to examine arterial distension using ultrasound systems. Typically the artery is imaged along the longitudinal plane and the distension at a selected location examined. The artery increases in diameter during systole, and reduces in diameter during diastole. Typically the overall distension is 10% of the diameter, or about 0.5 mm for a 5 mm diameter vessel.

The degree of arterial distension is related to the elasticity of the artery; stiff arteries will not stretch much, whereas elastic arteries will stretch more. It is possible to estimate an index of elasticity, called pressure strain elastic modulus, from distension and blood pressure.[15]

$$\text{Pressure strain elastic modulus} = \frac{\text{change in blood pressure}}{\text{fractional change in diameter}}$$

This provides an easy estimate of arterial stiffness, allowing applications in patients with, for example, abdominal aortic aneurysm.[16] The pressure strain elastic modulus is a measure of the structural stiffness of the artery and is dependent on the thickness of the arterial wall. It would be very desirable to measure the bulk modulus of the artery, also called the Young's modulus; however this requires knowledge of the wall thickness, which is difficult to measure using ultrasound imaging.

Measurement of wall motion on commercially available systems is slowly being introduced. These are aimed mainly at an assessment of flow-mediated dilatation. This is the phenomenon whereby the mean arterial diameter will increase slightly following a brief period of absent blood flow. Usually the brachial artery is considered and flow is stopped by inflating an arm cuff for a short period of time. The degree of diameter increase following cuff release is used as a measure of endothelial function. Studies over many years have shown that the overall diameter increase may be measured using ultrasound.[17,18]

Conclusions

The study of haemodynamics involves the application of the principles of fluid mechanics to blood flow in the circulation and provides an insight into the events which occur in both normal and diseased vessels. It is essential to have an understanding of these haemodynamic principles in order to be able to carry out Doppler examinations and to understand the findings which are obtained during the procedures.

REFERENCES

1. McDonald DA. *Blood flow in arteries*. London: Edward Arnold; 1974.
2. Caro CG, Pedley TJ, Schroter RC, et al. *The mechanics of the circulation*. Oxford: Oxford University Press; 1978.
3. Strackee J, Westerhof N. *The physics of heart and circulation*. Bristol: Institute of Physics; 1993.
4. Evans DH, McDicken WN, Skidmore R, et al. *Doppler ultrasound: physics, instrumentation and clinical applications*. Chichester: Wiley; 1989.
5. Taylor KJW, Burns PN, Wells PNT. *Clinical applications of Doppler ultrasound*. New York: Raven Press; 1995.
6. Holen J, Aaslid R, Landmark K, et al. Determination of pressure gradient in mitral stenoses with a non-invasive ultrasound Doppler technique. *Acta Med Scand* 1976;**199**:455–60.
7. Hoskins PR, Fleming A, Stonebridge P, et al. Scan-plane vector maps and secondary flow motions. *Eur J Ultrasound* 1994;**1**:159–69.
8. Stonebridge PA, Hoskins PR, Allan PL, et al. Spiral laminar flow in vivo. *Clin Sci* 1996;**91**:17–21.
9. Spencer MP, Reid JM. Quantitation of carotid stenosis with continuous wave (CW) Doppler ultrasound. *Stroke* 1979;**10**:326–30.
10. Murgo JP, Col MC, Westerhof N, et al. Manipulation of ascending aortic pressure and flow waveform reflections with the Valsalva manoeuvre: relationship to input impedance. *Circulation* 1981;**63**:122–32.
11. Adamson SL, Morrow RJ, Langille BL, et al. Site-dependent effects of increases in placental vascular resistance on the umbilical arterial velocity waveform in fetal sheep. *Ultrasound Med Biol* 1990;**16**:19–27.
12. Evans DH. Can ultrasonic duplex scanners really measure volumetric flow? In: Evans JA, editor. *Physics in medical ultrasound*. York: Institute of Physical Sciences in Medicine; 1986.
13. Gill RW. Measurement of blood flow by ultrasound: accuracy and sources of error. *Ultrasound Med Biol* 1985;**11**:625–41.
14. Hoskins PR. Accuracy of maximum velocity estimates made using Doppler ultrasound systems. *Br J Radiol* 1996;**69**:172–7.
15. Peterson LH, Jensen RE, Parnell J. Mechanical properties of aneurysms in vivo. *Circ Res* 1960;**8**:622–39.
16. Wilson KA, Lee AJ, Lee AJ, et al. The relationship between aortic wall distensibility and rupture of infrarenal abdominal aortic aneurysms. *J Vasc Surg* 2003;**37**:112–17.
17. Celermajer DS, Sorensen KE, Gooch VM, et al. Noninvasive detection of endothelial dysfunction in children and adults at risk of atherosclerosis. *Lancet* 1992;**340**:1111–15.
18. Sidhu JS, Newey VR, Nassiri DK, et al. A rapid and reproducible on line automated technique to determine endothelial function. *Heart* 2002;**88**:289–92.
19. Hammer S, Jeays A, MacGillivray TJ, et al. Acquisition of 3D arterial geometries and integration with computational fluid dynamics. *Ultrasound Med Biol* 2009;**35**:2069–83.

Chapter 3

The Carotid and Vertebral Arteries; Transcranial Colour Doppler

Paul L. Allan

The Carotid and Vertebral Arteries

CAROTID DISEASE AND STROKE

Stroke is a major cause of morbidity and mortality. In the United Kingdom, there are approximately 150 000 first strokes each year and some 53 000 deaths a year as a result of stroke; in the United States the equivalent figures are 795 000 strokes and 137 000 deaths each year. There are significant direct and indirect costs for society, in addition to the impact on the individuals and their families.[1]

ECST & NASCET

Two major trials have shown that endarterectomy for symptomatic patients with significant stenoses confers a significant advantage over medical management in terms of reducing morbidity and mortality.[1,2] The European Carotid Surgery Trial (ECST)[2] data showed that, during the follow-up period, there was an 18.6% reduction in the risk of ipsilateral major stroke for the surgical patients with stenoses >80% diameter reduction. The equivalent figure for the North American Symptomatic Carotid Endarterectomy Trial (NASCET)[3] study was a 17% reduction in the risk of ipsilateral stroke if surgery was undertaken in patients with >70% diameter reduction. The risk of surgically related death or stroke was 7% in ECST and 5.4% in NASCET and because of this small but real risk, endarterectomy for lesser degrees of stenosis, or in asymptomatic patients with stenosis, needs to be considered more carefully.

The two major trials used different methods for assessing the degree of carotid stenosis on arteriograms (Fig. 3-1), which resulted in a stenosis measured at 80% diameter reduction in ECST corresponding to a 50% diameter reduction by NASCET measurements. The ECST data were therefore reviewed using the NASCET criteria and this showed a similar 18.7% risk reduction in patients with a stenosis of 70–99% diameter reduction using the NASCET criteria.[4]

For symptomatic patients with less severe degrees of stenosis, endarterectomy is of marginal benefit, conferring an absolute risk reduction of 4.6% for patients with a 50–70% stenosis (NASCET) but no benefit for lesser degrees of stenosis.[5,6] For patients with asymptomatic stenoses >60% (NASCET), the absolute risk reduction from endarterectomy was only 3% over 3 years.[7]

The American Academy of Neurology reviewed the evidence from the various trials and has provided recommendations for the management of patients with carotid stenosis[8] (Box 3-1).

INDICATIONS FOR CAROTID ULTRASOUND

Ultrasound of the extracranial cerebral circulation is used predominantly in the assessment of patients with symptoms which might arise from disease in the carotid arteries, such as amaurosis fugax and transient ischaemic attacks (TIA), in order to identify those patients with significant carotid stenosis who will benefit from surgery. There are also other indications for which ultrasound of the neck vessels is of value and the main indications for ultrasound of the carotids are shown in Box 3-2.

1. ECST method

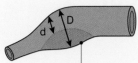

$$\frac{D-d}{D} = \% \text{ diameter stenosis}$$

Margin of bulb estimated
from arteriogram for D

Example

$$\frac{10-2}{10} = 80\% \text{ diameter stenosis}$$

2. NASCET method

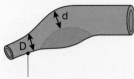

Diameter of ICA taken for D

Example

$$\frac{4-2}{4} = 50\% \text{ diameter stenosis}$$

3. Common carotid diameter method

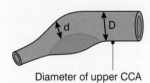

Diameter of upper CCA
is taken for D

Example

$$\frac{8-2}{8} = 75\% \text{ diameter stenosis}$$

FIGURE 3-1 Methods for estimating percentage diameter stenosis in arteriography.

BOX 3-1 INDICATIONS FOR CAROTID ENDARTERECTOMY

RECOMMENDATIONS OF THE AMERICAN ACADEMY OF RADIOLOGY[7]

Recommendation 1

- CE is effective for recently symptomatic patients (<6/12) with 70–99% ICA stenosis.
- CE should not be considered for symptomatic patients with <50% stenosis.
- CE may be considered for symptomatic patients with 50–69% stenosis if >5 year life expectancy and operative complication rate <6%.

Recommendation 2

- It is reasonable to consider CE for patients 40–75 years old with an asymptomatic stenosis of 60–99%, if life expectancy >5 years and surgical complication rate is <3%.

Recommendation 3

- No recommendation can be given regarding the value of emergency CE in patients with a progressing neurological deficit.

Recommendation 4

Patient variables should be considered:
- Women with 50–69% symptomatic stenosis do not show clear benefit from CE.

- Patients with hemispheric TIA/stroke show greater benefit from CE than those with retinal symptoms.
- Contra-lateral occlusion erases small benefit of CE in asymptomatic patients but in symptomatic patients, although there is increased operative risk, the benefit from CE remains.
- Patients having CE within 2/52 of TIA/mild stroke derive greater benefits.

Recommendation 5

- Patients undergoing CE should be treated with aspirin from before surgery until at least 3 months after surgery and indefinitely if there are no complications.

Recommendation 6

- There are no clear data to declare CE before or simultaneous with CABG to be superior.

Recommendation 7

- Patients with a severe stenosis (>70%) and a recent TIA/non-disabling stroke should have CE preferably within 2/52 of the last symptomatic event.
- There is insufficient evidence to support or refute CE within 4–6/52 of a moderate or severe stroke.

Cerebral Ischaemic Symptoms

There are many causes of cerebral ischaemic symptoms apart from disease at the carotid bifurcation. These include cardiac arrhythmias, hypotensive episodes, emboli and atheromatous disease elsewhere in the circulation between the heart and the intracerebral arterioles. Many of these can be treated with medical therapy but it is only the extracranial section of the carotid artery which is amenable to surgery, and it is for this reason that so much effort is devoted to the assessment of this area. The main aim is to classify patients into five main groups.

1. Those without significant disease.
2. Those with mild disease (<50% diameter reduction), who will benefit from medical therapy if they are symptomatic.
3. Those with more severe disease (50–70% diameter stenosis), who will be treated medically and may be followed to assess progression of disease, particularly if they are symptomatic.
4. Those patients with severe disease (>70% diameter reduction) who will benefit from surgery if they are symptomatic.
5. Those patients with a complete occlusion, who are therefore not candidates for surgery.

The relationship between the presence of carotid artery disease and the development of cerebral ischaemic symptoms is not straightforward and detailed discussion of this subject is beyond the scope of this book. However, patients who have suffered from temporary ischaemic symptoms, such as TIA, reversible ischaemic neurological deficits, or amaurosis fugax, are significantly more likely to suffer a stroke than asymptomatic subjects: 36% of patients who have a TIA will have an infarct within 5 years of the TIA, compared with an annual stroke rate of 1% for asymptomatic, elderly individuals.[9] Therefore it is reasonable to investigate patients with reversible ischaemic cerebral symptoms in order to identify those with a 70% or greater stenosis who will benefit from endarterectomy. Those with lesser degrees of stenosis can be treated medically and followed up; those who progress to more than 70% diameter stenosis can then be considered for surgery.

The situation regarding the examination of patients with asymptomatic carotid bruits is also complex. The authors, along with many people, would wish to know the status of their arteries if they were found to have an asymptomatic carotid bruit. However, a Cochrane Review of surgery for asymptomatic stenosis[7] concluded that 'for most people with a narrowing of the carotid artery which is not causing any symptoms a surgical operation carries a risk and has little benefit'. The review found that the absolute risk reduction from surgery on patients with >60% stenosis (NASCET) was only 1% a year, for centres with a surgical complication rate of <3%. More recent studies have concluded that as 'best medical therapy' continues to improve, surgery for asymptomatic carotid stenosis is no longer indicated.[10,11] Ultrasound will therefore have a role in the identification of those patients who might be considered for endarterectomy, in those centres which offer surgery. However, if there is a policy not to offer surgery to asymptomatic patients, then it might be argued that an ultrasound examination is unnecessary.

Atypical Symptoms

Some patients have unusual symptoms which may or may not be related to carotid disease. Atypical migraine, hyperventilation attacks and temporal lobe epilepsy may sometimes be difficult to diagnose and, in some patients, the possibility of carotid disease might be considered. Ultrasound is of value in excluding carotid disease as a cause of the symptoms in this group of patients, although some care must be given to patient selection to prevent large numbers of unnecessary examinations.

Patients at Risk of Perioperative Stroke

Arterial disease is usually a generalised process, although it affects different arterial territories to varying degrees. Therefore, patients undergoing surgery for conditions such as coronary artery disease, peripheral arterial disease and aortic aneurysms may also have significant carotid disease; there is concern that perioperative morbidity from strokes can be increased in these patients as a result of emboli or inadequate perfusion. Diabetics can also have severe arterial disease and are at risk from perioperative strokes when undergoing major surgery. A review of carotid artery disease and stroke during coronary artery bypass surgery[12] showed that patients without carotid disease had a <2% stroke rate and this only rose to 3% in patients with an asymptomatic stenosis >50%; it also drew attention to the role of aortic arch disease in the aetiology of strokes in coronary artery bypass graft patients. For patients with symptoms, ultrasound assessment of the carotids is valuable to allow decisions on modification to surgical bypass technique, or whether carotid endarterectomy should also be considered in addition to the surgery for the primary condition. However, this decision would depend on the relative urgency of the primary condition and many centres, whilst taking note of the carotid disease, will proceed with the main operation and consider subsequent endarterectomy in symptomatic patients.

Postendarterectomy Patients

Complications following endarterectomy can be divided into three groups based on the timing of the events.
1. Early occlusion due to thrombosis, occurring within the first 24–48 hours after the operation.
2. Stenosis developing over 12–18 months due to neointimal hyperplasia.
3. Recurrence of atheroma over a period of several years, resulting in restenosis.

Colour Doppler ultrasound provides a rapid and straightforward method for diagnosis of these complications.

Routine follow-up of asymptomatic patients is not justified by the pick-up rate for developing significant recurrent stenoses,[13] but any patient suffering symptoms related to the operated side should be examined by colour Doppler in the first instance.

Follow-Up of Carotid Stents

Carotid artery stenting is seen as a complementary technique to carotid endarterectomy and can be useful if endarterectomy is problematic or not feasible.

BOX 3-3 **CAUSES OF PULSATILE NECK MASSES**

- Normal but prominent carotid artery and bulb
- Ectatic carotid, brachiocephalic or subclavian artery
- Aneurysm of the carotid artery
- Carotid body tumour
- Enlarged lymph node adjacent to carotid sheath

Follow-up of stent patients with ultrasound allows early assessment of post-operative in stent restenosis and other complications.

Pulsatile Masses

Colour Doppler ultrasound provides a rapid technique for the assessment of pulsatile neck lumps. There is a variety of causes for these; the main ones are listed in Box 3-3.

Carotid Dissection

Dissection of the carotid artery may develop from a variety of causes.[14]
1. It may occur spontaneously, usually consequent upon atheromatous change.
2. It may result from the extension of an aortic arch dissection.
3. It may develop following trauma to the neck, such as occurs in whiplash injuries.
4. As a result of iatrogenic causes, such as carotid catheterisation.

Colour Doppler can be used to identify different flow patterns on either side of the flap, or the presence of a thrombosed channel, and monitor subsequent progress.

Epidemiological Studies and Monitoring of Therapy

The carotids provide a convenient window for the assessment of the whole arterial system. Patterns of development of atheroma vary in different arterial circulations. It was initially thought that changes in the carotids might allow some prediction of severity of disease in other vessels, such as the coronary arteries; in addition, their examination could also provide a method for assessing the rate of progression, or regression of disease, if treatment regimens were being investigated, or epidemiological studies were being performed. However, more recent consideration suggests that the value of using carotid disease as a marker of atherosclerosis lies more in refining the subject's classification based on other risk factors.[15,16]

By far the largest group of patients undergoing carotid ultrasound will fall into the first group of indications relating to the diagnosis of carotid atheroma and stenosis as a cause of cerebral ischaemic symptoms. In the end, the aim of the sonographer is to identify patients with carotid disease which may be the cause of their symptoms and to assess the severity of the disease, so that appropriate management decisions in relation to surgery or medical management can be taken.

ANATOMY AND SCANNING TECHNIQUE

The main steps in the examination are given in Box 3-4. The patient lies supine, with their neck a little extended by placing a pillow under their shoulders. The patient should be comfortable and excessive extension of the neck should be avoided. In addition, some patients with carotid or veretebral disease may find that neck extension compromises the flow of blood to the cerebral circulation, so if the patient appears to be asleep it is worth checking that they have not lost consciousness. Some patients may not be able to lie supine; if this is the case they can usually be examined adequately in a sitting position.

The examiner can sit beside the patient's thorax and scan the neck from this position, or sit at the patient's head and scan the neck from this location; this latter arrangement was favoured in the early days of carotid ultrasound as it was easier to obtain a standardised probe position, but it is no longer necessary with modern colour Doppler equipment. Furthermore, using this position at the head of the patient for carotid scanning during a general ultrasound list means that the couch and machine have to be moved around in the middle of the list, which is disruptive and time consuming.

A high-frequency transducer (7–14 MHz) is used[17] and the examination starts with a transverse scan of the carotid artery from as low in the neck as possible, to as high in the neck as possible behind the angle of the mandible. This approach will allow the depth and course of the vessels to be ascertained, together with the level of the bifurcation and the orientation of its branches (Fig. 3-2). In addition, areas of major disease will be identified and can be noted for further assessment.

Colour Doppler is then activated and the vessels are examined in the longitudinal plane, again from the lower neck upwards. Areas of abnormal flow are identified with colour Doppler, an initial assessment of their significance is made and the need to undertake a spectral examination can be considered. Just as importantly, areas of normal flow are seen, so that the normal segments of the vessel can be identified rapidly and excluded from further investigation. It may be necessary to try a variety of scan planes in order to see the bifurcation in some subjects; the normal approach is from an anterolateral or lateral direction but more posterior planes may be required and, in a

---

BOX 3-4 BASIC STEPS IN THE EXAMINATION

1. Transverse scan from low in the neck up to behind the angle of the mandible to locate bifurcation

2. Longitudinal colour scan to identify areas of abnormal flow and disease

3. Positive identification of the external carotid artery and internal carotid artery

4. Spectral Doppler

   (a) in normal vessels take readings from common carotid artery, internal carotid artery, external carotid artery

   (b) in abnormal vessels take readings from areas of disease in addition to standard readings from common carotid artery, internal carotid artery, external carotid artery

5. Examine the vertebral arteries

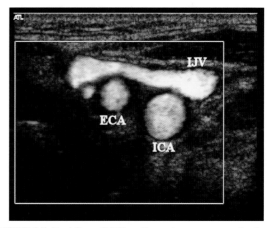

FIGURE 3-2 The left carotid bifurcation on transverse scanning from a lateral approach using power Doppler. The external carotid artery (ECA) and a small branch vessel lie anteriorly with the internal jugular vein (IJV) lying laterally, the internal carotid artery (ICA) lies behind the ECA.

few individuals, the approach may be from under the mastoid process and behind the sternomastoid muscle. In patients who have undergone recent carotid surgery, access can be problematical due to the skin incision and oedema of the soft tissues, so that a variety of approaches may need to be tried, or a lower-frequency transducer may be successful; sufficient information can usually be obtained to confirm flow in the vessel, or the absence of flow. Beards are not usually a problem but if they are particularly extensive and luxuriant they may interfere with access and sound transmission; liberal application of gel to exclude air between the hairs usually allows access to the carotids and other cervical structures, although there is some impairment of resolution.

Identification of the Internal and External Carotid Arteries

The common carotid artery on the right arises from the brachiocephalic artery behind the right sternoclavicular joint (Fig. 3-3), where the origin can usually be seen on ultrasound. On the left it usually arises directly from the aorta, so that its origin on the left cannot be seen on scanning from the neck. The level of the carotid bifurcation is usually at about the level of the upper border of the laryngeal cartilage but it may vary

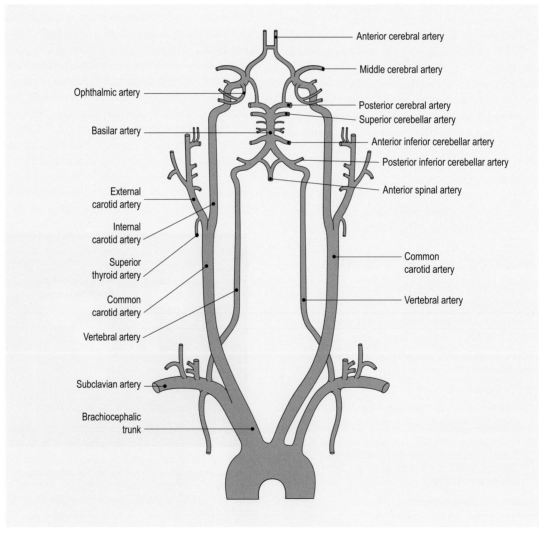

FIGURE 3-3 Carotid and vertebral arteries.

considerably. The two branches of the common carotid artery are the internal carotid artery and the external carotid artery. It is essential that they are identified positively, otherwise there is the possibility that disease in one vessel will be mistakenly attributed to the other, which may lead to further inappropriate investigations. The external carotid artery is usually the easier of the two branches at the bifurcation to recognise positively and the criteria to look for are listed in Box 3-5.

BOX 3-5 IDENTIFICATION OF THE EXTERNAL AND INTERNAL CAROTID ARTERIES

THE EXTERNAL CAROTID ARTERY
- Branches present
- Anterior position
- Waveform characteristics:
    High resistance pattern with relatively little diastolic flow
    Appears more pulsatile on colour Doppler
    Dichrotic notch is more prominent
- Positive 'temporal tap'

THE INTERNAL CAROTID ARTERY
- The other branch of the bifurcation
- Bulb at origin
- Posterior position and course angled posteriorly
- Less pulsatile waveform on colour Doppler with relatively high diastolic flow

The external carotid artery has branches just above the bifurcation (Fig. 3-4); the superior thyroid, ascending pharyngeal and lingual arteries may all arise from the external carotid artery below, or around, the level of the angle of the mandible.

The external carotid artery is nearly always the more anterior of the two branches. In one study it lay anteromedial to the internal carotid artery in 48.5% of bifurcations studied, anterior in 34.5% and anterolateral in 13%; other positions accounted for only 4% of vessels.[18]

The external carotid artery supplies the relatively high-resistance vascular bed of the facial muscles, pharynx, tongue and scalp. Therefore the external carotid artery has relatively less diastolic flow, which makes it appear more pulsatile on colour Doppler and to have a characteristic waveform on spectral Doppler with relatively low diastolic flow (Fig. 3-5A). In addition the dichrotic notch of the pulse wave is usually more prominent in the external carotid artery spectrum than in the internal carotid artery spectrum.

The superficial temporal artery is one of the terminal branches of the external carotid artery, and if this is tapped by a finger as it passes over the zygoma it will produce rapid, clear fluctuations in the waveform in the external carotid artery, whereas there is generally little or no effect in the ipsilateral common carotid artery or internal carotid artery (Fig. 3-4).

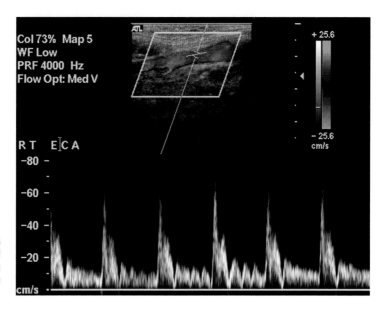

FIGURE 3-4 The external carotid artery showing a branch arising just above the bifurcation and fluctuations induced in the spectrum by tapping the superficial temporal artery at the level of the zygoma.

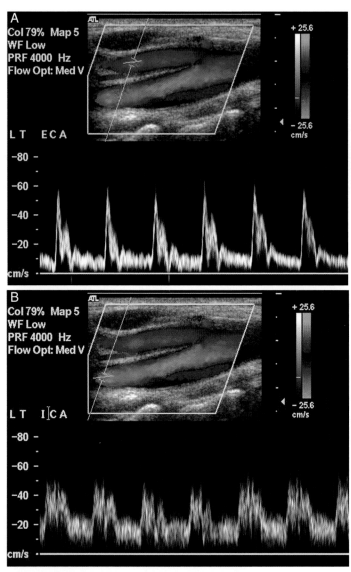

FIGURE 3-5 (A) The external carotid artery and the characteristic spectrum seen in normal vessels. There is relatively low diastolic flow and a prominent dichrotic notch compared with the spectrum from the internal carotid artery. (B) The internal carotid artery and its characteristic spectrum with more flow throughout diastole. The normal area of reversed flow in the carotid bulb is clearly visible.

Once the external carotid artery has been identified positively then it can be assumed that the other large vessel arising from the carotid bifurcation is the internal carotid artery. This vessel is nearly always the more posterior of the two branches and tends to run deeply and more posteriorly. It does not have visible branches at this level but the bulge of the carotid bulb is usually apparent in subjects without severe disease. Colour Doppler will show the normal area of reversed flow in the carotid bulb, sometimes referred to as the boundary layer separation zone. The spectrum from the internal carotid artery is less pulsatile and more sustained than that of the external carotid artery, with relatively high diastolic flow (Fig. 3-5B).

Diseased vessels may be more difficult to distinguish as plaques can obscure visual details; local

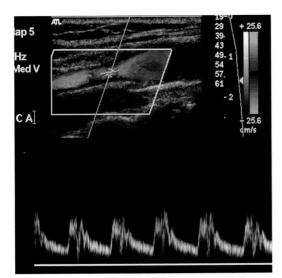

FIGURE 3-6 'Internalisation' of external carotid artery flow showing pan-diastolic flow as a result of an ipsilateral occlusion, or severe stenosis.

and remote disease can lead to alterations in the normal patterns of flow, so that distinction on the basis of the appearance of the waveform may be impossible; 'internalisation' of external carotid artery flow may be seen in patients with a severe stenosis or occlusion affecting the internal carotid artery and in whom external–internal collaterals around the meninges and cerebral circulation result in increased diastolic flow in the external carotid artery (Fig. 3-6). In addition some high bifurcations may be very difficult to see well enough to allow reliable assessment; in this situation scanning transversely with colour Doppler switched on may allow localisation of the internal and external carotid arteries, so that some spectral information can be acquired.

Standard Velocity Measurements

Once the bifurcation and its branches have been identified and assuming that no areas of significant disease are present, it is good practice to take peak systolic velocity measurements from the common carotid artery, the internal carotid artery and the external carotid artery in order to have a record of the examination. These are obtained using spectral Doppler from the upper common carotid artery 2–3 cm below the bifurcation; the internal carotid artery from 1 to

2 cm above the bulb, or as high as possible, in order to allow the normal bulbar turbulence to settle; and from the lower external carotid artery. For routine measurements the sample volume is set at about one-third of the total diameter and placed in the centre of the vessel in order to avoid the natural turbulence at the edge of the lumen and 'wall thump' from inclusion of the vessel wall in the sample volume. The Doppler angle is kept as low as possible, ideally in the range 45–60°; it is good practice to try to keep to a specific angle, such as 55° or 60°, in order to improve the reproducibility of results between examinations. For tight stenoses it is better to reduce the size of the sample volume, as this allows the area of the peak systolic flow signal to be better defined. Colour Doppler allows more accurate assessment of the direction of flow in a stenosis as this may not always be parallel to the walls of the vessel (Fig. 3-7). The precise final location of the sample volume is chosen using a combination of the audible Doppler signal and the spectrum so that the clearest, highest-frequency audible signal and the best spectral trace are obtained; in stenoses, the sample volume should be moved through the length of the stenotic segment in order to locate the peak signal. The gain for the spectral display is set to use the full grey scale without over- or under-saturation.

Measuring the Intima-Medial Thickness

This is not always required but should it need to be measured, for instance as part of a population survey, then it can be measured on an image of the distal common carotid wall where the echoes from the intima-media complex are most easily distinguished. The machine settings should be set to give a clear, uncluttered image of the vessel wall and the position of the transducer adjusted to show the characteristic double-line appearance of the vessel wall (Fig. 3-8). The image should be magnified as much as possible to make the measurement easier to perform. The intima-medial thickness (IMT) is best demonstrated in the upper common carotid artery on the posterior wall 1–2 cm below the bifurcation where the vessel is usually at right angles to the ultrasound beam. The internal carotid artery is more difficult to assess as the vessel slopes obliquely away from the transducer face in many cases. A minimum of three measurements over a 1 cm segment of the upper CCA are taken.

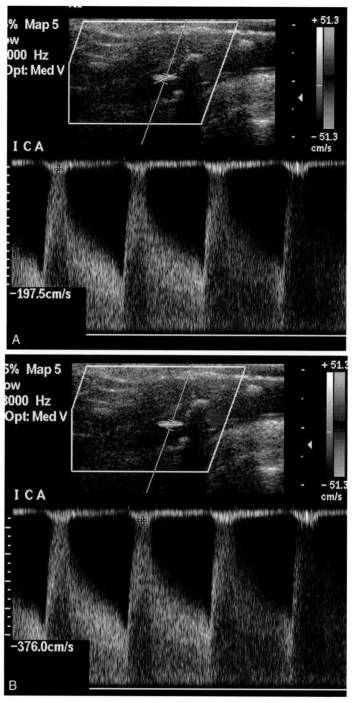

FIGURE 3-7 (A) The angle correction has been made aligning the cursor to the vessel wall resulting in a velocity estimate of approximately 2 m/s. (B) Using colour Doppler, the cursor is positioned along the line of the flow and results in a velocity of approximately 3.5 m/s.

The Vertebral Arteries

Once both carotids have been examined, the vertebral arteries are assessed. The vertebral artery on each side is the first branch of the subclavian artery (Fig. 3-3). It passes posteriorly and upwards to the vertebral foramen in the transverse process of the sixth cervical vertebra (V1 segment) (Fig. 3-9), and from there it passes upwards in the vertebral canal to the level of the axis (C2) (V2 segment). It emerges from the vertebral canal at C2, passing behind the lateral mass of the atlas (C1) to enter the skull through the foramen magnum (V3 segment) and runs anterior to the brain stem (V4 segment) to join with the vessel from the other side in front of the brain stem to form the basilar artery.[20]

The vertebral arteries are most easily located by placing the transducer longitudinally over the common carotid artery and angling it medially so that the vertebral bodies are identified; the transducer is then rotated laterally so that the transverse processes of the vertebrae and the spaces between them are

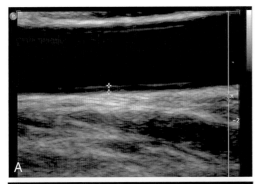
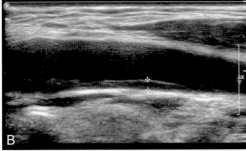
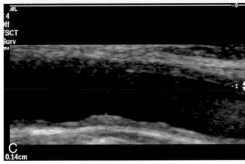

FIGURE 3-8 (A) A normal intima-medial thickness (IMT) of 0.7 mm measured in the upper common carotid artery. (B) Moderate thickening of the IMT at 1.2 mm (C) More marked intimal thickening of 1.4 mm.

Automated edge detection systems are available on some ultrasound systems but with careful attention to detail it is possible to measure the IMT manually with satisfactory, reproducible accuracy. The precise upper limit of the normal range is a matter of some discussion. IMT is known to vary with age, gender and race[16] but values of less than 0.8 mm correlate well with lack of coronary artery disease, whereas an increasing thickness above this level is associated with increasingly severe coronary artery disease, an increased risk of myocardial infarction and also stroke.[19]

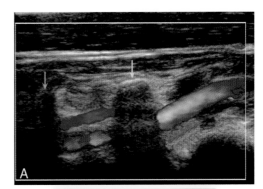
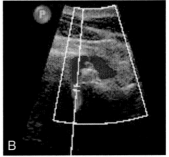

FIGURE 3-9 (A) The vertebral artery passing from its origin (V1 segment) to enter the vertebral canal and then running cranially (V2 segment) between the vertebral transverse processes (arrows). (B) The vertebral artery looping round the atlas (V3 segment).

visualised, the vertebral artery and vein may then be seen in these gaps. If the vertebral artery cannot be identified in the vertebral canal, it may be looked for in the lower neck as it passes backwards from the subclavian artery towards C6; or in the upper neck behind the mastoid process as it passes around the atlas (C1) and into the foramen magnum.

There may be marked variation in the size of the vertebral arteries and their relative contribution to basilar artery flow; when there is disparity of size, the left artery is usually the larger of the two and in 7–10% of individuals there are significant segments of hypoplasia, which result in the artery not being visible.[21] Clear visualisation of the vein but not the artery suggests that the artery may be either thrombosed or congenitally absent.

Colour Doppler makes assessment of flow direction in the vertebral arteries straightforward. They should have the same colour as the common carotid artery in front of them. Care needs to be taken in the diagnosis of reversed flow, particularly if the spectral Doppler trace has been inverted during the examination: if subclavian steal is suspected it is worth confirming that the machine is set up appropriately in order to avoid making an error.

ASSESSMENT OF DISEASE

Measurement of the Degree of Stenosis

Two types of information can be used to assess the degree of stenosis: direct measurement using the calipers on the machine; and velocity criteria derived from spectral Doppler.

Direct Visualisation and Measurement. If the stenosis and plaque can be seen clearly then it is possible to measure the calibre of the residual lumen and the original calibre of the vessel. Diameter reduction ratios, or area reduction ratios, are the usual methods for describing the reduction in vessel calibre; percentage residual lumen can also be used. Diameter measurements are generally a little quicker to perform but are slightly less representative of the stenosis, as they do not take account of variations in plaque thickness around the circumference of the vessel and there is the potential to underestimate, or overestimate, the degree of stenosis (Fig. 3-10). Care must be taken to

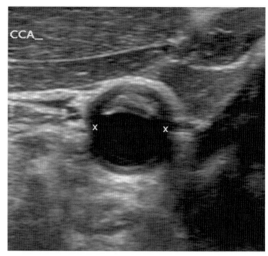

FIGURE 3-10 Transverse view of a plaque in the common carotid artery with asymmetrically located plaque. Note that an inappropriate longitudinal scan plane (x–x) could result in a significant underestimation of the degree of stenosis.

examine a diseased segment of vessel in both transverse and longitudinal views so that the distribution of plaque can be clearly assessed and the most appropriate diameter measurement can be made; this is usually the shortest diameter. Measuring stenoses by area reduction, although more time consuming, overcomes this problem with the eccentricity of the plaque being taken into account as the luminal and vessel areas are measured.

It is important that the type of measurement used is clearly defined as either a diameter reduction or an area reduction, because significant misunderstandings may occur in the interpretation of the results. For a given stenosis, a 50% diameter reduction corresponds to a 70% area reduction, so that misinterpretation of a 70% area stenosis as a diameter reduction will result in a significant overestimation in the assessment of calibre reduction, possibly leading to unwarranted surgery (Fig. 3-11). It is good practice always to define the value of a stenosis as either an area or a diameter reduction and this is essential if the measurement is in a different form from that normally used.

Most stenoses are relatively short in longitudinal extent, usually no more than a centimetre for the maximum degree of narrowing. Some patients, however, have longer segments of varying calibre reduction and it is important to remember that, although the

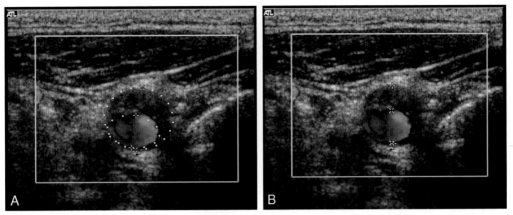

FIGURE 3-11 A stenosis measured with (A) an area-reduction calculation (measured as 62%) and (B) a diameter-reduction calculation (measured as 40%).

degree of pressure drop across a stenosis is related primarily to the reduction in radius, it is also related to the length of the stenosis. However, length has a much smaller effect, as the resistance is related to the first power of the length, rather than the fourth power of the radius (Poiseuille's Law):

$$R = \frac{8l\eta}{\pi r^4}$$

If the patient is being considered for endarterectomy, in addition to measuring the degree of stenosis, it is important to assess the level of the bifurcation, the length of the stenosed segment and the diameter of the internal carotid artery above the stenosis. The reason for this is that high bifurcations (<1.5 cm from the angle of the mandible), high distal extent of the stenotic segment (>2 cm above the bifurcation) and a small internal carotid artery (<0.5 cm), or a kinked internal carotid artery, can complicate surgery and prior warning will allow the appropriate surgical technique to be used. Ultrasound can predict these features satisfactorily and supplemental arteriography is not usually necessary.[22]

Doppler Criteria. In many cases the region of the stenosis is not seen clearly due to complex plaque structure and calcification. In these cases direct measurement cannot be used to quantify the degree of stenosis and Doppler criteria must be used. Over the years, much work has been done correlating Doppler findings with degrees of stenosis found on arteriography, or at surgery. It has been shown that carefully obtained Doppler criteria correspond well with the degree of stenosis, and values which allow the severity of internal carotid artery stenoses to be predicted have been developed. However, the literature can be confusing, with apparently widely varying velocities being quoted for specific levels of stenosis in the early days of duplex ultrasound: one study suggesting that a peak systolic velocity of >1.3 m/s was appropriate for diagnosis of a diameter stenosis of 60% or greater;[23] whilst another study proposed a velocity of 2.25 m/s for a 70% stenosis.[24] This apparent lack of consensus emphasises the fact that there was variation from one department to another depending on the equipment and technique used. Each department must therefore develop and audit criteria which they find work in their environment and complement the clinical criteria and practices used in their institution.

The peak systolic velocity, end-diastolic velocity and the ratio of peak systolic velocities in the internal and common carotid arteries (IC/CC systolic ratio) are the most useful measurements in general practice[25,26] (Fig. 3-12). Spectral broadening and filling in of the window under the spectrum are subjective, difficult to quantify and can be affected significantly by gain control settings; however, they do indicate abnormal flow if they are present. The IC/CC diastolic ratio can also be measured but this does not usually add to the information obtained from the three main criteria.

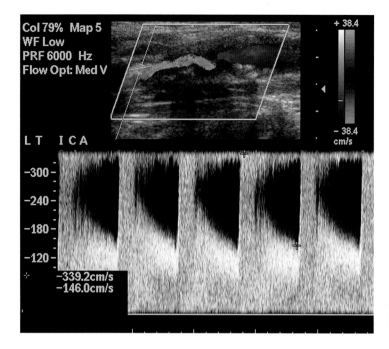

Col 79% Map 5
WF Low
PRF 6000 Hz
Flow Opt: Med V

+ 38.4

– 38.4
cm/s

LT   ICA

–300
–240
–180
–120

–339.2cm/s
–146.0cm/s

FIGURE 3-12 A stenosis of the internal carotid artery showing a peak systolic velocity in excess of 3.4 m/s and an end-diastolic velocity of 1.5 m/s. There is aliasing of the colour Doppler display.

The main levels which need to be distinguished are 50% diameter reduction, where blood flow starts to decline, and 70% diameter reduction, which is the level strongly associated with clinical symptoms and for which surgery will be considered. The values for the criteria which the authors have found to be useful in their practice to predict these levels of stenosis in the internal carotid artery are shown in Table 3-1 and are based on those reported by Grant et al.[25] and Oates et al.[26] It is important to remember that the peak systolic and diastolic values refer only to the internal carotid artery, not to the common carotid artery or external carotid artery. Furthermore, it should be borne in mind that physiological variations due to heart rate, cardiac output and contralateral occlusion may affect the velocities in a vessel, potentially leading to a false diagnosis of a pathologically high velocity, although these cases should be clarified by the use of the velocity ratios. It should also be remembered that peak velocities decline with very high degrees of stenosis (>90% diameter stenosis)[27] as discussed in Chapter 2.

Attempts have been made to use colour or power Doppler criteria to assess the severity of stenoses.[28,29] Direct measurement of the residual lumen based on

TABLE 3-1 Diagnostic Criteria for Doppler Diagnosis of Stenoses of 50% and 70%

Diameter Stenosis (%)	Peak Systolic Velocity ICA (m/s)	End-Diastolic Velocity ICA (m/s)	IC/CC Systolic Ratio
50	>1.25	>0.4	>2
70	>2.3	>1.0	>4

ICA, internal carotid artery; IC/CC, internal carotid/common carotid. From Grant et al.[25] and Oates et al.[26]

power or colour Doppler can be made but it is essential that care is taken with the gain settings to ensure that there is not any over- or underestimation of the residual lumen; this type of direct measurement will always be less accurate than measurements made on a good B-mode image but, for more severe degrees of stenosis (>50% diameter reduction), they can provide additional confirmatory information. For cases where a diagnosis must be made between 'subtotal', or 'near' occlusion and complete occlusion, then careful setting up of the colour and power Doppler modes is essential for reliable distinction (see below).

In addition to the direct measurement of the residual lumen demonstrated by the colour map, a cursor with angle correction can be placed over the colour map and used to provide an estimate of the mean velocity in the underlying pixel. This allows the mean velocities in a stenotic segment to be estimated. However, these correlate less well with the degree of stenosis than peak systolic or diastolic velocities. Although experienced operators can often get a good idea of the severity of a stenosis from the overall appearances and the colour map changes, it is always better to use the colour map to identify areas of abnormal flow and use this to position the sample volume for spectral Doppler analysis as it may sometimes be difficult to grade stenoses using colour findings alone (Fig. 3-13).

Effects of Disease Elsewhere

The velocities and flow characteristics seen in any given section of a vessel depend not only on local conditions but also on conditions elsewhere along the vessel, in other vessels connected to that vascular territory (Fig. 3-14A & B) and to other factors, such as heart rate, cardiac output and blood pressure (Box 3-6). The best example of this is vertebral or subclavian steal, where a proximal occlusion of the subclavian artery results in reversed flow in the ipsilateral vertebral artery.

Carotid occlusion can lead to an increase in the volume of blood flowing in the contralateral carotid artery. This is achieved primarily by the blood flowing more quickly, therefore there is the potential to mistakenly suggest that an increased velocity measurement is compatible with a degree of stenosis but review of the colour Doppler image should refute this impression in a non-diseased carotid. The use of ratios, mainly the IC/CC peak systolic ratio, helps identify the nature of increased velocities in both normal vessels and those with minor atheroma, as in these circumstances the velocity in both the common carotid artery and the internal carotid artery is increased and the ratio does not alter; whereas if there is significant local disease affecting the internal carotid artery, the velocity in this vessel is increased but the common carotid artery velocity is unchanged, so that the ratio is also increased.

In patients with bilateral severe carotid stenoses, when one side is stented or operated upon, the improvement in flow up the operated vessel will reduce flow up the contralateral carotid and this may result in a decrease in peak velocities on the untreated side that might lead to this stenosis being down-graded in severity. In one series of patients with bilateral significant stenoses on duplex scanning,[30] the stenosis on the non-operated side was reclassified as non-haemodynamically significant in 20% of cases. It is therefore necessary for these patients to be reassessed prior to any management decisions relating to the untreated artery.

Carotid Occlusion

Occlusion can affect the internal carotid artery (Fig. 3-15) or common carotid artery separately, or together. Occlusion of the common carotid artery does not always result in occlusion of the internal carotid artery, as sufficient blood flow may be provided by retrograde flow down the ipsilateral external carotid artery to maintain patency of the internal carotid artery. This pattern of abnormal flow may be quite confusing if it is not recognised but it is of clinical importance, as these patients can still suffer ischaemic events in the relevant internal carotid artery territory.[31] The opposite pattern of flow may be seen in a small number of patients with common carotid artery occlusion with reverse flow in the internal carotid artery on the side of the common carotid artery occlusion (a carotid steal phenomenon) and antegrade flow in the ipsilateral external carotid artery. If the lower margin of the occluded segment is above the level of the bifurcation then a characteristic pattern of forward and reverse flow ('stump thump') is seen in the patent residual lumen of the internal carotid artery (Fig. 3-15B).

If an occlusion of the internal carotid artery is suspected it is essential that care is taken to ensure that the Doppler settings on the machine are appropriate for locating any low-velocity, small-volume flow that may be present in a narrow residual lumen in the segment under investigation. Colour and power Doppler assessments of the vessel should be carried out with the system set for maximum sensitivity in order to identify any small residual lumen ('string sign' or pseudo-occlusion) (Fig. 3-16) or adjacent vessels that might confuse the situation.[32] Spectral Doppler should also be performed carefully at maximum

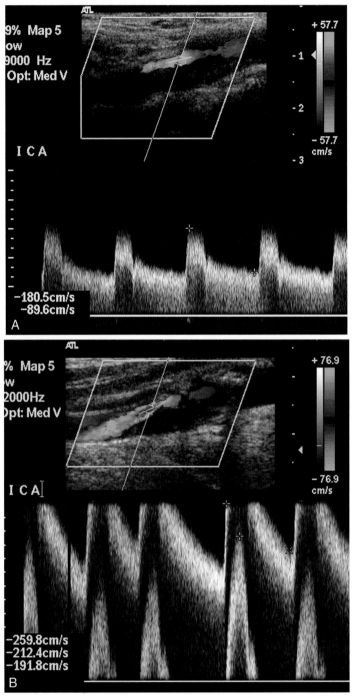

FIGURE 3-13 Similar appearances of two ICA stenoses on colour Doppler but spectral Doppler shows a peak systolic velocity of 1.8 m/s in (A) but a peak systolic velocity >4 m/s in (B).

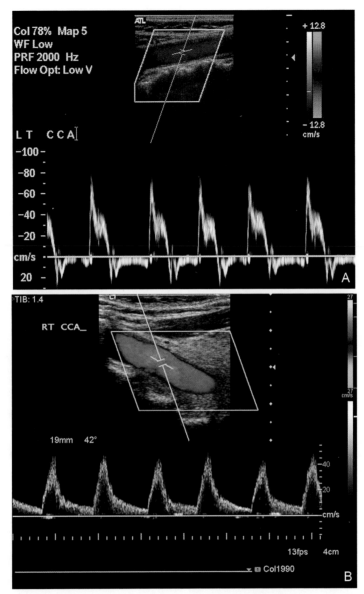

FIGURE 3-14 Common carotid waveforms (A) in a patient with aortic valve incompetence showing reversed diastolic flow on both colour and spectral Doppler; (B) in a patient with aortic valve stenosis showing delayed systolic acceleration.

sensitivity, although care must be taken to identify and exclude any waveforms arising from adjacent vessels. Conversely, colour Doppler or power Doppler may show the location of a residual channel in a vessel that was otherwise thought to be occluded; echo-enhancing agents are of value if there is any persisting uncertainty.

Occlusion of the internal carotid artery results in the reduction of diastolic flow in the ipsilateral common carotid artery, so that the common carotid artery waveform becomes more like that seen in the external carotid artery. Reduction of common carotid artery end-diastolic flow may therefore be an initial clue to the presence of an internal carotid artery occlusion,

BOX 3-6 **FACTORS AFFECTING THE WAVEFORM**

Local	Atheroma and plaques
	Tortuosity
Proximal	Common carotid artery origin disease
	Aortic valve disease
Distal	Carotid siphon disease
	Intracranial vessel disease
Remote	Contralateral carotid occlusion
Physiological	High cardiac output states

or a very severe stenosis.[33] Care should be taken, however, as the development of collateral channels between the external carotid artery and internal carotid artery circulations in the orbit and meninges can result in 'internalisation' of the external carotid artery flow with relatively high diastolic flow in the external carotid artery; this results in a mistaken impression of a patent internal carotid artery, if it is not recognised. The 'temporal tap' manoeuvre can usually clarify the situation. Occlusion of the carotid

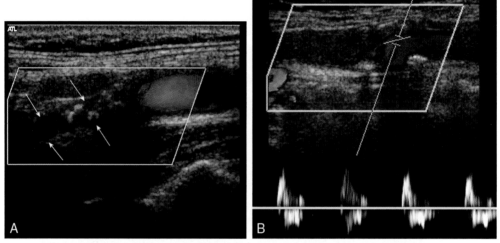

FIGURE 3-15 (A) An occluded internal carotid artery, the occluded lumen is indicated by the arrows. (B) characteristic low-velocity forward and reverse flow in the ICA just below an occlusion ('stump thump')

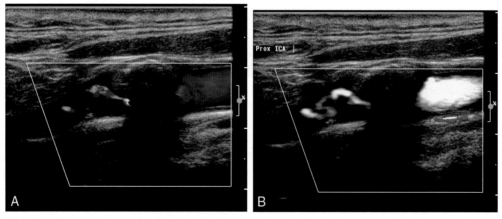

FIGURE 3-16 A thin residual channel on colour Doppler (A) and on power Doppler (B) which is more sensitive for weaker, slower signals and shows the tortuous residual lumen more clearly.

on one side may result in increased flow through the contralateral carotid vessels, as discussed earlier.

Recanalisation of an occluded carotid artery is not as rare as might be imagined.[34] One series followed eight patients with internal carotid artery occlusion with serial 6-monthly ultrasounds for a period of up to 8 years, all of the eight patients showed evidence of spontaneous recanalisation occurring between 6 and 96 months.[35]

If there is occlusion of both the internal carotid artery and external carotid artery then the ipsilateral common carotid artery also usually occludes. Before thrombosis occurs, however, a to-and-fro pattern of flow may be seen in the common carotid artery, which signifies that there is no net forward flow of blood up the vessel.

Plaque Characterisation

Much effort has been expended in attempting to classify atheroma and plaques on ultrasound, particularly in the carotids, where high-resolution ultrasound gives good images of many plaques. Steffen et al.[36] proposed a classification of plaque which takes account of the different types of plaque and its components (Fig. 3-17). Types 1 and 2 were predominant in symptomatic arteries, whereas types 3 and 4 were more

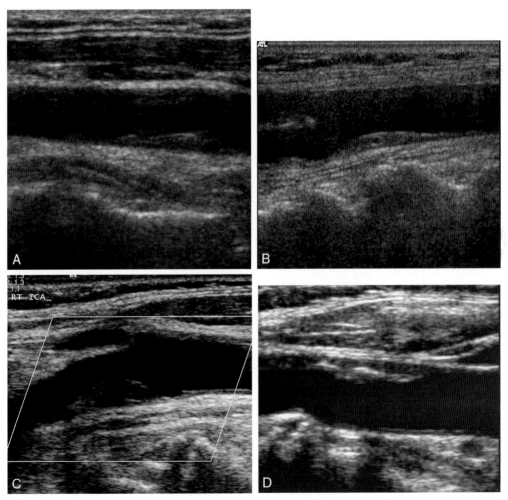

FIGURE 3-17 Different types of plaque seen on ultrasound. (A) Type 1, dominantly echolucent with a thin echogenic cap. (B) Type 2, substantially echolucent lesions with small areas of echogenicity. (C) Type 3, dominantly echogenic lesions with small areas of echolucency of <25%. (D) Type 4, uniformly echogenic lesions.

common in asymptomatic patients; these findings have been supported by other groups.[37–39] These studies suggest that the more friable, lipid-containing, soft plaques are more likely to result in plaque disruption and produce symptoms than firmer, more fibrous and coherent plaques.

The value of ultrasound in predicting the complications associated with plaques is more difficult to define. These complications include intraplaque haemorrhage, surface ulceration and adherent thrombus. The presence of intraplaque haemorrhage has been inferred from the presence of hypoechoic areas within the plaque. However, it is also possible that many of these areas are aggregates of lipid or necrosis, rather than areas of haemorrhage. Sometimes an ulcer in the plaque can be clearly seen (Fig. 3-18), but many plaques are irregular without being ulcerated and, conversely, an ulcerated plaque may not be identified on ultrasound. Thrombus adherent to the surface is suggested by an anechoic or hypoechoic area adjacent to the plaque surface on colour or power Doppler. It is important that the system is set up appropriately, otherwise the lack of colour on the image may be due to technical factors, rather than the presence of thrombus.

Some studies have shown a good correlation between the ultrasound appearances and those found at operation,[40,41] but the results from others have been less satisfactory, with poor prediction of ulceration or haemorrhage.[42,43] Another study from the Seattle group showed that there was no significant difference in plaque constituents between the endarterectomy specimens removed from symptomatic and asymptomatic patients with high-grade stenoses.[44] Visualisation of plaque type in high-grade (>60% diameter reduction) stenoses is usually inadequate to identify reliably plaque characteristics and the Seattle study would suggest that the degree of stenosis is the more important factor in this group of patients. However, if there is a good view of the diseased segment, the plaque can be described in terms of its type (1–4), extent (focal, diffuse, circumferential) and any obvious associated complications (ulceration, thrombus, haemorrhage). If visualisation is moderate or poor then discretion is necessary and only those features which are clearly seen should be noted. For example, it may be difficult to distinguish between a plaque ulcer and a gap between two adjacent plaques, or to decide if a colour void associated with the plaque surface is really due to adherent thrombus or to technical factors. Ulceration should only be diagnosed if the plaque and the ulcer are clearly seen, otherwise plaques should be described as smooth or irregular. It should be remembered that many diseased segments are not clearly seen due to the presence of calcification, which makes any attempt at plaque characterisation very difficult, or impossible.

In practical terms, a smooth, homogeneous, predominantly echogenic plaque is less likely to be associated with symptoms, whereas an irregular, heterogeneous or hypoechoic lesion is of greater concern. A stenosis of only 50% (diameter reduction) but with an unstable plaque type in a symptomatic patient might well be a matter of clinical concern and considered for surgery.

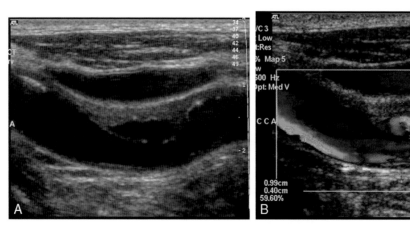

FIGURE 3-18 An ulcerated plaque. A thin rim is seen on the B-scan image (A) but colour Doppler (B) shows flow within the plaque.

Takayasu's arteritis is a condition of unknown aetiology which can affect the carotid arteries amongst other vessels. A cell-mediated auto-immune reaction is strongly implicated with granulomatous infiltration of the vessel wall leading to fibrosis and scarring, occasionally ectasia or aneurysm formation may be seen. The appearances on ultrasound reflect these changes with diffuse, homogeneous mural thickening (Fig. 3-19) with or without significant stenosis, dilatation or aneurysm formation.[45]

Pulsatile Masses

The main causes of pulsatile neck masses are given in Box 3-3. Normal but prominent carotids and ectatic carotid or subclavian arteries are easily identified using colour Doppler and do not usually require any further investigation.

Aneurysms of the carotid arteries can also be identified as they are in continuity with the artery. The majority arise following surgery but they may also occur following trauma, including whiplash neck injuries and biopsy of cervical masses. Pseudoaneurysms may also be seen. The flow in the aneurysm may be seen with colour Doppler, unless there is thrombosis of the lumen of the dilated segment. In some cases of aneurysm of the common carotid artery, it may be difficult to identify the internal carotid artery above the dilatation and care must be taken to establish whether it is patent or not; flow in the ipsilateral ophthalmic artery is not necessarily evidence of patency, as this may come from collateral filling via the circle of Willis. Aneurysms of the upper internal carotid artery may be difficult to identify with certainty, or the findings may be misinterpreted as a straightforward stenosis or dissection.[46]

Lymph nodes and other masses adjacent to the carotids will transmit pulsations and require distinction from intrinsic vascular lesions. This is not usually a problem, but occasionally a deposit will surround the carotid artery and, unless there is a previous history of malignancy, diagnosis can be difficult. Adherence to the carotid sheath can be assessed by gentle palpation and getting the patient to swallow so that relative movement between the mass and the carotid can be assessed.[47] Colour Doppler ultrasound also has an important role in defining the solid nature of a neck lump prior to biopsy and excluding a vascular lesion, such as an aneurysm.

Carotid body tumours are rare but can be diagnosed easily with ultrasound. Characteristically there is a hypoechoic mass between the two branches at the bifurcation, spreading them apart in a 'wine glass' deformity (Fig. 3-20). Colour Doppler shows a highly vascular lesion and the external carotid usually shows a low-resistance pattern of flow on spectral Doppler.[48]

Dissection of the Carotid Arteries

The ultrasound findings in this condition can vary considerably. The vessel may be occluded completely;

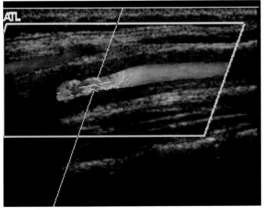

FIGURE 3-19 Takayasu's arteritis affecting a common carotid artery and showing diffuse intimal thickening and a more focal stenosis.

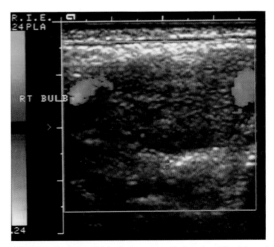

FIGURE 3-20 A carotid body tumour splaying apart the internal carotid artery and external carotid artery. Colour Doppler shows the abnormal tumour circulation.

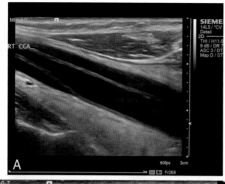

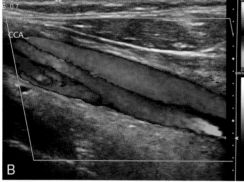

FIGURE 3-21 Dissection of the common carotid artery extending up from a dissection of the aortic arch (A). Colour Doppler (B) shows a peripheral channel with blood flowing towards the head (red) and an inner channel with blood flowing in the opposite direction (blue).

show a smooth tapering stenosis, with or without a recognisable haematoma/thrombosed false lumen being visible (Fig. 3-21); or a membrane with a double lumen may be seen with variable flow patterns in the two channels on either side.[49,50] Recanalisation of the occluded vessel is a recognised occurrence and occurs in up to 60% of cases.[51] Dissection of the vertebral arteries may also occur and is usually manifest as absent flow in the affected artery.[49]

Vertebral Arteries

Frequently only cursory attention is paid to the vertebral arteries, unless there are specific signs and symptoms pointing to a posterior fossa problem, when a more detailed examination of the vessels is required.[20] As noted previously, there are several variations of anatomy and size of the vertebral arteries which may affect the ultrasound findings; a further issue to be considered

is that disease affecting one artery may be compensated by the other side, or collaterals from the circle of Willis, so that blood flow to the posterior fossa circulation is maintained and local, unilateral vertebral artery disease is of little clinical significance. Nevertheless, some basic patterns of flow can be identified:

1. No flow detected in the region of the relevant vertebral artery means that the artery is either hypoplastic, absent, or thrombosed. Visualisation of the artery on B-mode without demonstrable flow within it on colour/power and spectral Doppler with the system set to maximum sensitivity suggests that it is thrombosed, or dissected.

2. Demonstration of a focal area of increased velocity at the origin of the vertebral artery (Fig. 3-22A), or at some point along its course between the subclavian artery and the foramen magnum, is consistent with a focal stenosis, the significance of which will depend on the clinical situation and the state of the contralateral vertebral artery. Visualisation of the vertebral artery is normally inadequate to make a reliable direct diameter reduction measurement feasible.

3. A 'tardus-parvus' waveform suggests a proximal stenosis; this should be sought by careful examination of the artery from the subclavian artery up to the foramen magnum (Fig. 3-22B).

4. The proximal vertebral artery waveform shows reduced or absent diastolic flow, implying a distal stenosis/occlusion (Fig. 3-23).

5. Reversed flow is consistent with subclavian steal syndrome. This occurs when there is an occlusion or tight stenosis of the proximal subclavian artery at its origin and blood supply to the arm is maintained by reversal of blood flow down the ipsilateral vertebral artery (Fig. 3-24).

6. A biphasic vertebral artery waveform may be seen in patients with a developing steal situation from slightly less severe subclavian stenoses (Fig. 3-25) and, in some patients, reversed flow may only occur with the arm in certain positions, or after a period of exercise; therefore scanning after a period of arm exercise, such as elbow flexions holding a book, or some other relatively heavy object, should be considered if a steal syndrome is suspected. Alternatively a pressure cuff can be inflated to occlude blood flow to the arm and then released after

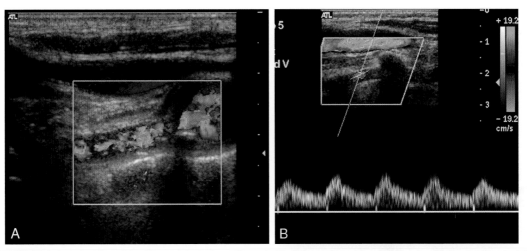

FIGURE 3-22 (A) A stenosis at the origin of the vertebral artery with marked turbulence shown on colour Doppler. (B) Spectral Doppler in the V2 segment shows a 'tardus-parvus' waveform with delayed systolic acceleration.

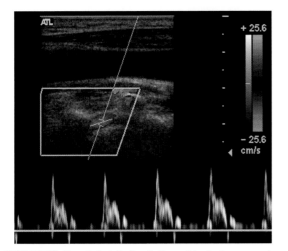

FIGURE 3-23 Absent diastolic flow in the vertebral artery suggests a severe stenosis distally.

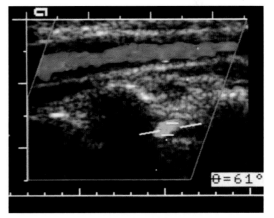

FIGURE 3-24 Reversed flow in the vertebral artery in a patient with a proximal left subclavian artery stenosis. The vertebral artery is the opposite colour (blue) from the common carotid artery.

2–3 min. The resulting reactive hyperaemia in the arm produces an increased demand for blood and reversal of flow in the relevant vertebral artery.

Reporting Carotid Ultrasound Examinations

Unlike an arteriogram, or magnetic resonance angiography (MRA) examination, there are no easily interpretable images from a Doppler examination as the outcome is a mixture of image assessment, Doppler parameters and clinical judgement. It is therefore sensible to standardise the information given in the report of a Doppler examination, to ensure that all necessary data are recorded.[17] The easiest way to do this is to record the data onto a standardised form, which can then be used in reaching management decisions about the patient, or comparing the Doppler examination with any associated MRA, computed tomography angiography (CTA), or arteriogram. The precise details will vary from centre to centre, depending on local preferences. The form used in our institution is shown in Figure 3-26. The main information which should be noted is given in Box 3-7.

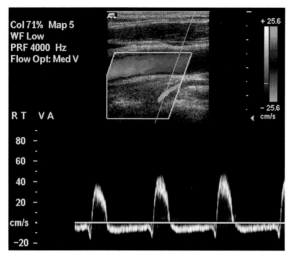

Col 71% Map 5
WF Low
PRF 4000 Hz
Flow Opt: Med V

ATL

+ 25.6

– 25.6
◄ cm/s

R T   V A

80 –
60 –
40 –
20 –
cm/s ·
–20 –

FIGURE 3–25 Biphasic flow in the vertebral artery of a patient developing a subclavian steal syndrome.

BOX 3-7 CAROTID EXAMINATION REPORT INFORMATION

- Patient demographic data etc.
- Patency of CCA, ICA, ECA
- Any variations of standard anatomy
- PSV, EDV for each CCA, ICA and ECA
- IC/CC peak systolic ratio for each side
- Estimate of degree of stenosis
- Description of any plaque clearly seen
  - Plaque type: lucent/echogenic/calcified
  - Plaque surface: smooth/irregular/ulcerated/thrombus
- Length of any stenosis
- Diameter of ICA above any stenosis
- Diagram of any stenosis giving an estimate of plaque disposition
- Level of the bifurcation in relation to angle of mandible on each side
- Vertebral arteries
  - Visualised/not visualised
  - Direction of flow
  - Any specific abnormalities identified in relation to the vertebral arteries

CCA, common carotid artery; ECA, external carotid artery; ICA, internal carotid artery; IC/CC, internal carotid/common carotid.

PROBLEMS AND PITFALLS IN CAROTID ULTRASOUND

Problems and pitfalls can arise from a variety of sources. These can be divided into those resulting from poor or faulty technique and those arising from pathological or physiological causes (Box 3-8). Technical aspects of setting up the system are discussed elsewhere (see Appendix) but other aspects which can lead to problems should be considered.

Long and Eccentric Lesions

The amount of pressure reduction across a stenosis is related primarily to the fourth power of the radius; however, as noted previously, it is also related to the length of the stenosis. This is not relevant for many stenoses, as they are relatively short, but some stenoses, particularly in the common carotid artery, may be longer. Therefore, whilst a 40% diameter stenosis extending over 5–8 mm length is not haemodynamically significant, a 40% diameter stenosis extending over 5–8 cm may well result in some reduction in pressure and a decrease in flow, resulting in cerebral perfusion problems in some circumstances, and this should be taken into account in the assessment of the patient.

Eccentric lesions may cause problems if the exact disposition of plaque around the circumference of the vessel is not appreciated (Fig. 3-10). Care should be taken to examine areas of disease transversely, as well as longitudinally, as discussed earlier. Another problem with eccentric lesions is that the high-velocity jet may emerge from the stenosis at an unusual angle that is not parallel to the vessel wall, as many people would assume; colour Doppler is useful in identifying these oblique jets and allows for a more accurate angle correction to be achieved (Fig. 3-7).[26]

Tortuous Vessels

Sharp twists in the course of a vessel result in changes to the pattern of blood flow in the lumen: blood on the outer margin flows faster than blood on the inside of the bend (Fig. 2-5); in addition, turbulence is generated, even if plaques are not present. Furthermore, assessing the angle of flow for calculation of velocity can be difficult, so that accurate, representative velocities are hard to define, especially if there is associated disease. Whenever possible, flow characteristics should be assessed as far as possible from the curved segment but if a measurement has to be made in a curved

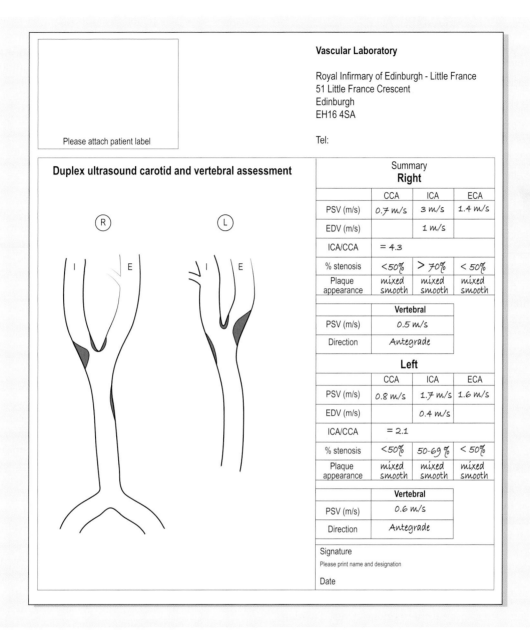

FIGURE 3-26 A specimen carotid examination report form. Digital report templates have also been developed for this purpose. (Courtesy of S-J Carmichael.)

segment, then the angle correction should be aligned to be parallel to the wall at that point.[26]

High-Grade Stenoses

In critical stenoses (>85% diameter reduction; see Chapter 2) velocity decreases; in addition, there is only a small volume of blood flowing through the narrow residual lumen. The signal strength is therefore poor and the Doppler shift is lower than might be expected. It is important to ensure that the machine is set up appropriately to detect these weaker, lower Doppler shifts, if they are not to be missed and a false diagnosis of occlusion reached (Fig. 3-16). The low flow distal to a very severe stenosis results in relative narrowing of

BOX 3-8 PROBLEMS AND PITFALLS

TECHNIQUE RELATED
- Incorrect Doppler sample volume position or size
- Doppler angle too large (>60–65°)
- Doppler settings too high for low-velocity, low-volume flow
- Good Doppler angles give poor images and vice versa

DISEASE RELATED
- Long lesions
- Eccentric lesions
- Tortuous vessels
- High-grade stenosis
- Lesions at the bifurcation
- Disease elsewhere in the vascular tree

the internal carotid artery lumen above the stenosis and this should be borne in mind when reporting these cases prior to carotid endarterectomy. The higher sensitivity of power Doppler and the increase in signal strength obtained with echo-enhancing agents are two developments which both individually and together improve the success of ultrasound in discriminating between an occlusion and a small residual lumen.[52]

Lesions at the Bifurcation

These can cause problems as a significant amount of plaque may be present in the bulb but, because of the relative dilatation of the lumen which is normally present here, this does not result in any narrowing of the flow channel between the common carotid artery and the internal carotid artery. Although this will not have any effect on the overall flow in the vessel, this disease may provide a source of emboli and may not be recognised if spectral criteria alone are used to identify stenotic segments, as there will not be a significant increase in velocity.[26]

Disease Elsewhere in the Vascular Tree

Vascular ultrasound allows direct assessment of much of the extracranial cerebral circulation from the clavicular region into the upper cervical area and disease in these segments can be measured directly. However,

changes in vessels remote from those under examination may affect the findings at any given point. As discussed previously, contralateral occlusion results in increased flow through the patent carotid with higher than normal velocities as a result of this increased flow. In patients with bilateral high-grade stenoses, an improvement in blood flow following surgery or stenting on one side will lead to a decrease in blood flow in the remaining stenosed vessel, which will reduce peak systolic velocities and may lead to a reclassification of the degree of stenosis.[30] Aortic valve disease (Fig. 3-14) or a common carotid artery origin stenosis on the left will not be visualised directly on carotid examination; the presence of disease in these areas can only be inferred from damping of the waveform with, or without, turbulence. Similarly disease more distal in the carotid siphon region will not be detected by cervical carotid examination.

CAROTID STENTS

Insertion of stents into stenotic segments of the common and internal carotid arteries is becoming increasingly recognised as an alternative to endarterectomy for treatment of significant extracranial carotid disease. Insertion of a stent affects the biomechanical properties of the arterial wall resulting primarily in increased stiffness; this means that velocity measurements from a non-stenotic stented segment will be higher than those from an equivalent unstented artery. Lal et al.[53] have proposed that a normal velocity through a stented segment can be up to 1.5 m/s; a 50% in stent restenosis is indicated by velocities ≥2.2 m/s; and an 80% in stent restenosis by velocities ≥3.4 m/s. In patients with bilateral severe stenoses, stenting or operating on one side should result in a change in blood flow in the non-operated artery so, as discussed previously, this means that a careful review of the current situation should be made before any conclusions are drawn or decisions made in relation to the other side.[30]

ACCURACY IN RELATION TO OTHER TECHNIQUES
Arteriography

Many studies have shown that spectral Doppler and colour Doppler have satisfactory accuracy in the diagnosis and assessment of disease when compared with arteriography. Some care must be taken when considering studies comparing the two techniques, as different types of angiography are used as the gold standard: direct carotid injection, arch injection, digital subtraction arteriography (DSA) and venous DSA have all been used. Different methods of measuring the degree of stenosis are also used (Fig. 3-1).[54] These will result in different estimations of the degree of stenosis for a bifurcation lesion depending on whether the diameter of the residual lumen is compared with the diameter of the common carotid artery, the diameter of the internal carotid artery, the estimated diameter at the bulb as calculated from calcification in the wall, or from the alignment of the vessels. There is also a degree of variation between different observers in the estimation of stenosis on arteriography, which may be up to 20%.[55] In addition, angiography has some intrinsic procedural risks arising from catheterisation and exposure to contrast and radiation. The risk of minor stroke from carotid arteriography has been reported to range from 1.3 to 4.5% and in the ACAS the combined neurological morbidity/mortality from arteriography in patients with haemodynamically significant stenoses was 1.2%.[56] A review of techniques used in the investigation of stroke patients reported a mortality of 1% and a disabling stroke rate of 4% from intra-arterial angiography.[57] In many centres, arteriography is now reserved for further assessment of complex cases, rather than as a primary diagnostic tool.

The overall performance of Doppler ultrasound compared with arteriography is good. Cardullo et al.[58] reviewed 16 spectral Doppler studies with 2146 Doppler–arteriogram comparisons; non-colour duplex Doppler had an overall sensitivity of 96%, specificity of 86%, positive predictive value of 89%, negative predictive value of 94% and accuracy of 91% for the diagnosis of a diameter stenosis greater than 50%. Subsequently, further studies have confirmed the value of colour Doppler with similar or better levels of accuracy and also its value in improving diagnostic confidence, clarifying difficult situations and reducing examination times. In particular the difficult distinction between a critical stenosis and a complete occlusion can be achieved in nearly all cases with the use of colour Doppler.[59]

Magnetic Resonance Angiography and Computed Tomography Angiography

Magnetic resonance angiography (MRA) and computed tomography angiography (CTA) are alternative methods for assessing the extracranial and intracranial cerebral circulation. These two techniques have an advantage over ultrasound in that they provide information on disease at the origins of the carotids and also in the intracranial circulation. However, they also have significant drawbacks. CTA requires injection of iodinated contrast agent, with the associated risks and exposes the patient to ionising radiation. In addition calcified plaque can impair assessment of diseased segments unless care is taken with image processing algorithms.

The two main MRA techniques are 'time of flight' (TOF) and contrast-enhanced MRA (CEMRA): they both 'image' the blood and infer the wall characteristics from the shape of the blood flowing in the vessel, whereas colour Doppler provides information on the wall of the vessel and any plaque, as well as the flowing blood. CEMRA is more recently developed and appears to have advantages in terms of sensitivity and specificity when compared with other 'non-invasive' techniques for carotid assessment (Table 3-2).[57] MRA is still limited

TABLE 3-2 Sensitivities and Specificities of Non-Invasive Imaging Tests for Different Degrees of Stenosis			
Stenosis Group	Imaging	Sensitivity (95% CI)	Specificity (95% CI)
70–99% (definitely operable)	US	0.89 (0.85–0.92)	0.84 (0.77–0.89)
	CTA	0.77 (0.68–0.84)	0.95 (0.91–0.97)
	MRA	0.88 (0.82–0.92)	0.84 (0.76–0.90)
	CEMRA	0.94 (0.88–0.97)	0.93 (0.89–0.96)
50–69% (possibly operable)	US	0.36 (0.25–0.49)	0.91 (0.87–0.94)
	CTA	0.67 (0.30–0.90)	0.79 (0.63–0.89)
	MRA	0.37 (0.26–0.49)	0.91 (0.78–0.97)
	CEMRA	0.77 (0.59–0.89)	0.97 (0.93–0.99)
0–49% & 100% (definitely not operable)	US	0.83 (0.73–0.90)	0.84 (0.62–0.95)
	CTA	0.81 (0.59–0.93)	0.91 (0.74–0.98)
	MRA	0.81 (0.70–0.88)	0.88 (0.76–0.95)
	CEMRA	0.96 (0.90–0.99)	0.96 (0.90–0.99)

From Wardlaw et al.[57]

to some extent by signal voids at relatively high velocities and artefacts can occur with patient movements such as swallowing. Earlier problems from signals arising in plaque haemorrhage and lipid deposits are less intrusive with modern equipment, sequences and processing algorithms. Another disadvantage of CTA and MRA, apart from exposure of the patient to contrast agents and radiation (CTA), is the significant amount of postprocessing and image manipulation required for an accurate assessment of the examination to be achieved. Although general data processing capacity and speeds have increased with modern computers, there is still a need to review several MR sequences, or undertake further workstation review of CTA and MRA exams in order to get a clear picture of the vessels, which add to the complexity of the examination and the time taken to reach a diagnosis.

Several authors have suggested that Doppler is satisfactory for initial screening of patients for carotid disease and for identification of patients requiring surgery in most cases but that CTA or MRA are useful additional tests which can be used instead of angiography if the ultrasound is inadequate or indeterminate, or if clinical uncertainty persists.[60–63]

Compared with arteriography, CTA and MRA, Doppler ultrasound is relatively cheap, rapid, non-invasive and accurate for the diagnosis of extracranial carotid disease. Whilst it will not provide information on siphon disease or aortic arch disease, this is not usually a significant problem in most patients in relation to the decision to perform an endarterectomy. If patients are being considered for stenting, then they will need an assessment of the aortic arch and carotid origins, normally by MRA or CTA. If a policy to operate on ultrasound alone is to be implemented then it is good practice to have a second operator scan the patient to confirm the assessment of the degree of stenosis[57] and the department/laboratory must ensure that scanning protocols and results are continuously reviewed, audited and validated with care taken to identify patients who will benefit from further imaging.

Transcranial Doppler of the Cerebral Circulation

The use of ultrasound to assess intracranial structures is not a new phenomenon. One of the first clinical applications of ultrasound as a diagnostic technique was in the assessment of midline intracranial structures with A-scan equipment. More recently, high-quality imaging and Doppler studies have been obtained in neonates through the patent fontanelles, or through the relatively thin bone of the neonatal skull. Transcranial Doppler was first described by Aaslid in 1982[64] and the technique of pulsed transcranial Doppler has subsequently been developed in many centres. This technique provides useful information on the direction and velocity of blood flow and the changes which may occur in these with various physiological, pharmacological or pathological conditions; it can also be used to monitor the intracranial circulation during carotid and other vascular surgical procedures.[65] However, it is a difficult technique to learn and to perform reliably as the vessels must be located without any imaging information.

Modern ultrasound equipment can now be configured to get some imaging detail and colour Doppler information from within the adult skull in many cases; best results are obtained with dedicated transducers and software. This allows localisation and positive identification of the major arteries and specific segments of these. The main problem is the bone of the skull vault, where it has been estimated that the attenuation can vary from 15–25 dB to 40–60 dB depending on the type and thickness of the bone for a single passage across the skull vault.[66] As the sound pulse has to pass through the skull on both the inward and outward segments of its passage, there is therefore considerable loss of energy. Power Doppler is of value in locating the vessels and the advent of intravascular ultrasound contrast agents has improved the signal-to-noise ratio significantly; it also makes the location of intracranial vessels more straightforward.[67]

TECHNIQUE

There are three potential sites of access for transcranial examinations in the adult: the transtemporal window, the suboccipital approach and the transorbital approach. The transtemporal window is used for assessment of the internal carotid arteries, the middle, anterior and posterior cerebral arteries. The window is located by applying liberal amounts of acoustic coupling gel to the hair and skin of the temporal region in front and above the external auditory meatus. Slowly moving the transducer around will allow the point of best transmission to be identified. In some 10% of subjects it may not be possible to get worthwhile images and Doppler signals;[68] there tends to be greater attenuation in older patients, females and Afro-Caribbean patients.[69]

The pituitary fossa and suprasellar cistern are the most recognisable structures in the transverse plane. Once these have been identified, colour Doppler can be used to locate the main arteries and the direction of flow in these vessels (Fig. 3-27). The ipsilateral middle cerebral artery is seen passing peripherally from the end of the internal carotid artery. It cannot often be seen in its entirety in a single scan plane and the transducer position must be varied to follow it out to the Sylvian fissure, where it turns posteriorly. The origin of the contralateral middle cerebral artery can also usually be identified. The proximal segments of the anterior cerebral arteries are also seen from the transtemporal approach. The direction of flow in the ipsilateral anterior cerebral artery is normally away from the transducer and flow is towards the transducer in the contralateral vessel. This arrangement will be altered if there is occlusion of the ipsilateral internal carotid artery and collateral flow through the anterior communicating artery is present. In this situation, flow in the anterior cerebral artery on the side of the occluded carotid will be reversed towards the transducer. The posterior cerebral arteries can be seen arising from the basilar artery and passing around the cerebral peduncles.

The suboccipital window is located by scanning transversely in the midline under the occipital bone. It is often better to position the transducer slightly to one side or the other of the midline as the nuchal ligament can interfere with the clarity of the image. The vertebral arteries can be seen passing around the atlas (Fig. 3-9B) and into the foramen magnum. The point where they join to form the basilar artery may be seen if it lies low enough in relation to the foramen magnum.

The transorbital approach is used in pulsed transcranial Doppler to assess the anterior cerebral arteries, but it is not very convenient for colour Doppler examinations as the transducers have a relatively larger footprint. Care must be taken, if this approach is used, to ensure that the transmit power is low in order to reduce the risk to the retina.

The major cerebral veins and venous sinuses are more difficult to demonstrate due to their anatomical locations and slow flow within them, but contrast agents have been reported to improve this situation.[67]

INDICATIONS

Transcranial colour Doppler has several advantages when compared with conventional transcranial Doppler. Visualisation of the intracranial anatomy allows rapid localisation and identification of specific vessels and specific segments of particular vessels. The colour Doppler signal allows rapid identification of flow patterns and direction, so compression studies are less necessary in order to assess collateral flow. The ability to perform angle-corrected velocity measurements produces more accurate readings and the ability to measure at specific sites allows better consistency for serial measurements.

Although still largely a research tool, the technique does have several potential applications. These were reviewed in 2004 by the American Academy of Neurology (Box 3-9).[70] In particular the ability to bring the ultrasound machine to the patient allows the technique to be used to monitor cerebral blood flow in a variety of cerebrovascular disorders, such as subarachnoid haemorrhage and stroke.

Conclusions

Colour Doppler ultrasound provides a useful technique for the assessment of the carotid and vertebral arteries in the neck. Careful attention must be paid to the standard techniques which are used for the examinations and each centre should use the Doppler criteria for stenosis that provide the most accurate and

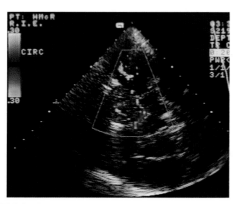

FIGURE 3-27 The anterior and middle cerebral arteries on transcranial colour Doppler ultrasound through the transtemporal window.

BOX 3-9 APPLICATIONS OF TRANSCRANIAL DOPPLER (TCD)

TCD is able to provide useful information and clinical utility is established

- Screening children with sickle cell disease to assess stroke risk
- Monitoring vasospasm after traumatic SAH

TCD is able to provide information but clinical utility compared to other diagnostic tools remains to be determined

- Evaluation of occlusive lesions of intracranial arteries in basal cisterns
- Confirming brain death

TCD is able to provide information but clinical utility remains to be determined

- Monitoring thrombolysis of acute MCA occlusions
- Detection of microembolic signals
- Monitoring during carotid endarterectomy and CABG
- Detection of impaired cerebral haemodynamics with severe extracranial ICA disease
- Detection of vasospasm after traumatic SAH
- Evaluation and monitoring of MCA territory infarctions

TCD is able to provide information but other diagnostic tests are typically preferable

- Detection of L → R cardiac and extracardiac shunts
- Evaluation of severe extracranial ICA disease

CABG, coronary artery bypass graft; ICA, internal carotid artery; MCA, middle cerebral artery; SAH, subarachnoid haemorrhage. From 'Assessment: Transcranial Doppler Ultrasonography', the American Academy of Neurology[70]

reproducible results in their experience. The availability of the technique has reduced the necessity for carotid arteriography in most departments. MRA and CTA continue to improve but ultrasound provides information on the nature of the plaque which is not available from these techniques.

REFERENCES

1. *Stroke Statistics.* 2009. British Heart Foundation and The Stroke Association. www.stroke.org.uk.
2. European Carotid Surgery Trialists' (ECST) Collaborative Group. Randomised trial of endarterectomy for recently symptomatic carotid stenosis: final results of the MRC European Carotid Surgery Trial (ECST). *Lancet* 1998;**351**:1379–87.
3. North American Symptomatic Carotid Endarterectomy Trial (NASCET) Collaborators. Benefit of carotid endarterectomy in patients with moderate or severe stenosis. *New Engl J Med* 1998;**339**:1415–25.
4. Rothwell PM, Gutnikov SA, Warlow CP. Reanalysis of the final results of the European Carotid Surgery Trial. *Stroke* 2003;**34**:514–23.
5. Rerkasem K, Rothwell PM. Carotid endarterectomy for symptomatic carotid stenosis. *Cochrane Database Syst Rev* 2011;(**4**).
6. Rothwell PM, Eliasziw M, Gutnikov SA, et al. Analysis of pooled data from the randomised controlled trials of endarterectomy for symptomatic carotid stenosis. *Lancet* 2003;**361**:107–16.
7. Chambers BR, Donnan GA. Carotid endarterectomy for asymptomatic carotid stenosis. *Cochrane Database Syst Rev* 2005;(**4**).
8. Chaturvedi S, Bruno A, Feasby T, et al. Carotid endarterectomy – An evidence based review. *Neurology* 2005;**65**:794–801.
9. Zwiebel WJ. Duplex sonography of the cerebral arteries: efficacy, limitations and indications. *AJR Am J Roentgenol* 1992;**158**:29–36.
10. Abbott AL. Medical (non-surgical) intervention alone is now best for prevention of stroke associated with asymptomatic severe carotid stenosis: results of a systematic review and analysis. *Stroke* 2009;**40**:e573–83.
11. Marquardt L, Geraghty OC, Mehta Z, et al. Low risk of ipsilateral stroke in patients with asymptomatic carotid stenosis on best medical therapy: a prospective, population based study. *Stroke* 2010;**41**:e11–17.
12. Naylor AR, Mehta Z, Rothwell PM, et al. Carotid artery disease and stroke during coronary artery bypass: a critical review of the literature. *Eur J Vasc Endovasc Surg* 2002;**23**:283–94.
13. Naylor AR, Merrick MV, Sandercock PAG, et al. Serial imaging of the carotid bifurcation and cerebrovascular reserve after carotid endarterectomy. *Br J Surg* 1993;**80**:1278–82.
14. Bassi P, Lattuada P, Gomitoni A. Cervical cerebral artery dissection: a multicenter prospective study (preliminary report). *Neurol Sci* 2003;**24**(Suppl. 1):S4–S7.
15. Touboul P-J, Hennerici MG, Meairs S, et al. Mannheim carotid intima-media thickness consensus (2004–2006). *Cerebrovasc Dis* 2007;**23**:75–80.
16. Hien-Tu N-T, Benzaquen BS. Screening for subclinical coronary artery disease measuring carotid intima media thickness. *Am J Cardiol* 2009;**104**:1383–8.
17. Tahmasebpour HR, Buckley AR, Cooperberg PL, et al. Sonographic examination of the carotid arteries. *Radiographics* 2005;**25**:1561–75.
18. Trigaux JP, Delchambre F, Van Beers B. Anatomical variations of the carotid bifurcation: implications for digital subtraction angiography and ultrasound. *Br J Radiol* 1990;**63**:181–5.
19. Simon A, Megnien J-L, Gilles C. The value of carotid intima-media thickness for predicting cardiovascular risk. *Arterioscler Thromb Vasc Biol* 2010;**30**:182–5.
20. Buckenham TM, Wright IA. Ultrasound of the extracranial vertebral artery. *Br J Radiol* 2004;**77**:15–20.
21. Berguer R, Kieffer E. The aortic arch and its branches: anatomy and blood flow. In: Kieffer E, Berguer R, editors. *Surgery of the arteries to the head.* New York: Springer Verlag; 1992. p. 5–31.
22. Wain RA, Lyon RT, Veith FJ, et al. Accuracy of duplex ultrasound in evaluating carotid anatomy before endarterectomy. *J Vasc Surg* 1998;**27**:235–42.

23. Bluth EI, Stavros AT, Marich KW, et al. Carotid duplex sonography: a multicentre recommendation for standardized imaging and Doppler criteria. *Radiographics* 1988;**8**:487–506.
24. Robinson ML, Sacks D, Perlmutter GS, et al. Diagnostic criteria for carotid duplex sonography. *AJR Am J Roentgenol* 1988;**151**:1045–9.
25. Grant EG, Benson CB, Moneta GL, et al. Carotid artery stenosis: gray-scale and Doppler US diagnosis – Society of Radiologists in Ultrasound Consensus Conference. *Radiology* 2003;**229**:340–6.
26. Oates CP, Naylor AR, Hartshorne T, et al. Joint recommendations for reporting carotid ultrasound investigations in the United Kingdom. *Eur J Vasc Endovasc Surg* 2009;**37**:251–61.
27. Spencer MO, Reid JM. Quantitation of carotid stenosis with continuous wave (CW) Doppler ultrasound. *Stroke* 1979;**10**:326–30.
28. Erickson SJ, Mewissen MW, Foley WD, et al. Stenosis of the internal carotid artery: assessment using colour Doppler imaging compared with angiography. *AJR Am J Roentgenol* 1989;**152**:1299–305.
29. Steinke W, Meairs S, Ries S, et al. Sonographic assessment of carotid artery stenosis. Comparison of power Doppler imaging and color Doppler flow imaging. *Stoke* 1996;**27**:91–4.
30. Sachar R, Yadav JS, Roffi M, et al. Severe bilateral carotid stenosis: the impact of ipsilateral stenting on Doppler-defined contralateral stenosis. *J Am Coll Cardiol* 2004;**43**:1358–62.
31. Belkin M, Mackey WC, Pessin MS, et al. Common carotid artery occlusion with patent internal and external carotid arteries: diagnosis and surgical management. *J Vasc Surg* 1993;**17**:1019–27.
32. Krieghauser JS, Patel MD, Nelson KD. Carotid pseudostring sign from vasa vasorum collaterals. *J Ultrasound Med* 2003;**22**:959–63.
33. Androulakis AE, Labropoulos N, Allan R, et al. The role of common carotid artery end-diastolic velocity in near or total internal carotid artery occlusion. *Eur J Vasc Endovasc Surg* 1996;**11**:140–7.
34. Meves SH, Muhs A, Federlein J, et al. Recanalisation of acute symptomatic occlusions of the internal carotid artery. *J Neurol* 2002;**249**:188–92.
35. Camporese G, Verlato F, Salmistraro G, et al. Spontaneous recanalization of internal carotid artery occlusion evaluated with color flow imaging and contrast arteriography. *Int Angiol* 2003;**22**:64–71.
36. Steffen CM, Gray-Weale AC, Byrne KE, et al. Carotid artery atheroma: ultrasound appearances in symptomatic and asymptomatic vessels. *Aust N Z J Surg* 1989;**59**:529–34.
37. Gronholdt ML, Nordestgaard BG, Schroeder TV, et al. Ultrasonic lucent plaques predict future strokes. *Circulation* 2001;**104**:68–73.
38. Golledge J, Cuming R, Ellis M, et al. Carotid plaque characteristics and presenting symptom. *Br J Surg* 1997;**84**:1697–701.
39. Geroulakos G, Ramaswami G, Niclaides A, et al. Characterization of symptomatic and asymptomatic carotid plaques using high resolution real-time ultrasonography. *Br J Surg* 1993;**80**:1274–7.
40. O'Donnell TF, Erdoes L, Mackey WC, et al. Correlation of B-mode ultrasound imaging and arteriography with pathologic findings at carotid endarterectomy. *Arch Surg* 1985;**120**:443–9.
41. Bluth EI, Kay D, Merritt CRB, et al. Sonographic characterization of carotid plaque: detection of haemorrhage. *AJR Am J Roentgenol* 1986;**146**:1061–5.
42. Ratliff DA, Gallagher PJ, Hames TK, et al. Characterisation of carotid artery disease: comparison of duplex scanning with histology. *Ultrasound Med Biol* 1985;**11**:835–40.
43. O'Leary DH, Holen J, Ricotta JJ, et al. Carotid bifurcation disease: prediction of ulceration with B-mode US. *Radiology* 1987;**162**:523–5.
44. Hatsukami TS, Ferguson MS, Beach KW, et al. Carotid plaque morphology and clinical events. *Stroke* 1997;**28**:95–100.
45. Gotway MB, Araoz PA, Macedo TA, et al. Imaging findings in Takayasu's arteritis. *AJR Am J Roentgenol* 2005;**184**:1945–50.
46. Rosset E, Albertini J-N, Magnan PE, et al. Surgical treatment of extracranial internal carotid artery aneurysms. *J Vasc Surg* 2000;**31**:713–23.
47. Mann WJ, Beck A, Schreiber J, et al. Ultrasonography for evaluation of the carotid artery in head and neck cancers. *Laryngoscope* 1994;**104**:885–8.
48. Barry R, Pienaar A, Pienaar C. Duplex Doppler evaluation of suspected lesions at the carotid bifurcation. *Ann Vasc Surg* 1993;**7**:140–4.
49. de Bray JM, Lhoste P, Dubaz F, et al. Ultrasonic features of extracranial carotid dissections: 47 cases studied by angiography. *J Ultrasound Med* 1994;**13**:659–64.
50. Logason K, Hardemark HG, Bärlin T, et al. Duplex scan findings in patients with spontaneous cervical artery dissections. *Eur J Vasc Endovasc Surg* 2002;**23**:295–8.
51. Steinke W, Rautenberg W, Schwartz A, et al. Non-invasive monitoring of internal carotid artery dissection. *Stroke* 1994;**25**:998–1005.
52. Sitzer M, Fürst G, Siebler M, et al. Usefulness of an intravenous contrast medium in the characterization of high-grade internal carotid stenosis with colour Doppler-assisted duplex imaging. *Stroke* 1994;**25**:385–9.
53. Lal BK, Hobson 2nd RW, Tofighi B, et al. Duplex ultrasound velocity criteria for the stented carotid artery. *J Vasc Surg* 2008;**47**:63–73.
54. Rothwell PM, Gibson RJ, Slattery J, et al. Prognostic value and reproducibility of measurements of carotid stenosis: a comparison of three methods on 1001 angiograms. *Stroke* 1994;**25**:2440–4.
55. Chikos PM, Fisher LD, Hirsch JH, et al. Observer variability in evaluating extracranial carotid stenoses. *Stroke* 1983;**14**:885–92.
56. Executive Committee for the Asymptomatic Carotid Atherosclerosis (ACAS) Study. Endarterectomy for asymptomatic carotid artery stenosis. *J Am Med Assoc* 1995;**273**:1421–8.
57. Wardlaw JM, Chappell FM, Stevenson M, et al. Accurate, practical and cost-effective assessment of carotid stenosis in the UK. *Health Technol Assess* 2006;**10**(30).
58. Cardullo PA, Cutler BS, Brownell Wheeler H. Detection of carotid disease by duplex ultrasound. *J Diagn Med Sonogr* 1986;**2**:63–73.
59. Lee DH, Gao FQ, Rankin RN, et al. Duplex and color Doppler flow sonography of occlusion and near occlusion of the carotid artery. *Am J Neuroradiol* 1996;**17**:1267–74.
60. Cinat ME, Casalme C, Wilson SE, et al. Computed tomography angiography validates duplex sonographic evaluation of carotid stenosis. *Am Surg* 2003;**69**:842–7.
61. Back MR, Rogers GA, Wilson JS, et al. Magnetic resonance angiography minimizes the need for arteriography after inadequate carotid duplex ultrasound scanning. *J Vasc Surg* 2003;**38**:422–30.
62. Herzig R, Burval S, Krupka B, et al. Comparison of ultrasonography, CT angiography and digital subtraction angiography in severe carotid stenoses. *Eur J Neurol* 2004;**11**:774–81.
63. Buskens E, Nederkoorn PJ, Buijs-Van Der Woude T, et al. Imaging of carotid arteries in symptomatic patients: cost-effectiveness of diagnostic strategies. *Radiology* 2004;**233**:101–12.

64. Aaslid R, Markwalder TM, Nornes H. Non-invasive transcranial Doppler ultrasound recording of flow velocity in basal cerebral arteries. *J Neurosurg* 1982;**57**:769–74.

65. Doblar DD. Intraoperative transcranial ultrasonic monitoring for cardiac and vascular surgery. *Semin Cardiothorac Vasc Anesth* 2004;**8**:127–45.

66. White DN, Curry GR, Stevenson RJ. The acoustic characteristics of the skull. *Ultrasound Med Biol* 1978;**4**:225–52.

67. Bauer A, Becker G, Krone A, et al. Transcranial duplex sonography using ultrasound contrast enhancers. *Clinl Radiol* 1996;**51** (Suppl. 1):19–23.

68. Ringelstein EB, Kahlscheuer E, Niggemeyer E, et al. Transcranial Doppler sonography: anatomical landmarks and normal velocity values. *Ultrasound Med Biol* 1990;**16**:745–61.

69. Halsey JH. Effect of emitted power on waveform intensity in transcranial Doppler. *Stroke* 1990;**21**:1573–8.

70. Sloan MA, Alexandrov AV, Tegeler CH, et al. Assessment: Transcranial Doppler ultrasonography. Report of the Therapeutics and Technology Assessment Subcommittee of the American Academy of Neurology. *Neurology* 2004;**62**:1468–81.

Chapter 4

The Peripheral Arteries

Paul L. Allan

Atheroma occurs to different degrees in different parts of an individual's cardiovascular system and the lower limb arteries are particularly prone to the development of atherosclerosis. Approximately 2% of adults in late middle age in Western countries have intermittent claudication[1] and each year in England and Wales around 50 000 patients are admitted to hospital with a diagnosis of peripheral arterial disease; 15 000 of these will require amputation.[2] There are many factors which may influence the development of disease and, in general terms, the prevalence of peripheral vascular disease detected by non-invasive procedures is about three times greater than the prevalence of intermittent claudication.[3] This chapter concentrates on the use of ultrasound in the assessment of disease in the lower limb arteries, as this is the area where most work is generated, but the value of ultrasound in the investigation of a variety of upper limb arterial disorders is also discussed.

Indications

Peripheral vascular disease

The main indications for performing Doppler ultrasound of the arteries of the upper and lower limbs are given in Box 4-1. The most common indication is the assessment of patients with ischaemic symptoms of the lower limb in order to determine if they are likely to benefit from angioplasty or a bypass graft. The ultrasound findings provide information on the extent and severity of disease; even in patients with limb-threatening ischaemia ultrasound is a useful first-line investigation that can provide the surgeon with all the information that is required for patient management. In many cases ultrasound will provide sufficient information for management decisions to be reached. In other cases, if further information is required, the subsequent magnetic resonance angiography (MRA)/computed tomography angiography (CTA)/arteriogram can be tailored appropriately. Ultrasound provides an accurate assessment of the major arteries which allows distinction between patients with significant peripheral arterial disease and those without. At the other end of the spectrum, patients with atypical symptoms that might be due to ischaemia can be examined to exclude the presence of significant arterial disease.

Bypass Grafts and Angioplasty

A variety of problems can occur with surgically inserted bypass grafts, especially in the first year after the operation. Ultrasound provides accurate information about any problems that may develop in relation to these bypass grafts. Similarly, patients in whom angioplasty has been undertaken can be followed with ultrasound to confirm residual patency, identify restenosis and assess improvements to flow following the procedure.

False Aneurysms and Other Pulsatile Masses

The assessment of pulsatile masses in relation to the arteries of the upper and lower limbs can be performed rapidly and easily using ultrasound. Aneurysms can be distinguished from non-vascular masses which lie adjacent to the artery. The complications of catheterisation procedures, including haematomas, arteriovenous fistulae and false or pseudoaneurysms, can be assessed and differentiated; in many cases, pseudoaneurysms can be treated under ultrasound control, thereby removing the need for a surgical procedure.

Haemodialysis Fistulae

Arteriovenous fistulae created for haemodialysis can be examined using ultrasound, allowing identification of complications associated with stenosis or occlusion, as well as estimation of blood flow through the shunt, particularly if this is thought to be inadequate or excessive (see Chapter 7).

Anatomy and Scanning Technique

ANATOMY – LOWER LIMB

The arteries of the lower limb arise at the bifurcation of the abdominal aorta (Fig. 4-1), the common iliac arteries run down the posterior wall of the pelvis and divide into the internal and external iliac arteries in front of the sacroiliac joint. The internal iliac artery continues down into the pelvis and is difficult to demonstrate with transabdominal ultrasound, although transvaginal or transrectal scanning will show some of its branches. The external iliac artery continues around the side of the pelvis to the level of the inguinal ligament, it lies anteromedial to the psoas muscle and is normally superficial to the external iliac vein.

The common femoral artery runs from the inguinal ligament to its division into superficial and deep femoral arteries in the upper thigh; this division is usually 3–6 cm distal to the inguinal ligament. The deep femoral artery, or profunda femoris artery, passes posterolaterally to supply the major thigh muscles. The importance of the profunda femoris lies in its role as a major collateral pathway in patients with significant superficial femoral artery disease. Several other branches arise from the external iliac, common femoral and profunda femoris arteries and occasionally one of these may be mistaken for the profunda femoris artery, especially if it is enlarged as a collateral supply.

The superficial femoral artery (also referred to as the femoral artery) passes downwards along the anteromedial aspect of the thigh lying anterior to the vein; in the lower third of the thigh it passes into the adductor canal, deep to sartorius and the medial component of quadriceps femoris. Passing posteriorly behind the lower femur it enters the popliteal fossa and becomes the popliteal artery, which lies anterior to the popliteal vein and gives off several branches, the largest of which are the superior and inferior geniculate arteries. Below the knee joint the popliteal artery divides into the anterior tibial artery and the tibioperoneal trunk, although the exact level of the division may vary; after 2–4 cm the latter divides into the posterior tibial artery and the peroneal artery.

The anterior tibial artery passes forwards through the interosseous membrane between the fibula and tibia. It then descends on the anterior margin of the membrane, deep to the extensor muscles on the anterolateral aspect of the calf (Fig. 4-2). At the ankle it passes across the front of the joint to become the dorsalis pedis artery of the foot which runs from the front of the ankle joint to the proximal end of the first intertarsal space where it gives off metatarsal branches and passes through the first intertarsal space to unite with the lateral plantar artery and form the plantar arterial arch.

The posterior tibial artery passes down the deep medial aspect of the calf to pass behind the medial malleolus, after which it divides into the medial and lateral plantar arteries of the foot; the lateral plantar artery joins with the dorsalis pedis artery in the plantar arch.

The peroneal artery passes down the calf behind the tibia and interosseous membrane and divides into several periarticular branches behind the ankle joint. The size of the calf arteries can be quite variable, the posterior tibial artery is the least variable in calibre but the anterior tibial and peroneal arteries may vary considerably in calibre and overall length in the calf. The arterial supply to the foot is not normally examined but if a bypass procedure to the pedal arteries is being considered then the dorsalis pedis and

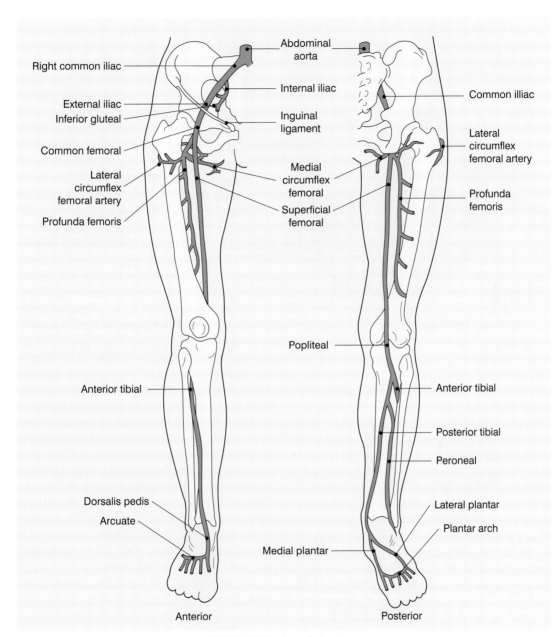

FIGURE 4-1 The lower limb arteries.

posterior tibial artery and its plantar branches should be assessed.

SCANNING TECHNIQUE – LOWER LIMB

A full scan of the lower limb arteries can be time consuming. In some cases a full scan from aortic bifurcation to the ankle or foot is required but in other cases the examination can be tailored to specific levels depending on the diagnostic information required. It is therefore useful if the diagnostic question can be clearly defined, so that the most appropriate examination can be performed.

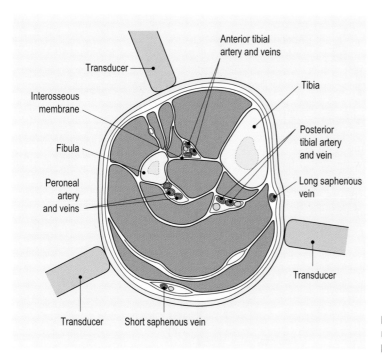

FIGURE 4-2 Cross-section of calf, showing major relations of calf arteries and the three main access points for demonstrating these vessels.

Common Femoral, Profunda Femoris and Superficial Femoral Arteries

The examination begins with the patient lying supine on the couch. The main steps in the examination are given in Box 4-2. A linear array transducer is used; usually 5–12 MHz depending on the performance of the ultrasound system and the build of the patient, lower frequencies may be required to examine the arteries in the adductor canal or in large patients. The distal external iliac/common femoral artery is located using colour Doppler as it leaves the pelvis under the inguinal ligament lateral to the femoral vein. Even if flow appears normal on colour Doppler and

BOX 4-2 BASIC STEPS IN THE EXAMINATION OF THE LOWER LIMB ARTERIES

1. Patient supine: scan common femoral, proximal profunda and superficial femoral artery down to adductor canal

2. Patient decubitus: scan adductor canal, popliteal artery to bifurcation and tibioperoneal trunk, scan posterior tibial and peroneal arteries

3. Patient supine: scan anterior tibial arteries. Scan iliac arteries and infrarenal aorta

there is no evidence of local disease, a spectral Doppler trace should be recorded, as changes in this may indicate the presence of significant disease proximally, necessitating a careful direct examination of the iliac vessels. The bifurcation of the common femoral artery into the profunda femoris and superficial femoral arteries is then examined using colour and spectral Doppler. The profunda femoris artery should be examined over its proximal 5 cm, especially in patients with severe superficial femoral disease, in order to assess the amount of collateral flow, or its potential value as a graft origin or insertion point.

The superficial femoral artery is then followed along the length of the thigh using colour Doppler. It is often better to move the transducer in sequential steps, rather than sliding it down the thigh, as most machines require a few frames of sampling at each position to provide a steady image. In addition, the moving transducer generates colour Doppler noise over the image, obscuring vascular details. Doppler spectra are obtained as necessary at points of possible disease. Even in the absence of colour Doppler abnormalities, it is good practice to obtain routine spectral assessments from the superficial femoral artery in the upper, middle and lower thigh, in order to confirm that there is no alteration in the waveform that might suggest disease. Sometimes the artery is difficult to see on colour or power Doppler as the signals are weak or absent. In these cases the artery may be visible by virtue of calcified plaques in the wall of the vessel. Alternatively, the superficial femoral vein, lying behind the artery, can be used as a guide to the position of the artery and spectral Doppler used to demonstrate the presence or absence of arterial flow. Echo-enhancing agents can be used if there is any continuing uncertainty concerning the patency of the artery.

There are three indirect signs of significant disease which might be apparent during the examination and which should prompt a careful review if a cause for these changes has not been identified.

1. Colour Doppler may show the presence of collateral vessels in the muscles of the thigh (Fig. 4-3A).
2. Collateral vessels may be seen leaving the main artery (Fig. 4-3B).
3. The character of the spectral waveform may show a change between two levels, indicating a segment of disease somewhere between the two points of measurement.

The Adductor Canal and Popliteal Fossa

The patient is then turned into a lateral decubitus position so that the medial aspect of the leg being examined is uppermost (Fig. 4-4). This position is better than the prone position as it allows access in continuity to the lower superficial femoral artery, the adductor canal area, the popliteal region and the medial calf. The region of the adductor canal must be examined with great care as it is a site where a short-segment stenosis or occlusion may be present,

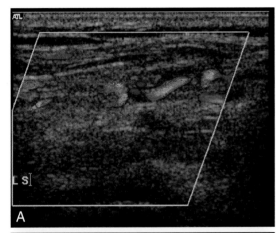

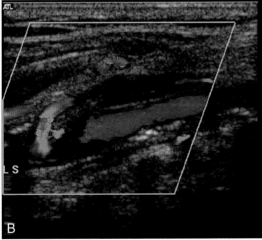

FIGURE 4-3 (A) Collateral vessels in the muscles of the thigh. (B) A larger collateral vessel joining the lower superficial femoral artery.

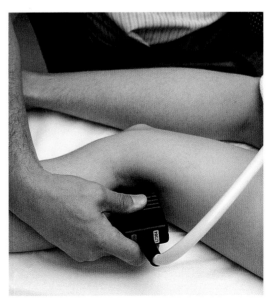

FIGURE 4-4 The position of the patient for examination of the adductor canal and popliteal fossa.

and this section of the vessel can be difficult to visualise as it passes deep to the thigh muscles. In some cases the use of a lower scanning frequency may help visualisation. The superficial femoral artery is examined as far down as it can be followed on the medial aspect of the thigh; the popliteal artery is then located in the popliteal fossa and followed superiorly. In difficult cases a mark can be put on the skin of the medial thigh to show the lowest segment of vessel visualised in the supine position; the popliteal artery is then followed superiorly in the decubitus position until the transducer reaches the level of the skin mark, ensuring that the vessel has been examined in continuity. The popliteal artery is then examined and followed down to the point of division into the tibioperoneal trunk and anterior tibial artery.

Calf Arteries

The complexity of the assessment of the calf arteries depends on the clinical situation. If the examination is to exclude significant proximal disease that would benefit from angioplasty or bypass grafts, then it is usually sufficient to assess the three calf arteries at the upper and mid-calf level, recording whether they are patent or not, in order to provide some assessment of the state of the distal run-off. In other cases a more detailed examination is required to clarify changes seen on MRA/arteriography, or if a distal insertion point for a bypass graft is being sought. The increased sensitivity of power Doppler is useful in detecting weak signals from small or diseased but patent vessels.

The posterior tibial artery is usually the easier of the two branches of the tibioperoneal trunk to locate. Often it can be located by placing the transducer in a longitudinal position on the medial aspect of the mid-calf area behind the tibia, using colour or power Doppler to show the course of the vessel, which can then be followed up and down the calf. In obese or oedematous legs, or if blood flow is impaired by disease, the posterior tibial artery and the other calf arteries may be difficult to locate. Scanning with colour Doppler in the transverse plane using some angulation towards the head or feet may show the relative positions of the posterior tibial and peroneal arteries. Alternatively, the associated veins can be used to identify the region of the relevant artery: squeezing the foot or lower calf will augment flow in the deep veins,

allowing these to be identified in either a longitudinal or transverse scan plane. The posterior tibial artery can also be located as it passes behind the medial malleolus, where its position is constant, and then followed back up the leg.

The peroneal artery runs more deeply down the calf than the posterior tibial artery, lying closer to the posterior aspect of the tibia and the interosseous membrane. It can be examined from several approaches: firstly from a posteromedial approach similar to that used for the posterior tibial artery; secondly, it can often also be seen from the anterolateral approach used for the anterior tibial artery as it runs behind the interosseous membrane (Fig. 4-2); thirdly, a posterolateral approach may be of value in some cases.

The anterior tibial artery is examined from an anterolateral approach through the extensor muscles lying between the tibia and fibula. The two bones can be identified on transverse scanning and the interosseous membrane located passing between them. The anterior tibial artery lies on the membrane and can be located using colour Doppler in either the longitudinal or transverse plane. It usually lies nearer the fibula than the tibia (Fig. 4-2).

The foot vessels are not usually examined but the dorsalis pedis artery may be examined in front of the ankle joint before it passes deep to the metatarsals; this is indicated if the artery is being considered for the insertion of a femorodistal graft.

The advent of power Doppler and echo-enhancing agents has extended the role of ultrasound in the assessment of vascular disease. In the proximal lower limb and iliac vessels, the location of the vessel and confirmation of occluded segments has been made easier and, in the distal part of the leg, they make assessment of the smaller vessels of the calf and foot easier. However, more work is required to evaluate further their role.[4]

Iliac Arteries

Examination of the iliac vessels is carried out as part of a general survey of the lower limb arteries, or if the clinical picture suggests a need to confirm or exclude disease affecting these vessels, or if the Doppler findings at the groin suggest the likelihood of significant proximal disease. The ease with which they can be visualised depends on the build of the patient and the amount of bowel gas present. It is usually necessary to use a 3–5 MHz transducer for satisfactory visualisation. Some examiners will prepare patients for iliac Doppler examinations with laxatives and low-residue diets if it is considered likely that these vessels will be examined, although most centres do not do this routinely.

The external iliac artery can be followed up from the groin for a variable distance; the vein, lying behind the artery, can be used to identify the probable location of the artery if this is not apparent. Colour or power Doppler may also help locate the vessel, even if it is not visible on the real-time image. Superiorly, the common iliac artery can be identified arising at the aortic bifurcation and then followed distally. Firm pressure with the transducer will displace intervening amounts of bowel gas to a large extent, although care must be taken not to compress the artery and produce a false impression of a stenosis. The internal iliac artery may be seen arising from the common iliac artery and passing deeply into the pelvis. This is a useful landmark as visualisation of the internal iliac artery origin, on tracking both the external iliac artery upwards and the common iliac artery downwards, means that the iliac arteries have been examined in their entirety.

The orientation of the iliac vessels as they pass round the pelvis and the use of sector or curved-array transducers can lead to problems with beam–vessel geometry and obtaining satisfactory angles of insonation. However, careful attention to positioning the transducer will usually allow an appropriate angle to be obtained.

ANATOMY – UPPER LIMB

The subclavian arteries arise from the brachiocephalic trunk on the right (Fig. 4-5) and directly from the arch of the aorta on the left; however, there is considerable normal variation in the patterns of their origination. The origin of the right subclavian artery can be examined behind the right sternoclavicular joint, where the brachiocephalic trunk divides into the right common carotid artery and the subclavian artery. The origin of the left subclavian artery from the aortic arch cannot be demonstrated, although the more distal segments can be seen as on the right side. The subclavian artery on each side runs from its point of origin to the outer

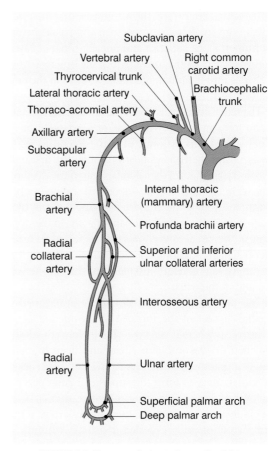

FIGURE 4-5 The upper limb arteries on the right.

border of the first rib where it becomes the axillary artery; the subclavian vein lies in front of the artery. The main branches of the subclavian artery are the vertebral arteries, the thyrocervical trunk, the internal thoracic (mammary) artery and the costocervical trunk.

The axillary artery runs from the lateral border of the first rib to the outer, inferior margin of the pectoralis major muscle. It gives rise to several branches which supply the muscles around the shoulder; the largest of these are the thoracoacromial trunk, the lateral thoracic artery and the subscapular artery.

The brachial artery passes down the medial aspect of the upper arm to the cubital fossa below which it divides into the radial and ulnar arteries; the point of division sometimes lies higher in the upper arm. Apart from muscular branches, the main branches of the brachial artery are the profunda brachii artery, which is given off in the upper arm and passes behind the humerus; the superior and inferior ulnar collateral arteries arise from the lower part of the brachial artery. It divides into the ulnar and radial arteries in the antecubital fossa.

The radial artery runs down the radial (lateral) aspect of the forearm to the wrist, where it passes over the radial styloid process, and over the lateral aspect of the carpus. It then passes down through the first interosseous space to form the lateral aspect of the deep palmar arch. It also has a superficial branch which anastomoses with the equivalent branch of the ulnar artery to form the superficial palmar arch. In the upper forearm the radial artery gives off the radial recurrent artery, which anastomoses with the profunda brachii artery, and several muscular branches in the forearm and at the wrist.

The ulnar artery passes down the anterior ulnar (medial) aspect of the forearm to the medial aspect of the wrist, where it runs over the flexor retinaculum and then divides into superficial and deep branches which anastomose with the equivalent branches of the radial artery to form the superficial and deep palmar arches. It gives off recurrent ulnar arteries below the elbow and the common interosseous artery, which forms anterior and posterior divisions, running on either side of the interosseous membrane.

SCANNING TECHNIQUE – UPPER LIMB

A 7–12 MHz transducer may be used in most cases for examining the arteries in the upper limb, as there is less tissue to penetrate than in the leg. The patient lies in a supine position with their head turned away from the side being examined, the arm is abducted with the elbow flexed and the back of the hand resting on the pillow by the patient's head, so that the axilla and medial aspect of the upper arm can be examined. Alternatively, the arm can be abducted and supported on a suitable shelf, or by asking the patient to hold onto a suitable part of the ultrasound machine. The distal brachiocephalic artery on the right and the mid-subclavian artery on the left can be visualised from a supraclavicular approach by angling the transducer down towards the mediastinum from above the medial clavicle and sternoclavicular joint. The subclavian arteries on both sides are seen behind the subclavian vein as they run up to cross the first rib. In patients with possible arterial compression syndromes, the artery is examined with the arm in various positions so that any narrowing or occlusion may be demonstrated.

The artery beyond the first rib is best examined from below the clavicle and followed distally. It can be followed in continuity as it runs deep to the pectoralis muscles through the axilla and into the medial aspect of the upper arm; from here it can be tracked down to the cubital fossa. The division of the artery into the two main forearm branches usually occurs below the cubital fossa and each branch can be followed to the wrist; if either the radial or the ulnar artery is difficult to trace down from the elbow, then the vessel should be sought at the wrist and followed back up the forearm.

Assessment of Disease

The assessment of lower limb atheroma is more complex than for the carotids as the potential for collateral supply around stenoses or occlusions is very much greater. The distinction must be made between haemodynamically significant disease and clinically significant disease. Two individuals may have the same degree of stenosis in their superficial femoral artery, but an 80% diameter reduction which develops acutely will be significantly symptomatic, whereas the same degree of stenosis developing over a period of time, allowing collateral channels to open, may be much less disabling. The findings on Doppler must therefore not be considered in isolation but in the light of the full clinical picture.

Colour Doppler allows the rapid identification of normal and abnormal segments of vessel. In addition, some stenoses may show a colour Doppler tissue 'bruit' due to the tissue vibrations set up by the blood passing through the stenosis. It is valuable to relate the level of any diseased segments demonstrated on ultrasound to bony landmarks which can be seen on angiography; this allows the appearances on the two examinations to be compared and confirm that the abnormality on the arteriogram is at the level of the lesion seen on ultrasound or vice versa. The groin skin crease corresponds to the superior pubic ramus and can be used for lesions in the upper part of the thigh; the upper border of the patella can be used for lesions in the lower part of the thigh; and the tibiofemoral joint space for popliteal lesions.

Some patients will show extensive diffuse disease along much, or all, of the superficial femoral artery but do not show any specific, localised stenoses. It is important to note this appearance, as the overall haemodynamic effect may be severe enough to produce a significant pressure drop along the vessel, thereby reducing limb perfusion, although this pattern of disease is not suitable for angioplasty. Other patients may have several stenoses along the length of the vessel, each of which is not haemodynamically significant but the effects of these are additive, so that there is still a significant drop in perfusion pressure distal to the affected segment.[5]

In addition, the presence of serial stenoses can affect the estimation of the degree of a distal stenosis, if this is not recognised. A significant proximal stenosis or occlusion will result in a drop in perfusion pressure and velocity which makes application of the peak systolic velocity (PSV) and peak velocity ratios, the usual criteria for quantifying a stenosis, problematical.[6] Power Doppler and echo-enhancing agents may allow an estimate of severity of the distal stenosis but if there is clinical doubt, other imaging should be considered.

The same principles apply to the assessment of disease in the upper limb, but the type and distribution of disease in the arm is different from that seen in the leg. Ischaemic symptoms in the arm may be the result of compression, embolic occlusion, or vasospasm and are less frequently due to localised atheroma.

The main diagnostic criteria which are of value in the assessment of lower limb atheroma are direct measurement of the stenosis, PSV ratios and waveform changes.

DIRECT MEASUREMENT

Direct measurement of a stenosis is often quite difficult in the lower limb arteries as these are relatively small, and it may be difficult to see the lumen clearly in the deeper parts of the thigh, particularly if there is disease present. However, direct measurement of a stenosis may be possible in the lower external iliac, common femoral, profunda femoris and upper superficial femoral arteries. Measurement of the diameter reduction is performed after assessment of plaque distribution in both longitudinal and transverse planes, so that the most appropriate diameter is selected. When a segment of stenosis or occlusion is detected the length of the affected segment should be measured, as this will be relevant to the suitability of the lesion for angioplasty; segments of disease, particularly occlusions, longer than 10 cm will not normally be considered for percutaneous treatment.[7]

PEAK VELOCITY RATIOS

Direct measurement of a stenosis is often not possible in the lower limb and the severity of the stenosis must then be estimated from the change in peak systolic velocity produced by the stenosis. Normal velocities in the lower limb arteries at rest are approximately 1.2 m/s in the iliac segments, 0.9 m/s in the superficial femoral segments and 0.7 m/s in the popliteal segment.[8] Various criteria have been put forward for the quantification of lower limb arterial stenosis. Those of Cossman et al.[9] have produced satisfactory results in our department and have the advantage of being easy to remember (Table 4-1). These criteria are based on the PSV at the stenosis and the ratio of the PSV at the stenosis compared with the velocity 1–2 cm upstream in a non-diseased segment. Colour Doppler allows the position and direction of peak velocity flow in the stenosis to be identified and the sample volume can be placed appropriately, final adjustments of position being performed by listening to the pitch of the frequency shift as the sample volume is moved through the stenosis. A further velocity measurement is then made in a 'normal' segment of artery 1–2 cm upstream from the stenosis and the ratio calculated (Fig. 4-6).

TABLE 4-1 Velocity Criteria for the Assessment of Lower Limb Stenoses		
Percentage Stenosis	Peak Systolic Velocity (m/s)	Velocity Ratio
Normal	<1.5	<1.5:1
0–49	1.5–2.0	1.5–2:1
50–75	2.0–4.0	2–4:1
>75	>4.0	>4:1
Occlusion	–	–

From Cossman et al.[9]

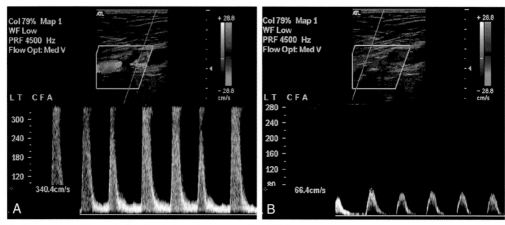

FIGURE 4-6 Measurement of the peak systolic velocity ratio at a stenosis. (A) Velocity at the stenosis is 3.4 m/s. (B) Velocity above the stenosis is 0.66 m/s, giving a ratio of approximately 5.

WAVEFORM CHANGES

The normal waveform in the main arteries of the resting lower limb has three components; four, or occasionally five, may be seen in fit young individuals. These represent the pressure changes which occur in the resting lower limb arteries during the cardiac cycle. First there is the rise in pressure and acceleration of blood flow at the onset of systole. There is then a short period of reversed flow as the pressure wave is reflected from the constricted distal arterioles. This is followed by a further period of forward flow produced by the elastic compliance of the main arteries in diastole (Fig. 4-7A). These changes are discussed in more detail in Chapter 2.

Exercise modifies this pattern by reducing the peripheral resistance. This results in the reversed component being lost and increased diastolic flow throughout the cardiac cycle (Fig. 4-7B). It is for this reason that ultrasound examination of the lower limb arteries should be performed in patients who have not had significant exercise of the leg muscles for about 15 min. Conversely,

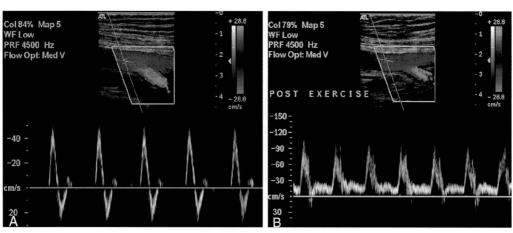

FIGURE 4-7 The normal femoral artery waveform. (A) In a limb at rest three components are visible. Aliasing in the profunda artery is due to the lower insonation angle giving a higher Doppler shift, not a focal stenosis. (B) Following exercise there is increased flow throughout diastole as a result of peripheral dilation. Note that the PRF scale has been increased in B to accommodate the higher peak systolic velocity.

examination after exercise, or reactive hyperaemia, may be used in order to 'stress' the lower limb circulation and reveal stenoses which are not significant at rest, when blood flow is relatively low, but which become apparent with the higher volumes flowing when the distal circulation to the muscles opens up.[10]

Disease in the vessel at the point of measurement, above it or below it, can affect the waveform, and if the vessel cannot be visualised in continuity then a change in the waveform between two points is indicative of disease. The two main features which may be altered are the overall shape of the waveform and the degree of spectral broadening as a result of flow disturbance;[8] the major changes are shown in Box 4-3 and illustrated in Fig. 4-8. Proximal disease above the point of measurement results in loss firstly of the third and then of the second components of the waveform, as the normal passage of the pressure wave along the artery is impaired. This interference with the passage of the pulse wave along the vessel is also manifest by the slowing of the systolic acceleration time. The width of the first, systolic complex is increased and the overall height is decreased. These changes result in 'damping' of the waveform, which is most marked when there is a proximal occlusion. The turbulence generated beyond a stenosis shows in the spectrum as spectral broadening and its presence therefore also indicates proximal disease, although not its severity, as mild turbulence may be due to a minor stenosis close by, or a more severe stenosis further away. The spectral broadening may be seen throughout the spectrum if the stenosis is close to the point of measurement; as the distance from the stenosis increases, the spectral broadening is seen in the postsystolic deceleration phase only.

BOX 4-3 WAVEFORM CHANGES ASSOCIATED WITH DISEASE IN THE LOWER LIMB

- Loss of third and then second phase of the waveform
- Increased acceleration time
- Widening of the systolic complex
- Damping of the waveform
- Spectral broadening
- Absent flow in occlusion

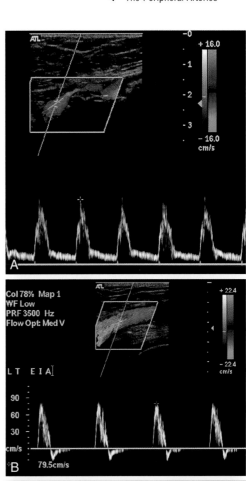
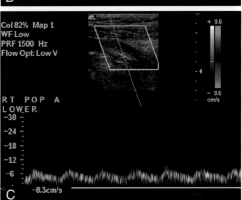

FIGURE 4-8 Abnormal lower limb artery waveforms. (A) Loss of reverse flow and diastolic flow due to distal disease producing peripheral dilatation; a large plaque impinges on the lumen. (B) Broadening of the waveform and turbulence secondary to a proximal stenosis. (C) Damped waveform in the popliteal artery secondary to a proximal occluded segment.

The disturbance of flow created by a stenosis may take several centimetres to resolve. The spectral broadening is lost and the systolic forward flow component is regained, but the reverse component and third component are much less likely to reappear distal to disease. In addition, if the distal limb is ischaemic, this will result in dilatation of the capillaries and increased flow throughout diastole. The presence of some, or all, of these changes requires that the vessel be carefully examined proximally to identify their source.

The presence of distal disease will also affect the waveform, resulting in increased pulsatility, with reduced diastolic flow, evident from the loss of the third component; in addition, the peak systolic velocity is reduced. This situation is most often seen at the origin of a superficial femoral artery with significant distal disease, although the precise changes are variable, depending on the degree of obstruction and the capacity of any collateral channels.[11]

ASSESSMENT OF AORTOILIAC DISEASE

The clinical findings, or the appearances of the waveform at the groin, may suggest the presence of significant disease in the aortoiliac segments.[12] The best method for assessment of these segments is by direct visualisation with colour Doppler and measurement of velocities as for the leg vessels. Satisfactory examinations have been reported in up to 90% of cases with careful scanning and preparation.[13] The main indirect indicators of significant iliac artery disease are spectral broadening, due to the turbulence set up by the stenosis, and widening of the systolic complex as a result of the stenosis slowing the systolic acceleration. As noted earlier, power Doppler and echo-enhancing agents show promise in improving visualisation and assessment using ultrasound.[4]

REPORTING THE EXAMINATION

The findings from a Doppler examination of the peripheral arteries are best reported on a diagram (Fig. 4-9) of the relevant arterial tree. The level and extent of any stenoses can be indicated on this, together with blood flow velocities at areas of stenosis and the standard sites of measurement. Non-visualised areas should also be indicated. For patients with bypass grafts, the location of the graft can be sketched in and relevant velocities indicated.

Arterial Bypass Grafts

A variety of bypass grafts may be employed to alleviate ischaemic symptoms (Box 4-4). Autologous vein is the preferred material and usually the long saphenous vein is used, although other veins may occasionally be employed. Synthetic materials [polytetrafluoroethylene (PTFE), Goretex, or Dacron] may be used if the long saphenous veins are unsuitable or unavailable. Infrainguinal femorodistal grafts are the commonest type of procedure; several problems may occur which result in graft failure (Table 4-2) and there has been much discussion about the possible benefits from programmes of graft surveillance in the postoperative period and whether these improve long-term patency rates, or not.[14]

The timing of graft failure is related to the cause of the problem. Failures occurring within 6–8 weeks of surgery are usually due to technical problems arising from the surgery; 3–5% of grafts fail at this stage, approximately 25% of all graft failures. Failures developing in the period beginning 3 months and extending to 2 years after surgery are usually due to neointimal hyperplasia; 12–37% of grafts fail during this period, approximately 70–80% of all graft failures; most of these will occur in the first 12 months. Beyond 2 years after surgery the usual cause of failure is progression of atherosclerosis, either in the native vessels or in the graft itself.[15] In addition to graft stenosis or occlusions, other problems may occur, including dehiscence at the origin or insertion and false aneurysm formation, arteriovenous fistulae, infected collections and compression or kinking.

The theory behind surveillance programmes is that they will identify grafts at risk before they fail and allow remedial action to be taken to maintain patency and function. The timing of the surveillance scans is based on this time scale for problems. An early scan 4–6 weeks after the operation is performed, subsequently a scan is done at 3 months and then at 3-monthly intervals until the end of the first year. It is not usually necessary to continue beyond this if no cause for concern exists, as the majority of failures will occur in the first year. However, if there are particular reasons for concern, such as mild or moderate stenosis (velocity ratio >2), then surveillance can be extended as appropriate. Surveillance programmes have been shown by some authors to be beneficial in terms of enhanced graft patency and limb survival

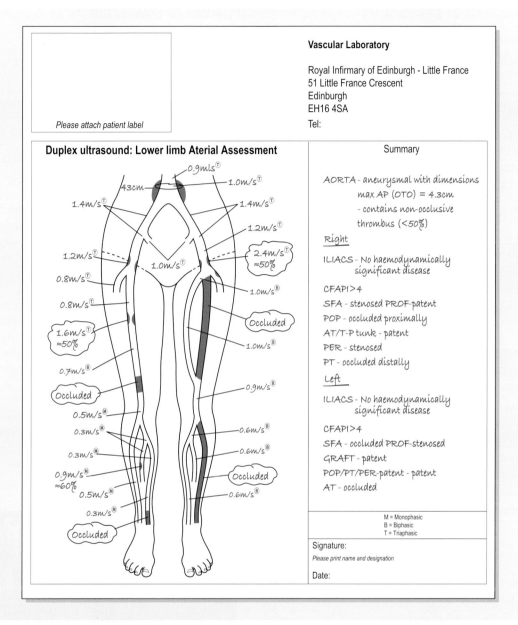

FIGURE 4-9 An example of a diagram that can be used for reporting arterial and lower limb bypass graft examinations. The findings from an arterial examination are shown on the right leg and from a bypass graft examination on the left leg. (Courtesy of S-J Carmichael.)

rates.[16] However, Lane et al. in a review of 42 studies[14] noted that the evidence that surveillance programmes improved amputation/limb salvage rates, or the patient's quality of life overall was not yet available. Their recommendations were that a duplex scan 6 weeks after surgery might identify grafts at risk which would benefit from surveillance but that those grafts without signs of concern at 6 weeks could be best managed with clinical follow up, together with ankle/brachial pressure measurements, with duplex scanning

BOX 4-4 TYPES OF BYPASS GRAFT

TYPES OF GRAFT

Aorto-iliac

Iliofemoral

Femoropopliteal – may arise from external iliac artery rather than common femoral artery

Femorodistal – to calf vessels or dorsalis pedis

Femorofemoral crossover

Axillofemoral

MATERIALS USED FOR GRAFT

Vein

In situ vein

Reversed vein

Synthetic

Dacron

Polytetrafluoroethylene (PTFE)

Gore-Tex

TABLE 4-2   **Causes of Graft Failure**

Intrinsic	Extrinsic
Stenosis	Inflow disease progression
Proximal or distal anastomosis	Outflow disease progression
Mid-graft	Clamp injury
Diffuse myointimal hyperplasia	Thromboembolism
Aneurysm	Hypercoagulation states
Anastomotic	Sepsis
Mid-graft	

Haemodynamic failure occurs when the graft is patent but the limb remains ischaemic.

being undertaken if there were clinical concerns. It is recognised that further Level 1 evidence is required to clarify the role of surveillance one way or the other.

The situation is more straightforward for synthetic grafts. Several studies have shown that synthetic grafts are more likely to fail without warning signs being demonstrated on Doppler,[17,18] and Lane et al. found no evidence to support duplex surveillance of prosthetic femoro-distal grafts.[14] Symptomatic grafts, however, should always be examined, as a treatable lesion may be demonstrated prior to complete graft thrombosis and failure.

TECHNIQUE OF EXAMINATION

It is of value if the request for a graft assessment gives details of the surgery and the type of graft inserted; ideally, a diagram of the course of the graft should be provided. For a femoro-distal graft the examination should begin at the groin and the graft located; transverse scanning is helpful with identification of the graft origin. Once located the graft should be followed up to its point of origin from the native artery. The majority of grafts are femoropopliteal and run from the common femoral artery, or lower external iliac artery, to the upper or lower popliteal artery; occasionally the graft may originate from deeper in the pelvis, lower down the superficial femoral artery, or from the profunda femoris artery. The native artery above the graft is assessed and the velocity of blood flow measured with spectral Doppler. The origin of the graft is then examined carefully and any increase in velocity, or disturbance of flow, noted (Fig. 4-10).

The graft is followed down the length of the thigh. Most grafts run along the medial aspect of the thigh; however some grafts, particularly repeat grafts, may follow unusual courses, even crossing the thigh to run down the lateral aspect of the leg. Velocity measurements are obtained at any point of disturbed flow; if no disturbance is present, two to three velocity measurements are taken along the length of the graft to ensure that there is satisfactory flow.

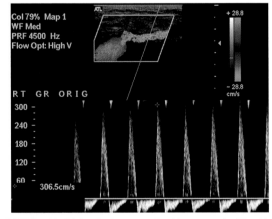

FIGURE 4-10 Origin of a femoropopliteal bypass graft with a high velocity of 3.06 m/s.

At the graft insertion, the flow above, at and below the anastomosis is examined, any significant changes in the velocities should be assessed as possible signs of stenosis. Some care must be taken in the interpretation of velocity increases at both the origin and insertion of grafts, as moderate changes may be the result of disparity in size between the graft and the native vessel and therefore not pathological in origin, particularly at

the distal insertion, if this is into a relatively small calf artery or the dorsalis pedis artery.

Synthetic grafts are relatively straightforward to assess, as any problems usually occur at the origin or insertion, rather than along the length of the graft. Vein grafts, however, can develop problems at any point along their length, particularly at sites of avulsed valves or tied perforating veins (Fig. 4-11). Stenoses can occur

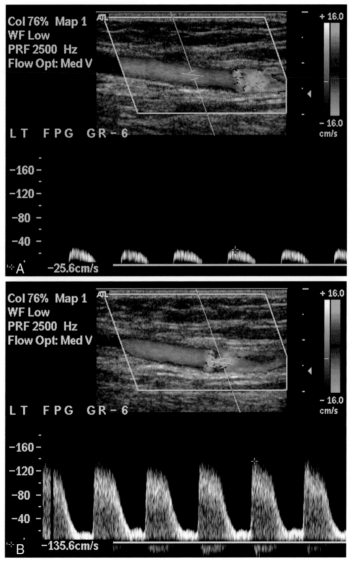

FIGURE 4-11 A stenosis in an in situ vein graft. The slight dilatation of the vessel at the level of the stenosis indicates that this is the site of an avulsed valve. The velocity above the stenosis (A) is only 0.25 m/s but increases to 1.35 m/s at the stenosis (B); a velocity ratio of 5.4.

secondary to surgery, or as a result of intimal hyperplasia, which can be stimulated by the turbulence at an irregularity in the vein wall. In situ vein grafts may also have persistent arteriovenous communications if a perforating or superficial communicating vein has been overlooked during the operation. These may be quite small but their presence should be suspected if there is a rapid, unexplained drop in velocity along the graft, or if pulsatile venous flow is seen in the common or superficial femoral veins. Scanning transversely along the line of the in situ graft makes it easier to identify these communicating vessels and demonstrate their course.

A note should also be made of any collections seen along the track of the graft. In the postoperative period these are usually small collections of serous fluid, haematomas, or small lymphoceles; normally these resorb over a few weeks (Fig. 4-12A). If infection is suspected (Fig. 4-12B) then a fine needle (20–22 G) can be used to perform a diagnostic aspiration, although care should be taken not to introduce infection into a sterile collection.

If an occluded graft is demonstrated but the leg is asymptomatic then it is worth checking if the patient has had more than one bypass procedure, as a second, patent graft may be present elsewhere in the leg.

Other bypass procedures that may be performed include aorto-external iliac or femoral grafts, axillofemoral grafts, femoro-femoral (crossover) grafts. These use synthetic grafts and do not usually enter into graft surveillance programmes, although an ultrasound scan may be requested if there are clinical concerns. Distal lower limb grafts to the lower calf arteries, or dorsalis pedis artery, are also performed.

FEATURES OF A GRAFT AT RISK

The main features which suggest that a graft is at risk of failing are shown in Table 4-3. There is good correlation between these criteria and the incidence of subsequent graft failure. The finding of a fall in the ankle/brachial pressure index of more than 0.15 in addition to the presence of a stenosis of more than 70%, or low mean graft velocity, is a strong indicator of a graft at risk.[19] Gibson et al.[20] found that there was a significantly higher incidence of graft failure if there was a graft-related stenosis with a velocity ratio >3.5 and a mean graft PSV of <50 cm/s, calculated from velocities obtained at non-stenotic points along the length

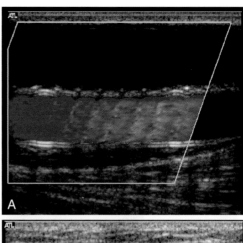

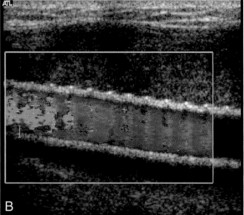

FIGURE 4-12 (A) A small trans-sonic lymphocele around a femoropopliteal bypass graft; (B) an infected fluid collection around a synthetic graft showing low-level echoes within the fluid.

TABLE 4-3 **Doppler Criteria for Graft Stenosis and Grafts at Risk**	
Direct measurement of stenosis	Moderate >50% diameter stenosis Severe >70% diameter stenosis
Peak systolic velocity changes	>1.5 m/s = 50–70% diameter stenosis >2.5 m/s >70% diameter stenosis
End diastolic velocity	>1.0 m/s >70% diameter stenosis
Velocity ratio	>2.5 >50% diameter stenosis >3.5 >70% diameter stenosis
Peak systolic velocity	<50 cm/s in narrowest segment

of the graft. However, they found that a low mean graft velocity by itself without an associated stenosis was not associated with graft failure.

Other abnormalities which may be seen in relation to a bypass graft are a false aneurysm at the origin or insertion due to dehiscence of the anastomosis (Fig. 4-13), or an arteriovenous fistula.

False Aneurysms

These are usually straightforward to diagnose on colour Doppler ultrasound, although occasionally there may be some difficulty if there is also a large

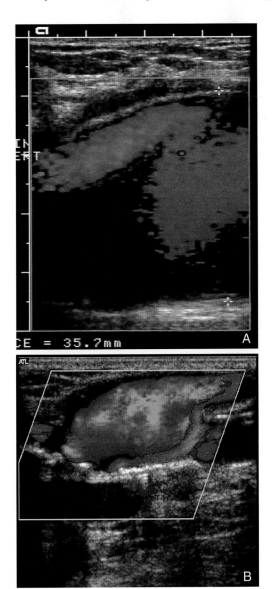

FIGURE 4-13 (A) Dehiscence at the insertion of a graft into the lower popliteal artery; (B) aneurysmal dilatation at the origin of a bypass graft.

haematoma present. The incidence of femoral false aneurysms increased as more interventional procedures were carried out through femoral puncture sites; rates of 0.2–0.5% after diagnostic arteriography and 2–8% following coronary artery angioplasty and stent placement have been reported.[21] Newer, improved techniques for sealing vascular puncture sites and radial/brachial access have led to some improvement in these figures. The characteristic appearance is a hypoechoic area which shows swirling blood flow on colour Doppler (Fig. 4-14A). It is important that the relationship of the aneurysm to the femoral artery is identified to ensure that any therapeutic thrombin injection is made into the aneurysm and not the artery. This may be difficult to define in the presence of a significant haematoma; in these cases identification of the artery above and below the haematoma and tracking back to the aneurysm area will allow some assessment of the relationships to be reached. Spectral Doppler of the track between the artery and the aneurysm, or at the aneurysm neck, shows a characteristic 'to-and-fro' flow signal as blood flows in during systole and out during diastole (Fig. 4-14B). Rarely, a false aneurysm may be associated with an arteriovenous fistula passing from the cavity to an adjacent vein. The clue to the presence of the fistula is the loss of the 'to-and-fro' flow in the track from the artery, with only forward flow being shown, which increases towards end-diastole. The need for intervention to treat a false aneurysm needs careful consideration: thrombin injection, surgery and possibly ultrasound-guided compression are all recognised treatments but it should be remembered that a significant proportion of pseudo-aneurysms will thrombose spontaneously within 2–3 weeks; in one surgical series, 86% of 147 patients managed conservatively showed spontaneous thrombosis of their false aneurysms, or arteriovenous fistulae, within a mean period of 23 days.[22]

ULTRASOUND-GUIDED TREATMENT OF FALSE ANEURYSMS

Thrombin Injection

Bovine thrombin and, more recently, human thrombin are now available in many centres and the treatment of choice for most false aneurysms is injection of human thrombin directly into the aneurysmal sac

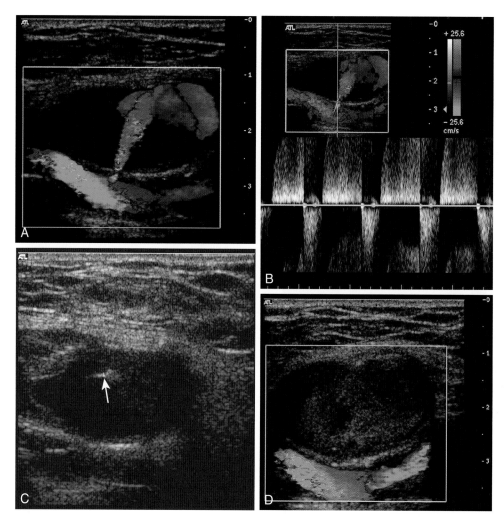

FIGURE 4-14 (A) A false aneurysm showing a patent lumen on colour Doppler; (B) the characteristic 'to-and-fro' flow on spectral Doppler; (C) tip of the needle for thrombin injection seen within the false aneurysm; (D) thrombosed false aneurysm following treatment with thrombin.

under ultrasound control. In the great majority of cases, this will produce immediate and complete thrombosis of the false aneurysm within a few seconds. When the needle tip is positively identified within the aneurysm (Fig. 4-14C), the thrombin solution is injected into the lumen of the aneurysm through a 22–25 G needle attached to an insulin type of syringe (1 mL) to allow careful titration of the amount injected; normally 400–1000 IU of thrombin will be sufficient to produce thrombosis within 20–30 s (Fig. 4-14D). Care should be taken to keep the needle away from the neck of the false aneurysm

to reduce the risk of thrombin refluxing into the artery and down the limb; similarly wide necked aneurysms have a higher risk of thrombin escaping. Following the procedure the patient should stay on bed rest for 1–3 h with regular review of the distal circulation in the affected limb and most centres undertake a check ultrasound examination at 24 h. In some cases a small residual region of continuing flow may require a second injection. One study of 101 false aneurysms showed 95% primary success rate after a single injection and 98% after a second injection in three cases; only two patients required surgical repair.[21] Sheiman and Mastromatteo[23] looked at the reasons for failure in a small series of false aneurysms undergoing thrombin injection; they found that arterial laceration of >8 mm was the cause of failure in four out of five cases and local infection the most likely cause in the remaining patient.

Bovine thrombin may produce allergic responses in the patient and induce antibodies to native clotting factors; therefore, it is better to use human-derived thrombin if this is available. Contraindications to thrombin injection include ischaemic skin changes over a large aneurysm, local infection, evidence of nerve compression, or evidence of an arteriovenous fistula. Thrombin injection is reported to have worked satisfactorily after failed compression therapy in patients on full antiplatelet and anticoagulation therapy.[24]

There have been reports of the successful treatment of false aneurysms in other sites by thrombin injection; these include aneurysms in relation to haemodialysis access sites, an anterior tibial artery pseudoaneurysm that developed after a tibial osteotomy and a common carotid artery pseudoaneurysm that developed following an unsuccessful central venous line insertion.[25]

Ultrasound-Guided Compression

If suitable thrombin preparations are not available, then treatment of false aneurysms using ultrasound-guided compression might be considered. The ability of colour Doppler to demonstrate flowing blood in the aneurysm and track allows the operator to apply graded compression using pressure from the transducer, so that flow into the aneurysm is stopped, whilst allowing flow to continue down the native artery. This allows the aneurysm and track to thrombose and therefore remove the need for surgery.[26] There are, however, some circumstances where it is recognised that compression is unlikely to succeed and direct referral for surgery should be considered; these are shown in Box 4-5. The most common contraindications for compression are the age of the aneurysm and warfarin therapy; if it has been present for more than 7–10 days then the track will have started to develop an endothelium and the surrounding tissues are less compliant, so that adequate compression becomes difficult.

BOX 4-5 CIRCUMSTANCES WHEN COMPRESSION OF A FALSE ANEURYSM IS LESS LIKELY TO SUCCEED

- Aneurysms more than 7–10 days old
- Associated infection
- Severe pain/discomfort
- Large haematoma
- Aneurysms above the inguinal ligament

The procedure is quite time consuming for the operator and uncomfortable for the patient, so it is better to give some analgesia to the patient prior to the commencement of prolonged compression. The aneurysm and its track are identified and compression is applied by pressing the transducer increasingly firmly down on these until flow in them has ceased but flow is still present in the native artery. This degree of pressure is then maintained for 10–15 min before being released slowly. If flow is still seen in the lumen, compression is reinstated for a further period of 10 min before again gently relaxing the pressure. These cycles of compression and relaxation are repeated until all flow in the aneurysm lumen has stopped. Usually the lumen of the aneurysm thromboses in an irregular fashion from the outside inwards, until complete obliteration is achieved. In one large series,[26] the average time for successful treatment of a simple unilocular aneurysm was 43 min (SD ± 40 min) and 69 min (SD ± 54 min) for complex multiloculated lesions. Another large series showed a 72% primary success rate using compression in 297 false aneurysms, 7/12 patients who underwent a second compression episode had successful occlusion giving a secondary success rate of 74%.[27] Following successful obliteration the patient is scanned after 24 h to confirm that the aneurysm remains occluded (Fig. 4-14D). A variety of mechanical compression devices have also been proposed but results with these are variable.

OTHER PULSATILE MASSES

Aneurysms

Aneurysms of the lower limb arteries may occur in isolation, or as multiple lesions. They are more common in the popliteal arteries but may be found elsewhere in the legs or, more rarely in the upper limb arteries. As with aortic aneurysms they can enlarge over a period of time; their size and rate of enlargement can be followed with ultrasound. Their main clinical significance is that they can act as a source of emboli to the distal lower limb, or may thrombose leading to acute ischaemia.

Cystic Adventitial Disease

This is a rare condition in which fluid-filled cysts are found in the wall of the artery, usually the popliteal artery, or superficial femoral artery in the adductor canal. The aetiology of these cysts is unclear and various theories, including repeated trauma, ectopic synovial tissue, or a congenital abnormality linking the cyst to the adjacent knee joint space or to adjacent tendons, have been proposed.[28] Signs and symptoms of ischaemia can be variable and confusing.[29] Ultrasound is useful in diagnosis as it will show the narrowing of the lumen, together with the associated cystic lesion producing the stenosis (Fig. 4-15).

Brachial Compression Syndromes

Thoracic outlet syndrome, or compression of the subclavian artery as it crosses the first rib, may be due to

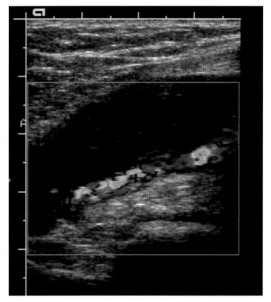

FIGURE 4-15 Cystic adventitial disease of the popliteal artery. The cystic component is seen above the patent lumen.

congenital fibrotic bands at the insertions of the anterior and middle scalene muscles, or to compression associated with a cervical rib. The accompanying vein is also usually affected. Some degree of compression may be seen in up to 20% of normal subjects. The compression is often positional, typically occurring when the arm is elevated above the head, so various positions of the arm and shoulder may need to be assessed. Sometimes the symptoms only occur with the patient in a particular position such as standing or lying down. Usually the diagnosis is straightforward on clinical grounds, with the pulse in the affected arm disappearing when the arm is in the appropriate position. However, in some cases the diagnosis, or the cause, is less clear cut and colour Doppler can be used to image the subclavian artery as the arm is moved into various positions with the patient supine or erect. The transducer is usually placed in the supraclavicular position but scanning under the clavicle may be useful, particularly when the arm is fully elevated. Careful examination of the artery as it passes over the first rib may show changes in the waveform as the vessel is compressed (Fig. 4-16). Sometimes access to the subclavian artery in the region of the first rib can be difficult. In these cases, scanning the axillary artery whilst the arm is put in different positions will show any changes in velocity or waveform resulting from arterial compression. A rebound increase in velocity may be noted in the distal arteries on release of compression.[30]

POPLITEAL ARTERY COMPRESSION

In cases of suspected entrapment of an artery or graft in the adductor canal or popliteal fossa, direct examination of the vessel is often restricted by the limited access to the popliteal fossa with the knee flexed. However, careful examination of the lower popliteal artery or posterior tibial artery with the knee in different positions of flexion will demonstrate changes in the arterial waveform resulting from compression. Athletes may get compression of the popliteal artery between the lateral femoral condyle or upper tibia and the hypertrophied gastrocnemius, or soleus and plantaris muscles. This can be demonstrated on Doppler ultrasound by scanning with the foot in a neutral position and then in a position of active plantar flexion.[31]

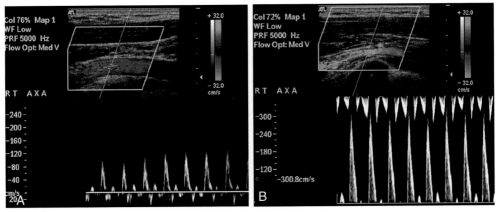

FIGURE 4-16 Compression of the subclavian artery as the arm is elevated/abducted. At rest flow in the axillary artery is approximately 1 m/min; (B) showing narrowing of the artery as it crosses the first rib as the position of the arm is changed. The velocity increases to 3 m/min.

Rarely, athletic patients may get iliac artery compression from a bulky psoas muscle on strenuous exercise. Scanning following a period of exercise shows turbulence, tissue bruits and very high local velocities in the inguinal area.

Accuracy in Relation to Other Techniques

The gold standard for the assessment of the accuracy of Doppler ultrasound is usually arteriography but with modern computed tomographic arteriography (CTA) and magnetic resonance arteriography (MRA) techniques more widely available, diagnostic arteriograms are performed much less frequently. The reservations on the accuracy of arteriography, which are discussed in Chapter 3 on carotids, are also applicable to peripheral arterial disease. Cossman et al.[9] compared colour Doppler with arteriography in 84 limbs, from the iliac to lower popliteal segments, using the criteria discussed earlier. For the detection of stenoses greater than 50%, they found an overall sensitivity of 87% (156/180 segments), specificity of 99% (444/449), accuracy of 95% (600/629), positive predictive value of 96% and negative predictive value of 95%. For the diagnosis of arterial occlusion the overall sensitivity was 81% (76/94), with specificity of 99% (463/466), accuracy of 96% (539/560), positive predictive value of 95% and negative predictive value of 96%.

Polak[32] reviewed five studies performed between 1989 and 1992, including the study by Cossman et al.[9] Colour Doppler was compared to arteriography

and the overall sensitivity for the detection of a stenosis greater than 50% was 87.5% (316/361 segments), for an occluded segment the sensitivity was 92.6% (403/435), and the overall specificity for the identification of normal segments was 97% (1247/1282). These studies have assessed femoropopliteal disease; accurate assessment of infrapopliteal crural vessel disease with duplex is a little more difficult, although a sensitivity of 77% has been reported[33] but if information on these vessels is clinically important then arteriography should be considered if there are any reservations about the duplex examination.

Similar, positive results have been obtained for duplex in upper limb disease with 79% sensitivity, 100% specificity and 99% accuracy for haemodynamically significant (50–70%) stenoses and 98% sensitivity, 99% specificity and 99% accuracy for occlusion being reported by Tola et al.[34] who compared duplex ultrasound with intra-arterial digital subtraction angiography (DSA) in 578 upper limb arterial segments.

CTA and MRA have now largely replaced catheter arteriography for diagnostic examinations of the peripheral arteries. CTA now provides high-resolution images of the arteries which can be reviewed in 3D and manipulated on workstations. It can be used on individuals for whom MRI is contra-indicated, or people who are claustrophobic. The disadvantages of CTA are that vascular calcifications can interfere with accurate visualisation; anaphylactic reactions to iodine or nephrotoxicity in patients with impaired renal function; and exposure to ionising radiation.[35]

TABLE 4-4A	**Sensitivity of Non-Invasive Imaging Techniques for >50% Stenosis**				
	No. of studies	**No. of patients**	**No. of segments**	**Sensitivity**	**Specificity**
CE–MRA	7	279	4837	95.1% (91.9–99.5%)	92.3% (63.7–99.2%)
2D TOF MRI	5	287	2668	87.9% (78.5–93.5%)	85.1% (73.9–89.1%)
CTA	6	245	4270	92.7% (88.9–98.8%)	90.3% (83.3–97.4%)
Duplex US	7	369	5633	89.1% (79.7–97.6%)	95.0% (88.5–99.0%)

Adapted from Collins et al.[36]

TABLE 4-4B	**Sensitivity of Non-Invasive Imaging Techniques for Occlusion**				
	No. of studies	**No. of patients**	**No. of segments**	**Sensitivity**	**Specificity**
CE–MRA	6	244	4529	93.7% (84.7–100%)	99.0% (97.0–99.8%)
2D TOF MRI	4	245	2290	87.0% (76.9–100%)	94.2% (85.1–98.3%)
CTA	5	195	3530	95.0% (88.6–100%)	99.5% (98.8–100%)
Duplex US	7	379	5588	87.9% (73.7–94.3%)	98.4% (96.1–100%)

Adapted from Collins et al.[36]

MRA can be carried out using several sequences and techniques. The most frequently used are time of flight and contrast-enhanced examinations. Contrast-enhanced studies (3D CE-MRA) provide the better sensitivity but there is a small risk of inducing nephrogenic systemic fibrosis (NSF) in a small number of susceptible individuals. The disadvantages of MRA are those common to all MR examinations, so the technique is not suitable for all patients.[35]

A review comparing studies on the detection of peripheral vascular disease using duplex, CTA, MRA (TOF) and CE-MRA (Table 4.4), showed that 3D CE-MRA has the highest sensitivity for detection of 50% stenosis;[36] whereas CTA has a small advantage for the detection of occlusion. However, duplex ultrasound shows satisfactory performance and has advantages in availability and cost of equipment, although it has to be recognised that the results depend significantly on the skill and expertise of the operator. A more detailed review looking at economic aspects of the four imaging techniques suggests that duplex ultrasound is the most cost-effective technique for evaluation of a whole leg but, if analysis is limited to a section of the leg (above or below the knee) then TOF MRA is the most cost-effective diagnostic strategy.[37]

Conclusions

Providing that the examination is performed carefully by a skilled operator, Doppler ultrasound provides a relatively cheap and an accurate technique for the assessment of many patients with disease or previous surgery to the peripheral arteries, particularly in the lower limbs. In symptomatic patients it can be used as a first-line test to identify those patients without significant disease, those patients who may benefit from angioplasty and patients who are likely to require surgical bypass. In many centres, ultrasound is now used alone prior to surgery, with CTA or MRA used to clarify the situation in problematic cases. Power Doppler and echo-enhancing agents will increase the diagnostic sensitivity of Doppler ultrasound and the need for arteriography in many cases should be substantially reduced.

REFERENCES

1. Fowkes FGR. Epidemiology of atherosclerotic disease in the lower limbs. *Eur J Vasc Surg* 1988;**2**:283–91.
2. Department of Health and Social Security, Office of Population Censuses and Surveys . *Hospital Inpatient Enquiry*. London: HMSO; 1988.
3. Leng GC, Evans CJ, Fowkes FGR. Epidemiology of peripheral vascular diseases. *Imaging* 1995;**7**:85–96.

4. Eiberg JP, Hansen MA, Jensen F, et al. Ultrasound contrast-agent improves imaging of lower limb occlusive disease. *Eur J Vasc Endovasc Surg* 2003;**25**:23–8.

5. Bergamini TM, Tatum CM, Marshall C, et al. Effect of multilevel sequential stenosis on lower extremity arterial duplex scanning. *Am J Surg* 1995;**169**:564–6.

6. Allard L, Cloutier G, Guo Z, et al. Review of the assessment of single level and multilevel arterial occlusive disease in lower limbs by duplex ultrasound. *Ultrasound Med Biol* 1999;**25**:495–502.

7. Whyman MR, Allan PL, Gillespie IN, et al. Screening patients with claudication from femoropopliteal disease before angioplasty using Doppler colour flow imaging. *Br J Surg* 1992;**79**:907–9.

8. Jäger KA, Ricketts HJ, Strandness Jr DE. Duplex scanning for evaluation of lower limb arterial disease. In: Bernstein EF, editor. *Noninvasive diagnostic techniques in vascular disease*. St Louis: CV Mosby; 1985. p. 619–31.

9. Cossman DV, Ellison JE, Wagner WH, et al. Comparison of contrast arteriography to arterial mapping with color-flow duplex imaging in the lower extremities. *J Vasc Surg* 1989;**10**:522–9.

10. van Asten WN, van Lier HJ, Beijnevald WJ, et al. Assessment of aortoiliac obstructive disease by Doppler spectrum analysis of blood flow velocities in the common femoral artery at rest and during reactive hyperaemia. *Surgery* 1991;**109**:633–9.

11. Zierler RE. Duplex and color-flow imaging of the lower extremity arterial circulation. *Semin Ultrasound CT MR* 1990;**11**:168–79.

12. Sensier Y, Bell PR, London NJ. The ability of qualitative assessment of the common femoral Doppler waveform to screen for significant aorto-iliac disease. *Eur J Vasc Endovasc Surg* 1998;**15**:357–64.

13. Rosfors S, Eriksson M, Hoglund N, et al. Duplex ultrasound in patients with suspected aortoiliac occlusive disease. *Eur J Vasc Surg* 1993;**7**:513–17.

14. Lane TRA, Metcalfe MJ, Narayanan S, et al. Post-operative surveillance after open peripheral arterial surgery. *Eur J Vasc Endovasc Surg* 2011;**42**:59–77.

15. Mills JL. Mechanisms of graft failure: the location, distribution and characteristics of lesions that predispose to graft failure. *Semin Vasc Surg* 1993;**6**:78–91.

16. Fasih T, Rudol G, Ashour H, et al. Surveillance versus nonsurveillance for femoro-popliteal bypass grafts. *Angiology* 2004;**55**:251–6.

17. Dunlop P, Sayers RD, Naylor AR, et al. The effect of a surveillance programme on the patency of synthetic infrainguinal bypass grafts. *Eur J Vasc Endovasc Surg* 1996;**11**:441–5.

18. Hoballah JJ, Nazzal RM, Ryan SM, et al. Is color duplex surveillance of infrainguinal polytetrafluoroethylene grafts worthwhile? *Am J Surg* 1997;**174**:131–5.

19. Bandyk DF. Essentials of graft surveillance. *Sem Vasc Surg* 1993;**6**:78–91.

20. Gibson KD, Caps MT, Gillen D, et al. Identification of factors predictive of lower extremity vein graft thrombosis. *J Vasc Surg* 2001;**33**:24–31.

21. Maleux G, Hendrickx S, Vaninbroukx J, et al. Percutaneous injection of human thrombin to treat iatrogenic femoral pseudoaneurysms: short- and midterm ultrasound follow-up. *Eur Radiol* 2003;**13**:209–12.

22. Toursarkissian B, Allen BT, Petrinec D, et al. Spontaneous closure of selected pseudoaneurysms and arteriovenous fistulae. *J Vasc Surg* 1997;**25**:803–8.

23. Sheiman RG, Mastromatteo M. Iatrogenic femoral pseudoaneurysms that are unresponsive to percutaneous thrombin injection: potential causes. *Am J Roentgenol* 2003;**181**:1301–4.

24. Gorge G, Kunz T. Thrombin injection for treatment of false aneurysms after failed compression therapy in patients on full dose antiplatelet and heparin therapy. *Catheter Cardiovasc Interv* 2003;**58**:505–9.

25. Gershin E, Karram T, Gaitini D, et al. Percutaneous ultrasonographically guided thrombin injection of iatrogenic pseudoaneurysms in unusual sites. *J Ultrasound Med* 2003;**22**:809–16.

26. Coley BD, Roberts AC, Fellmeth BD, et al. Postangiographic femoral artery pseudoaneurysms: further experience with US-guided compression repair. *Radiology* 1995;**194**:307–11.

27. Eisenberg L, Paulson EK, Kliewer MA, et al. Sonographically guided compression repair of pseudoaneurysms: further experience from a single institution. *Am J Roentgenol* 1999;**173**:1567–73.

28. Flanigan DP, Burnham SJ, Goodreau JJ, et al. Summary of cases of adventitial disease of the popliteal artery. *Ann Surg* 1979;**189**:165–75.

29. Cassar K, Engeset J. Cystic adventitial disease: a trap for the unwary. *Eur J Endovasc Surg* 2005;**29**:93–6.

30. Wadhwani R, Chaubal N, Sukthankar R, et al. Color Doppler and duplex sonography in 5 patients with thoracic outlet syndrome. *J Ultrasound Med* 2001;**20**:795–801.

31. Baltopoulos P, Filippou DK, Sigala F. Popliteal artery entrapment syndrome: anatomic or functional syndrome? *Clin J Sports Med* 2004;**14**:8–12.

32. Polak JF. Peripheral arterial disease. Evaluation with color flow and duplex sonography. *Radiol Clin North Am* 1995;**33**:71–90.

33. Karacagil S, Lofberg AM, Granbo A, et al. Value of duplex scanning in evaluation of crural and foot arteries in limbs with severe lower limb ischaemia – a prospective comparison with angiography. *Eur J Vasc Endovasc Surg* 1996;**12**:300–3.

34. Tola M, Yurdakul M, Okten S, et al. Diagnosis of arterial occlusive disease of the upper extremities: comparison of color duplex sonography and angiography. *J Clin Ultrasound* 2003;**31**:407–11.

35. Cao P, Eckstein HH, De Rango P, et al. Management of critical limb ischaemia and diabetic foot. Clinical practice guidelines of the European Society for Vascular Surgery. Chapter 2: Diagnostic methods. *Eur J Vac Surg* 2011;**42**(Suppl. 2):S13–S32.

36. Collins R, Burch J, Cranny G, et al. Duplex ultrasonography, magnetic resonance angiography and computed tomography angiography for diagnosis and assessment of symptomatic, lower limb peripheral arterial disease: a systematic review. *BMJ* 2007;**334**:1257–65.

37. Collins R, Cranny G, Burch J, et al. A systematic review of duplex ultrasound, magnetic resonance angiography and computed tomography angiography for the diagnosis and assessment of symptomatic, lower limb peripheral arterial disease. *Health Technol Assess* 2007;**11**(20).

Chapter 5

The Peripheral Veins

Paul L. Allan

The peripheral veins may be affected by a variety of disorders which can be assessed by ultrasound. Deep vein thrombosis (DVT) and thromboembolic disease are the most common indications for investigation of the peripheral veins but venous insufficiency and vein mapping are also reasons for examining the veins. Anderson et al.[1] found an average annual incidence of 48 initial cases, 36 recurrent cases of DVT and 23 cases of pulmonary embolus per 100 000 population in the Worcester DVT study. The prevalence of varicose veins and chronic venous insufficiency is more difficult to quantify, but it has been estimated that 10–15% of males and 20–25% of females in an unselected Western population over 15 years of age have visible tortuous varicose veins; 2–5% of adult males and 3–7% of females have evidence of moderate or severe chronic venous insufficiency, with a point prevalence for active ulceration of 0.1–0.2%.[2]

Indications

The indications for ultrasound of the venous system are shown in Box 5-1. The most frequent indication for ultrasound of the veins is for the investigation of possible DVT in the lower limb and, occasionally, in the upper limb – especially if there have been central venous catheters inserted for intensive care monitoring, chemotherapy, dialysis or parenteral feeding. Similarly, indwelling femoral catheters are prone to induce thrombosis and patients should be examined early if this is suspected. Ultrasound provides a non-invasive, reliable method for examining the venous system, particularly with respect to the diagnosis, or exclusion, of dangerous proximal thrombus in symptomatic patients.[3] The results for asymptomatic thrombus in the lower limbs are less encouraging and this should

be recognised when using ultrasound to screen for DVT in asymptomatic patients.[4]

Recurrence of varicose veins following surgery can pose many problems for the clinician trying to clarify the venous anatomy. Colour Doppler can be used instead of venography and varicography in most cases and may be the only examination required to define the anatomy and function in patients with recurrent varicose veins.[5]

The impact of postphlebitis syndromes and chronic venous insufficiency is a rather larger problem than is apparent from its relatively low clinical profile. In one large epidemiological study of 4376 subjects, 62% had some evidence of varicose veins; signs of chronic insufficiency were present in 22%.[6] Varicography shows perforator veins which are obviously incompetent and some incompetent superficial and deep venous segments, but ultrasound has the advantage that the segments of the deep and superficial systems can be examined and the direction of blood flow within each segment can be demonstrated. In addition, it is less unpleasant for the patient and allows multiple assessments to be performed without discomfort. The main disadvantage is that it is fairly time-consuming, particularly in complex cases, and requires a significant degree of expertise in order to perform examinations efficiently.

The superficial veins of the legs and, occasionally, the arms may be used for bypass grafts for the coronary or lower limb arteries. If there is any doubt about their suitability as a conduit following previous varicose vein surgery, or in terms of their calibre, ultrasound can be used to assess the diameter and length of vein available. In addition, the sonographer can map out the course of the vein to allow easier harvesting.

It may be difficult occasionally to locate a suitable vein for central venous cannulation, particularly in patients who have had multiple previous central venous lines, such as intensive care or chemotherapy patients. Ultrasound can be used to clarify the location and patency of potentially suitable veins and, in difficult cases, the puncture may be made under direct ultrasound visualisation.

Anatomy and Scanning Technique

The anatomy of the venous system in the limbs is more complex and variable than that of the arteries. The components and nomenclature of the lower limb veins were reviewed by a consensus group in 2002 and their recommendations are used here.[7] The meanings of the terms 'proximal' and 'distal' may cause confusion as the veins start at the periphery and blood flows centrally towards the heart so that 'upstream' is peripheral and 'downstream' is central, which is the opposite from the situation in the arteries. The convention is that proximal describes locations nearer the heart and distal refers to points further from the heart; these terms are used in this way in this chapter.

ANATOMY – LOWER LIMB

The veins of the lower limb are divided into deep and superficial systems. These are linked by a variable number of perforator veins which carry blood from the superficial to the deep systems (Fig. 5-1).

The Deep Veins

The anatomy of the lower limb veins is rather variable. Generally the veins accompany the arteries but their number may vary and the communications with other veins along the way can show a variety of patterns; however, a general arrangement is usually apparent. In the calf there are veins running with the main arteries: the posterior tibial, peroneal and anterior tibial veins; there are usually two, occasionally three veins with each artery (Fig. 5-2). In addition there are veins draining the major muscle groups in the posterior calf. These are seen in the upper calf as they pass upwards to join the other deep veins in the lower popliteal region; the gastrocnemius and soleal veins are the largest of these. The gastrocnemius vein is the more superficial and may be mistaken for the small saphenous vein; clues to its true identity are that it is usually accompanied by the artery to the muscle and it can be followed distally down into the muscle rather than outwards to lie subcutaneously on the fascia around the calf, which is the position of the small saphenous vein.

The calf veins join to form the popliteal vein, or veins – there may be two, or sometimes three channels, especially if there is a dual superficial femoral vein. The popliteal vein runs up through the popliteal fossa, lying more posterior and usually medial to the artery. As well as the veins from the calf and calf muscles, it is joined by the small saphenous vein at the saphenopopliteal junction.

The popliteal vein becomes the femoral vein at the upper border of the popliteal fossa; rarely, the popliteal vein runs more deeply to join with the profunda femoris vein. The femoral vein passes through the femoral canal and runs up the medial aspect of the thigh, posterior to the femoral artery to join with the profunda femoris vein (which can alternatively be called the deep femoral vein) in the femoral triangle below the groin; the profunda femoris vein drains the thigh muscles. The confluence of the femoral and profunda femoris veins to form the common femoral vein is normally a little more caudal than the bifurcation of the common femoral artery into the femoral and profunda femoris arteries. The femoral vein may have significant segments of duplication (Fig. 5-3) along its length in up to 25–30% of subjects,[8,9] these dual segments may have a variable relation to the artery, so that they may be overlooked unless care is taken in the examination of the thigh veins with both transverse and longitudinal views being obtained.

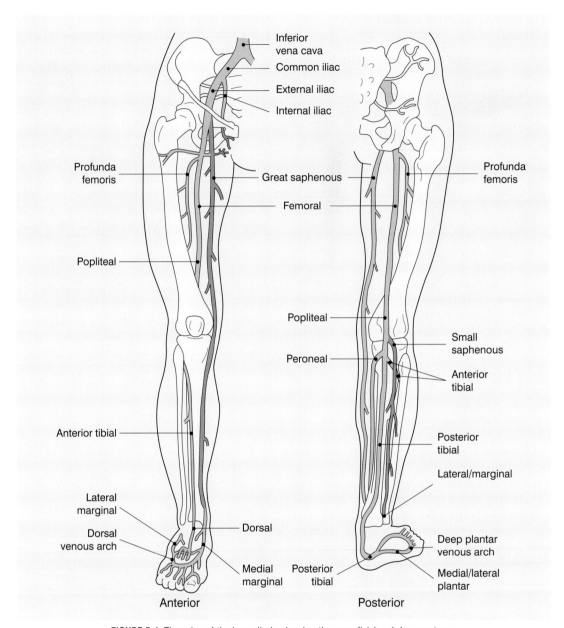

Inferior
vena cava

Common iliac

External iliac

Internal iliac

Profunda
femoris

Great saphenous

Femoral

Profunda
femoris

Popliteal

Popliteal

Small
saphenous

Peroneal

Anterior
tibial

Anterior tibial

Posterior
tibial

Lateral/marginal

Lateral
marginal

Dorsal

Dorsal
venous arch

Deep plantar
venous arch

Medial
marginal

Posterior
tibial

Medial/lateral
plantar

Anterior

Posterior

FIGURE 5-1 The veins of the lower limb, showing the superficial and deep systems.

In the pelvis and groin, the anatomy is generally consistent. The femoral vein and profunda femoris vein join to form the common femoral vein, which lies medial to the common femoral artery. The common femoral vein is joined by the great saphenous vein at the saphenofemoral junction; the appearance of the common femoral vein, great saphenous vein and the common femoral artery in transverse section is sometimes referred to as the 'Mickey Mouse' view (Fig. 5-4). The common femoral vein is also joined by veins from the muscles around the hip. These veins are variable in size and number, occasionally one of these is large

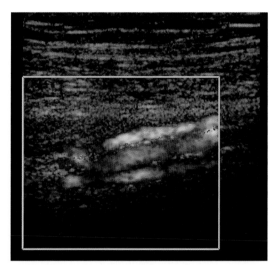

FIGURE 5-2 Power Doppler showing paired deep calf veins running with the artery.

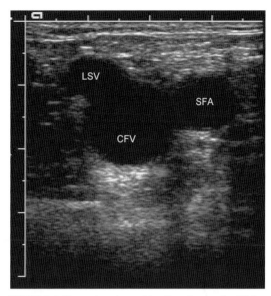

FIGURE 5-4 The saphenofemoral junction showing the 'Mickey Mouse' view.

enough to be confused with the great saphenous vein or profunda femoris vein but careful attention to the anatomy should clarify the situation. The common femoral vein becomes the external iliac vein after it has passed under the inguinal ligament, and then it passes posteriorly along the posterior pelvis, running alongside the external iliac artery. The internal iliac vein, which drains the pelvic structures, joins with the external iliac vein deep in the pelvis to form the common iliac vein (Fig. 5-5). The two common iliac

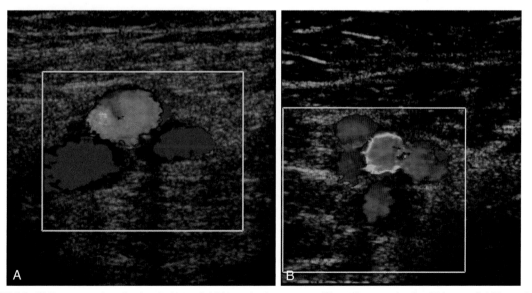

FIGURE 5-3 (A) Transverse view showing dual superficial femoral vein segments; (B) another example of multiple superficial femoral vein segments showing a central artery (aliased colour signal seen as red) with four venous channels adjacent to it.

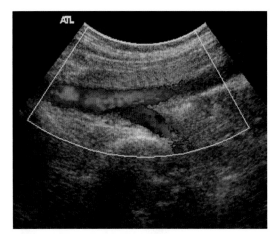

FIGURE 5-5 The confluence of the internal and external iliac veins forming the common iliac vein.

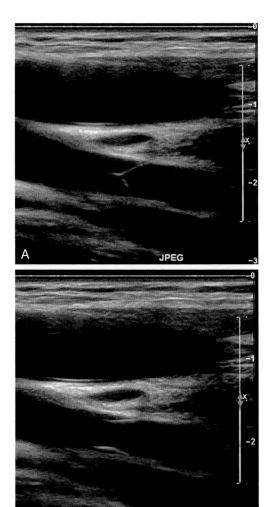

FIGURE 5-6 Normal valves in the profunda femoris vein; (A) valves shut, (B) valves open.

veins then join at the level of the aortic bifurcation to form the inferior vena cava, which normally passes cranially on the right side of the aorta. The left common iliac vein passes behind the right common iliac artery just distal to this confluence. In a small number of individuals this confluence does not occur and the two common iliac veins continue cranially as dual inferior venae cavae; this reflects the arrangement of paired cardinal veins in the embryo.

The deep veins have a series of valves along their course (Fig. 5-6). These are somewhat variable in their number and location. They are most numerous in the veins below the knee; in the thigh, the femoral vein usually has one just below the confluence with the profunda femoris vein and at several levels below this. The iliac veins, in contrast, have relatively few valves;[10] rarely a valve may be seen in the inferior vena cava.

The Superficial Veins

The two main superficial venous channels in the lower limb are the great and small saphenous veins. The great saphenous vein arises from the medial aspect of the dorsal venous arch of the foot and passes in front of the medial malleolus to run up the medial aspect of the calf and knee into the thigh. In the upper thigh, the great saphenous vein curves laterally and deeply to join the common femoral vein just below the inguinal ligament. The great saphenous vein has two components in the calf: the posterior division passes up from the medial malleolus and communicates with the perforator veins; the anterior division usually joins the posterior division just below the level of the knee joint. Duplication of the great saphenous vein can be seen in the thigh in up to 50% of people,[11] this usually takes the form of parallel channels. The great saphenous vein receives many superficial tributaries and is connected to the deep veins by perforating veins; some of these tributaries in the thigh can be quite prominent and may be mistaken for the main vein if their true nature is not recognised. In the region of the saphenofemoral junction the great saphenous vein receives several tributaries draining the groin, lower abdominal wall and perineum. These veins are of significance in the recurrence of varicose veins following high ligation, as they provide a network of collateral channels which may bypass the resected segment.

The small saphenous vein arises from the lateral aspect of the dorsal venous arch of the foot, passing below and behind the lateral malleolus to run up the posterolateral aspect of the calf to the popliteal fossa, where it passes through the deep fascia to join the popliteal vein. Classically, it enters the lateral aspect of the popliteal vein at the level of the popliteal skin crease, or within a few centimetres above this but the level of the confluence can be quite variable. It can be distinguished from the posterior muscle venous sinuses as it does not have an accompanying artery and it is seen to lie within the fascial triangle in the posterior thigh defined by the deep muscular fascia and the superficial fascia (Fig. 5-7). Occasionally there is a thigh extension of the small saphenous vein, passing upwards to join the profunda femoris vein in the lower thigh – a Giacomini vein.[12] Burihan and Baptista-Silva[13] dissected 200 adult cadaver legs and reported 20 different patterns of termination of the small saphenous vein. In 27.5% of legs the small saphenous vein terminated in the principal deep vein of the leg (popliteal or lower femoral vein), in 25% of legs the small saphenous vein, or a branch arising from it, communicated with the great saphenous vein. In the remaining legs, there was a wide variety and combination of communications with other veins, including the deep femoral vein, the mid-thigh perforator vein, muscular veins and even the inferior gluteal vein in three legs. Other studies have shown that Giacomini veins can be affected by varicose disease with reflux either upwards or downwards in the thigh to the greater and lesser saphenous veins respectively.[14]

The Perforating Veins

The perforating veins connect the superficial veins to the deep veins. They are numerous and very variable in both size and location. In the past, they were often known by eponymous designations[15] but with the revised nomenclature they are now identified by their anatomical location – for example: medial, lateral, or anterior ankle perforator – full details are given in the consensus statement on venous nomenclature.[7] They

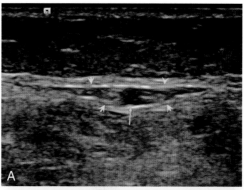

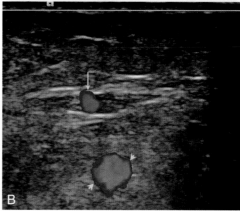

FIGURE 5-7 (A) The small saphenous vein (arrow) in the posterior calf lying in the fascial triangle (arrowheads) formed between the superficial fascia and the deeper muscular fascia; (B) colour Doppler showing the small saphenous vein (arrow) and a muscle vein (arrowheads) deep to the fascia which might be mistaken for the SSV if its location is not recognised.

are normally less than 5 mm in diameter and blood flows inwards from the superficial to the deep systems.

SCANNING TECHNIQUE – LOWER LIMB

The technique varies depending on the clinical indication. The most common indication is the diagnosis or exclusion of DVT in the lower limb. This section therefore concentrates on this aspect and variations in technique for other indications will be dealt with in subsequent sections (Box 5-2). A 7–10 MHz linear transducer will normally provide sufficient penetration, although in large or oedematous thighs a lower frequency may be required. It is important to ensure that the system is set up for the slower velocities found in veins, rather than the significantly higher arterial velocities.

BOX 5-2 BASIC STEPS IN THE EXAMINATION FOR THROMBOSIS

1. Patient sitting on couch/trolley: compression of common femoral vein, superficial femoral vein from groin to adductor canal
2. Colour Doppler with augmentation, examine common and superficial femoral veins
3. Patient decubitus, or with leg elevated: compression and Doppler examination of popliteal vein(s)
4. Patient sitting, if possible, with legs dependent: examine the calf veins with compression and colour Doppler
5. Patient supine: examine iliac veins if thrombus suspected in these

It is advantageous if there is a tilting couch available so that the patient can be moved from the horizontal to various degrees of head-up elevation as necessary. In the absence of a tilting couch it is better if the patient can be examined with the thorax higher than the legs, as this produces some distension of the lower limb veins, which makes them easier to identify and the assessment of compression more straightforward.

There are three components to the ultrasound examination of the veins for DVT: imaging, Doppler and compression. Thrombus may be seen in the vein, Doppler may show abnormal, or absent, flow signals and compression refers to the fact that a normal vein is easily compressible – light pressure with the transducer will obliterate the lumen of the vein, whereas thrombus in the lumen will prevent apposition of the walls. Two points should be noted in relation to compression: first, compression should be performed in the transverse plane (Fig. 5-8) for the reason that if it is done in the longitudinal plane a thrombosed vein may disappear as it is no longer in the scan plane, rather than because it has been compressed. Second, fresh thrombus is soft and gelatinous, so that firm pressure can produce a degree of compression, which may give a false impression of patency. The use of colour Doppler will clarify this situation. A further reason for scanning in the transverse plane is that dual segments of the superficial femoral vein will be identified more reliably.

The examination begins at the groin, where the common femoral vein is located on a transverse scan and compressed. Compression is then repeated at intervals of 3–5 cm down the length of the thigh to the adductor canal. At this point the superficial femoral vein is difficult to compress from an anterior approach as it is well supported by the bulk of the anterior thigh muscles. Compression is better achieved in this region by placing a hand behind the medial thigh and pushing up with the fingers against the transducer. The scan plane is then changed to longitudinal and the vein examined with colour Doppler, or power Doppler, as the transducer is moved up the thigh. If the iliac veins are not being formally examined it is useful to obtain a spectral waveform in quiet respiration from the

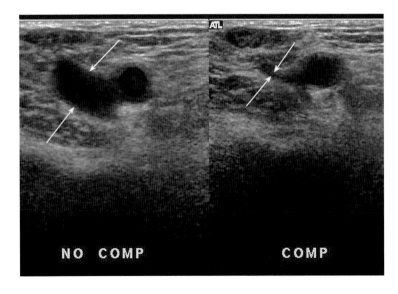

FIGURE 5-8 Normal compression: the lumen of the vein (arrows) is completely obliterated by pressure from the transducer.

common femoral vein to confirm cardiac and respiratory flow variation being transmitted down patent iliac veins from the chest. Squeezing the calf gently will augment flow and allow easier detection of areas of flow or thrombosis; alternatively, the patient can be asked to plantar-flex their toes, which results in calf muscle contraction and emptying of the calf veins. Colour Doppler is often sufficient, in conjunction with the findings on compression, to confirm or exclude a diagnosis of DVT (Fig. 5-9). If there is any doubt then a spectral assessment will allow a better appreciation of damped flow, absent respiratory variation and impaired augmentation.

Once the thigh veins have been examined the patient is turned into a lateral position, with the medial aspect of the leg being examined uppermost, so that the popliteal veins can be examined. Again, compression and colour Doppler are used to assess the veins. Some patients, particularly postoperative hip patients, may not be able to move into a decubitus position. In these cases the popliteal veins can be examined with the knee partially flexed up off the couch, with external rotation, if possible, so that the transducer can be positioned in the popliteal fossa; a curved array can be of benefit in gaining access in this situation. Alternatively, the leg can be elevated and supported off the couch by an assistant. In addition to the popliteal vein, the main muscular veins draining soleus and gastrocnemius should be assessed, especially if there is pain and tenderness associated with the posterior calf muscles (Fig. 5-10).

The calf veins can be examined after the popliteal vein with the patient in the decubitus position on a tilted couch, or in the supine position with the knee flexed up off the mattress, if the patient is relatively immobile. Alternatively, the patient can sit on the couch with their legs over the side so that the dependent calf veins are well distended. The posterior tibial and deeper peroneal vessels are most easily located by

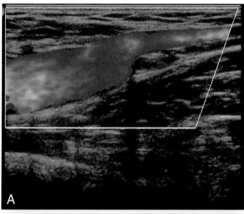

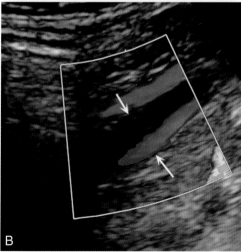

FIGURE 5-9 The common femoral vein showing (A) complete colour fill-in across the vein lumen in a normal vein: (B) only a small residual lumen in a partially thrombosed vein.

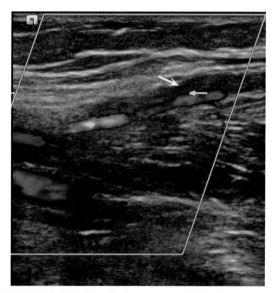

FIGURE 5-10 Thrombosis in the gastrocnemius vein (arrows). The popliteal vein was patent.

scanning in the transverse plane from the medial side of the calf and identifying the arterial signals on colour Doppler (Fig. 4-2). These veins may also be located on a longitudinal scan; again the arterial signal provides a useful guide to the position of the veins. If there are difficulties identifying the posterior tibial veins at the mid-calf level then scanning the lower calf just above the medial malleolus, where the vessels are superficial and constant in location, may be of value; the posterior tibial vessels can then be followed back up the calf with augmentation of flow as necessary in order to assess patency. In the mid- and lower calf, squeezing the calf can produce motion artefacts from movement of the calf muscles which obscure the flow signals from the veins; in these cases, squeezing the foot will produce adequate augmentation of flow. The anterior tibial veins are examined from an anterolateral approach: scanning transversely, the tibia, fibula and interosseous membrane are identified. The anterior tibial vessels are found on the superficial aspect of the interosseous membrane, although it should be noted that these veins are rarely involved in DVT in isolation from the other calf veins. The peroneal veins may also be visualised deep to the interosseous membrane in many patients from this anterolateral aspect, allowing their examination if they have not been identified from a posteromedial approach; a posterolateral approach is also of value in identifying the deeply situated peroneal veins in some patients.

The iliac veins are examined by following the external iliac vein upwards from the common femoral vein into the pelvis. A 3–5 MHz transducer is usually necessary for adequate penetration. Firm pressure may be required to displace bowel gas. This may produce narrowing or effacement of the more superficial segments of vein, resulting in an absence of signal and a possible false diagnosis of occlusion. If the pelvic veins are difficult to trace superiorly then the common iliac vein can usually be identified just distal to the inferior vena cava and aortic bifurcation; this can then be followed peripherally. In some patients it is impossible to identify the deeper pelvic portion of the iliac veins; however, if there is a patent external iliac vein which shows respiratory variation with good augmentation and a patent upper common iliac vein, then it is highly unlikely that there is significant thrombus in the invisible segment. Transvaginal scanning will show the deeper pelvic veins and may be considered if there is a need to visualise these vessels directly. In thinner patients, or patients with good pelvic access, the proximal internal iliac vein may be seen joining the external iliac vein in the pelvis (Fig. 5-5). The inferior vena cava is examined if thrombus is seen extending into this vessel. It is important, whenever thrombus is diagnosed in a leg vein, that the proximal extent of the clot is identified, as this may have a significant impact on management decisions in relation to anticoagulation therapy, or the placing of a filter.

In pregnant women in the later part of pregnancy, the uterus will lie on the iliac veins in the supine position and compress them, thus reducing flow and impairing augmentation in the lower limb veins. This can be alleviated by asking the patient to turn into a semi-decubitus position, with the side being examined uppermost, so that the uterus falls away, allowing better flow in the pelvic veins. An alternative is to examine the patient standing, as the uterus moves forward away from the iliac veins in this position.

ANATOMY – UPPER LIMB

The veins of the upper limb are also divided into deep and superficial groups (Fig. 5-11). The deep veins are usually paired and accompany the arteries: the radial, ulnar and brachial veins; with the axillary, subclavian and brachiocephalic veins more centrally. There is a variable pattern of communicating veins between the deep veins and between the deep and the superficial veins. The superficial system is more variable than in the leg but there are usually two main vessels: the cephalic vein on the radial aspect of the arm and the basilic vein on the ulnar side. These communicate at the cubital fossa by way of the median cubital vein and they also communicate with the deep brachial veins at this level. The basilic vein pierces the deep fascia on the medial aspect of the mid-upper arm to join the brachial veins and this combined venous channel becomes the axillary vein when it enters the axilla. The cephalic vein passes more cranially along the lateral aspect of the biceps. At the level of pectoralis major it turns medially and deeply to pierce the clavipectoral fascia below the clavicle and joins the upper axillary vein. The axillary vein also receives other tributaries from the region of the shoulder joint and the lateral chest wall.

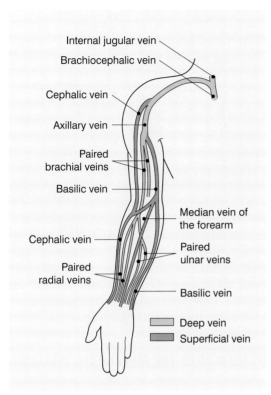

Internal jugular vein

Brachiocephalic vein

Cephalic vein

Axillary vein

Paired brachial veins

Basilic vein

Cephalic vein

Median vein of the forearm

Paired ulnar veins

Paired radial veins

Basilic vein

☐ Deep vein
☐ Superficial vein

FIGURE 5-11 The veins of the upper limb, showing the main superficial and deep veins.

The axillary vein becomes the subclavian vein as it crosses the first rib, where it lies in front of the artery; the main tributary of the subclavian vein is the external jugular vein. The subclavian vein on both sides joins with the internal jugular vein behind the medial end of the clavicle to form the brachiocephalic vein, which is also known as the innominate vein.

SCANNING TECHNIQUE – UPPER LIMB AND NECK

Examination of the upper limb veins is normally performed with the patient supine and the arm abducted to about 90°; the patient may require some support for the arm, or they can be asked to hold onto some suitable part of the ultrasound machine beside them. A transducer frequency of 7–12 MHz can be used. The examination begins above the sternoclavicular joint, where the distal brachiocephalic vein can be assessed and the confluence with the internal jugular vein examined, particularly if central lines have been inserted. The subclavian vein is examined from above and then below the clavicle; it is seen lying in front of the subclavian artery as it runs over the first rib. The axillary vein is then followed across the axilla into the upper arm, from where the brachial veins can be examined down to the elbow. The veins below this are not usually examined unless there is some specific reason, such as the presence of a dialysis shunt. Augmentation of flow is obtained by manual compression of the forearm, or upper arm; alternatively, asking the patient to clench their fist will increase venous flow. If there is a suspicion of a possible venous compression syndrome, the arm veins can be examined with the limb in different positions of abduction; comparison of flow on the two sides can be of value.

The internal jugular vein runs in the carotid sheath from the jugular foramen in the base of the skull down to join with the subclavian vein; it lies superficial to the carotid artery. There may be significant variation in size between the two sides. It is normally compressed easily by pressure from the transducer, so a light touch is required. Flow in the vein is influenced significantly by right heart activity, so colour Doppler will show variable forward and reverse flow, with spectral Doppler showing the 'a', 'c' and 'v' waves of the jugular pulse. Respiratory variation will also be seen, with increased forward flow during inspiration when intrathoracic pressure is negative and slowing during expiration when the intrathoracic pressure is positive. Flow can therefore be modified by respiratory manoeuvres such as deep inspiration, or a Valsalva.

Diagnosis of Deep Vein Thrombosis

Clinical diagnosis of DVT is inaccurate and clinical scoring systems, such as the Wells Score (Box 5-3), have been introduced and refined to stratify risk more accurately.[16] In addition measurements of serum D-dimer can be used to further refine the selection of patients more likely to have a DVT who will benefit from an ultrasound scan.[17] Patients with a low probability for DVT should have a D-dimer estimation. If this is negative, they are highly unlikely to have a DVT and do not require scanning; if the D-dimer is positive, or the patient has an intermediate or high probability score for DVT, then a scan should be performed. D-dimer levels are less useful in patients with many pre-existing

BOX 5-3 **PRETEST PROBABILITY FOR DEEP VEIN THROMBOSIS (DVT)**

• Active cancer (patient receiving treatment for cancer within previous 6 months, or currently receiving palliative treatment)	+1
• Paralysis, paresis, or recent plaster immobilisation of the lower extremities	+1
• Recently bedridden for 3 days or more, or major surgery within the previous 12 wks requiring general or regional anaesthesias	+1
• Localised tenderness along the distribution of the deep venous system	+1
• Entire leg swollen	+1
• Calf swelling at least 3 cm larger than that on the asymptomatic side (measured 10 cm below tibial tuberosity)	+1
• Pitting oedema confined to the symptomatic leg	+1
• Collateral superficial veins (non-varicose)	+1
• Previously documented deep vein thrombosis	+1
• Alternative diagnosis at least as likely or greater than that of DVT	−2

A score of two or higher indicates that the probability of deep vein thrombosis is likely; a score of less than two indicates that the probability of deep vein thrombosis is unlikely. In patients with symptoms in both legs, the more symptomatic leg is used.

From Wells et al.[16]

BOX 5-4 **CAUSES OF A RAISED D-DIMER**

• Deep vein thrombosis	• Malignancy
• Liver disease	• Trauma
• High rheumatoid factor	• Pregnancy
• Inflammation	• Recent surgery

conditions, or who have recently undergone surgery as false positives are more common (Box 5-4).

The diagnosis of normal or thrombosed veins is based on the compressibility of the veins, the appearance of the veins and the changes which occur to the spectral and colour Doppler findings. The main changes associated with DVT are shown in Box 5-5. The lower limb is examined for possible thrombosis much more frequently than the upper limb, although the principles and features described are also applicable to the arm veins.

BOX 5-5 **SIGNS OF DEEP VEIN THROMBOSIS**

• Absent or reduced compressibility
• Thrombus in the vein: static echoes, incomplete colour fill-in, expansion of the vein
• Static valve leaflets
• Absent flow on spectral or colour Doppler
• Impaired or absent augmentation of flow
• Loss of spontaneous flow and respiratory variation
• Increased flow in collateral channels

COMPRESSIBILITY

As noted above, a normal vein is easily compressible with only mild to moderate pressure from the transducer, so that the lumen is completely obliterated. A vein filled with thrombus will be held open (Fig. 5-12), although it must be remembered that fresh thrombus has the consistency of jelly, so that it can be compressed to some extent by strong pressure.

APPEARANCES OF THE VEIN AND THE VEIN LUMEN

The lumen of a normal vein is usually anechoic and, on colour Doppler, the whole lumen of the vein should be filled with colour, particularly on augmentation of flow. Although fresh thrombus is anechoic, or hypo-echoic, it becomes increasingly echogenic as it matures. In addition fresh thrombus has a tendency to expand the vein and make it look rounder and fuller than a normal vessel.[18] This is accentuated at the upper end of the thrombus where the patent lumen above the clot may be relatively poorly filled with blood due to the distal obstruction by the thrombus (Fig. 5-13).

Fresh thrombus is not particularly adherent to the vein wall, so that some blood may be seen around the periphery of the clot in the vein on colour Doppler. Another appearance which may be seen in early thrombosis is that of a thin tail of thrombus extending up the vein from its origin and lying free in the lumen of the vein (Fig. 5-14). Older thrombus becomes increasingly echogenic, adherent to the vein wall and contracts as it becomes more organised and fibrotic. This may result in the vein being reduced to a relatively small echoic structure that may be difficult to locate. Alternatively, the thrombus may retract to one side of the vein, resulting in an asymmetric lumen on colour Doppler.

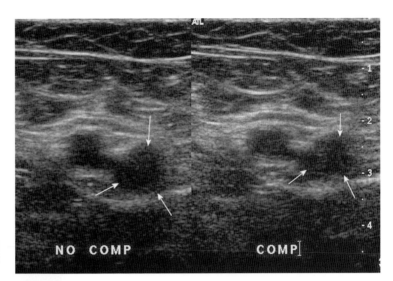

FIGURE 5-12 Positive compression test, the thrombosed vein (arrows) does not change calibre on compression with the transducer.

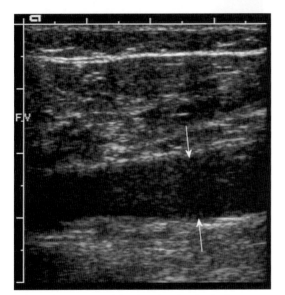

FIGURE 5-13 A vein containing thrombus: low-level echoes are seen in the clot (arrows), the patent lumen above the thrombus is narrower than the thrombosed segment.

An exception to the rule that flowing blood is not echogenic is seen in pregnancy, or any other situation where there is slow venous flow and a tendency to hyperviscosity. In these individuals faint, mobile echoes are seen moving up the vein on real-time imaging; these accelerate on augmentation of flow. These echoes are produced by clumps, or aggregates of red cells, and do not usually cause any significant difficulties in diagnosis.

Normal valves may be seen moving gently in the currents from blood passing them, particularly in the larger thigh veins (Fig. 5-6). One of the earliest sites of deep vein thrombus formation is in the sinus above a valve cusp, so that apparent rigidity or fixation of a cusp should raise the suspicion of possible early DVT and a careful examination of the area should be undertaken.

The walls of a normal vein are smooth and unobtrusive. Following recanalisation after a DVT, they become irregular, thickened and echogenic; calcification may also occur in a small number of cases.

SPECTRAL DOPPLER FINDINGS

Spontaneous Flow and Respiratory Variation

Even at rest and with some head-up tilt there should still be spontaneous flow along the vein which shows some respiratory variation or phasicity, particularly in the proximal leg veins. This variation is produced by the intra-abdominal pressure changes on respiration and is the opposite of the changes found in the jugular vein and arm veins. On inspiration the diaphragm descends and the intra-abdominal pressure rises; this results in decreased flow from the leg veins into the abdomen. On expiration the intra-abdominal pressure decreases and flow from the legs increases. Similarly, if the patient holds their breath, flow in the leg veins slows and may cease until the patient relaxes, when there is relatively high flow from the legs. As well as

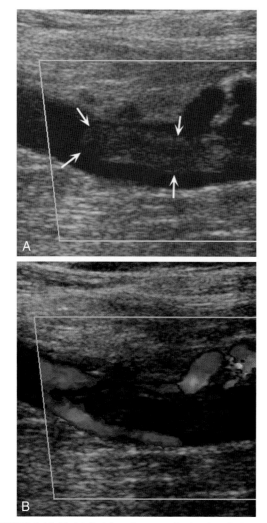

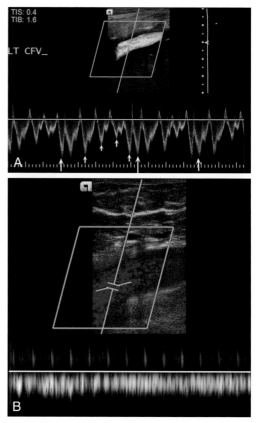

FIGURE 5-15 Spectral Doppler traces from different common femoral veins: (A) Prominent cardiac pulsation or periodicity (small arrows) and respiratory variation or phasicity (large arrows); (B) Flattened trace in a patient with segmental iliac vein thrombosis.

FIGURE 5-14 (A) A tail of thrombus extending up the vein (arrows) which is not sufficiently large to produce any obstruction to flow and could be overlooked if visualisation of this area was poor; (B) power Doppler image of the same thrombus showing flow around it.

changes in flow secondary to respiration, there is also variation of flow secondary to cardiac contractions (Fig. 5-15A). Respiratory variations in flow are sometimes referred to as phasicity and cardiac variations as periodicity.

If there is thrombus occluding the vein there will not be any flow detected in the vein lumen at the level of the thrombus. Sometimes thrombosis is segmental, with a segment of iliac vein or superficial femoral vein

occluded but with patent veins below this level; there is a higher incidence of this in pregnant patients and patients with pelvic tumours. Patent segments below the thrombus may show some slow antegrade flow, particularly if collateral channels are adequate, but this does not show any respiratory or cardiac variation and the augmentation response is damped (Fig. 15-15B).

Augmentation

Normal venous flow is slow and can be improved by compression distal to the point of assessment. There are various techniques for achieving this which are discussed further in the section on chronic venous insufficiency, but for the assessment of possible DVT manual compression of the calf is usually sufficient. The muscles of the calf are squeezed rapidly and firmly in order to propel blood up the veins. In a normal venous system there will be a rapid rise and fall in the frequency shift; whereas if there is a thrombosed segment in the veins, this will increase resistance to flow with damping, or absence, of the augmentation response (Fig. 5-16). It should be remembered that increased resistance to flow anywhere in the vein above the point of compression will result in impaired augmentation and the thrombus may be above or below the point of examination. Therefore, the demonstration of impaired augmentation should lead to a careful search for thrombus in that limb; particularly in the calf or iliac segments. The squeeze of the calf muscles should not be violent, or excessive, as patients will often have tender or painful calves; in addition there is a small potential risk of dislodging a fresh friable thrombus, producing a pulmonary embolus. The risk of this is small and reports of this type of event are few.[19]

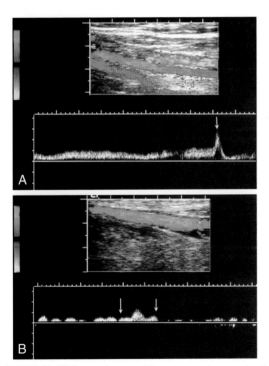

FIGURE 5-16 (A) A normal augmentation response to squeezing the calf; there is a rapid rise and fall in the velocity of blood past the transducer (arrow). (B) Abnormal augmentation, with damping of the response as a result of thrombus impeding the flow of blood up the vein (arrows).

Flow in Collateral Channels

When the normal venous channels are occluded, blood may be seen in collateral veins. In the acute stage, intramuscular channels will not have developed significantly but increased velocity and flow may be seen in the two saphenous veins, or the profunda femoris vein, which provide pre-existing collateral pathways. Over a period of several weeks the intramuscular venous channels will develop and these may be apparent on colour Doppler; therefore their presence indicates a thrombus of some age, rather than fresh thrombus, unless there has been rethrombosis in a segment of clearing clot.

DISTINCTION OF ACUTE FROM CHRONIC THROMBUS

The features which suggest older, rather than fresh, thrombus are given in Table 5-1. However, it is not always possible to define the age of a thrombus and, in these cases, the management of the patient must be based on the clinical picture.

Fresh thrombus is hypoechoic or anechoic. It may not be attached to the wall around the whole circumference of the vein but if it fills the vein, the vein is a little expanded (Fig. 5-13).[18,20] Increased flow may be detected in the profunda femoris vein, or saphenous veins. As thrombus matures it becomes increasingly echogenic and starts to contract as it becomes organised. Longitudinal studies of thrombosed veins show that some 64–75% of veins will recanalise completely, or in part, by 1 year after thrombosis,[21] although valvular incompetence will be found at some level in the majority of these.[22] The remaining veins will show varying degrees of recanalisation, with a thickened irregular wall around an uneven lumen (Fig. 5-17);

TABLE 5-1 Distinction between Acute and Chronic Thrombus

Acute	Chronic
Anechoic or hypoechoic	Increasingly echogenic
Expansion of the vein	Contraction of the vein
Some compression possible	Incompressible
Thrombus 'tail' in lumen	Clot adherent around the wall of the vein
Absent or minimal collaterals	Collateral channels in the tissues

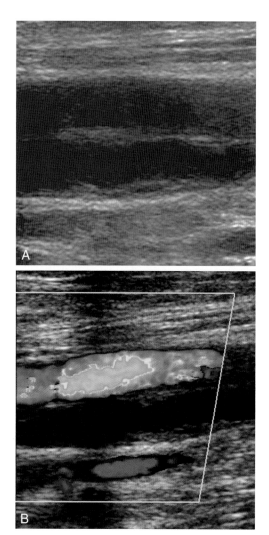

FIGURE 5-17 Recurrent venous thrombosis: (A) a recanalised superficial femoral vein with irregular walls; (B) colour Doppler shows no evidence of flow indicating hypoechoic fresh thrombus in the residual lumen.

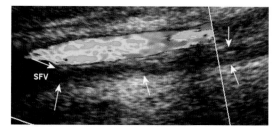

FIGURE 5-18 Chronic thrombosis showing a narrow fibrotic superficial femoral vein.

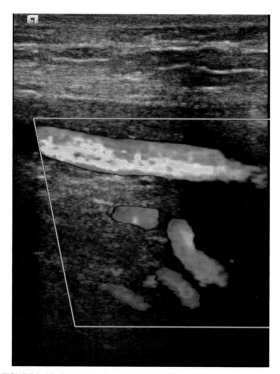

FIGURE 5-19 Collateral channels behind the lower superficial femoral artery in a patient with an occluded femoral vein.

or remain as fibrotic, permanently occluded structures (Fig. 5-18). Abnormal collateral venous channels will develop in the soft tissues around any segments which are significantly obstructed for any length of time (Fig. 5-19).

UPPER LIMB AND JUGULAR VEIN THROMBOSIS

The same principles apply to examination of the upper limb and neck veins. Lack of compressibility of the deep veins of the arm and neck and/or absence of flow on colour or power Doppler are diagnostic of thrombosis (Fig. 5-20). The larger, more proximal veins, such as the axillary and subclavian, cannot be compressed due to their location; diagnosis of thrombosis in these vessels will therefore depend on careful assessment using colour or power Doppler (Fig. 5-21). Indirect signs of thrombosis include loss of respiratory phasicity or cardiac variation, which indicates proximal occlusion and are useful if central vein (innominate

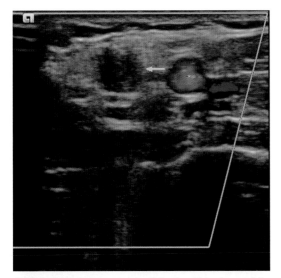

FIGURE 5-20 Transverse view of the brachial artery and its accompanying veins; one of the veins is thrombosed (arrow).

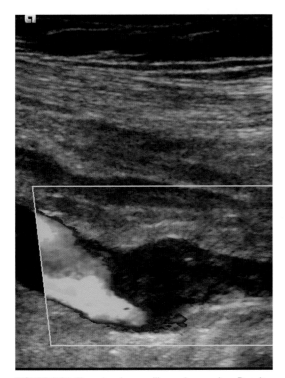

FIGURE 5-21 Thrombus in an axillary vein on colour Doppler.

or superior vena cava) thrombosis is suspected. Respiratory phasicity can be modified by asking the patient to breathe deeply, hold their breath or perform a Valsalva manoeuvre. Comparison with the other side may be helpful, assuming that this is normal.

Baarslag et al.[23] compared colour Doppler with venography and found 82% sensitivity and 82% specificity for the diagnosis of upper limb DVT; 63% of the patients who had thrombosis had an associated malignant disease and in 14% of those with thrombosis this was associated with an in-dwelling central venous catheter in patients without malignant disease. There is a low risk of clinically significant pulmonary embolus from upper limb DVT; in one series of 65 patients with arm vein thrombosis, none of the patients were found to have symptomatic pulmonary emboli.[24]

Problems and Pitfalls in the Diagnosis of Deep Vein Thrombosis

Some of these have been discussed already; however, the value of ultrasound as a technique for the diagnosis of DVT depends on the operator performing a careful, complete examination, being aware of potential pitfalls and recognising when a less than adequate examination has been performed. The main problem areas which should be remembered are shown in Box 5-6.

Inadequate Visualisation. The essential requirement for a satisfactory examination is good ultrasound access to the veins of the limb. Many patients with a possible diagnosis of DVT have swollen or oedematous legs; this situation is aggravated if the patients are also obese. If visualisation is poor then it is possible to miss significant thrombus unless the situation is recognised and appropriate care is taken with the examination

BOX 5-6 PROBLEMS AND PITFALLS IN THE DIAGNOSIS OF DEEP VEIN THROMBOSIS

- Swollen/oedematous/fat legs
- Dual thigh and popliteal veins
- Non-occlusive thrombus
- Segmental calf vein thrombus
- Segmental iliac vein thrombus
- Pregnant patients

and machine settings, as well as with the selection of an appropriate transducer.

Duplicated Venous Segments. Dual segments of femoral vein may be overlooked unless they are actively sought with transverse scanning. If they are not recognised, then one component may be patent and seen on colour Doppler, whereas the other component may contain thrombus and be overlooked (Fig. 5-22).

Non-occlusive Thrombus. Similarly, non-occlusive thrombus may be missed if the vein is not seen adequately. If there is only a small amount of thrombus in the vein then good flow signals will be obtained on spectral and colour Doppler and the presence of the thrombus may not be recognised (Fig. 5-14). This is particularly important in obese or oedematous legs.

Isolated Calf Vein Thrombus. The calf veins are multitudinous in number and variable in their anatomy. Even with a careful, patient, time-consuming examination it is difficult to exclude completely the presence of a small segmental thrombus in a calf vein or muscular sinus (Fig. 5-10, Fig. 5-23). In a mobile patient with a little calf tenderness or swelling this is not a problem, as the body's normal thrombolytic mechanisms will probably clear this. However, in a patient who is immobile following surgery or a stroke,

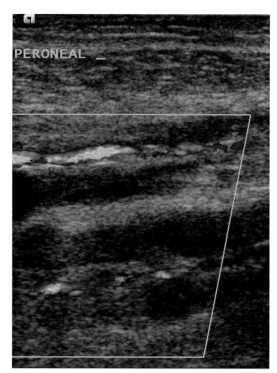

FIGURE 5-23 Calf vein thrombosis: Flow is seen in the posterior tibial and peroneal arteries but not in the accompanying veins.

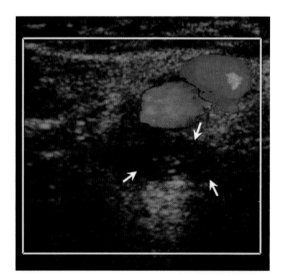

FIGURE 5-22 Dual superficial femoral vein segments; the more posterior segment (arrows) is thrombosed and could be overlooked.

a small segmental calf thrombus indicates that the clotting cascade has been activated and there is a possibility that this small thrombus may increase in size, resulting in a significant, occlusive thrombus. Therefore a follow-up scan should be considered in these patients in order to identify any progression of thrombus from the calf. A study by Labropoulos et al.[25] reviewed 5250 patients; isolated calf vein thrombus was found in 4.8% (282 limbs in 251 patients). In these patients, variable patterns of involvement of the calf veins were demonstrated with the soleal veins involved in 20% of cases, gastrocnemius veins in 17%, peroneal veins in 15% and the posterior tibial veins in 12%; in 64% of these positive cases, only a single vein group was involved.

A review by Scarvelis et al.,[26] discussing the management of patients with deep vein thrombosis, comments that only 1–2% of patients who have a negative initial ultrasound will be confirmed to have a proximal DVT upon serial testing, so serial examinations are not cost-effective. However, whilst re-scanning should not be a routine expectation, it should be considered in cases with a high clinical probability or clinical concern and an initial negative scan.

Asymptomatic Thrombus. The accuracy of Doppler in the detection of asymptomatic thrombus is less impressive than that for symptomatic thrombus,[4,27,28] and the technique is therefore generally inadequate as a screening tool for the detection of asymptomatic thrombus. This is probably because asymptomatic thrombi are more likely to be small and non-occlusive; in addition, there is a higher incidence of distal thrombi in the calf veins, which may be more difficult to demonstrate with ultrasound.[3]

Segmental Iliac Vein Thrombus. The external and common iliac veins may not be demonstrated in their entirety due to obesity or overlying bowel gas. Care must be taken to exclude segmental iliac vein thrombosis (Fig. 5-24), especially if this is a possibility following pelvic surgery; although it is rare for iliac thrombosis not to include the common femoral vein, segmental iliac thrombosis can occur and should be sought in patients with a good clinical picture for DVT but a negative scan of the femoral and popliteal veins. An indicator of segmental iliac thrombosis is loss of cardiac and respiratory variation (Fig. 5-15) and an impaired augmentation response in the common femoral vein. In some patients segmental iliac vein thrombosis may be associated with a structural web or spur in the left common iliac vein wall at the point where it is crossed by the right common iliac artery – May–Thurner syndrome.[29] The internal iliac veins are difficult to assess but any thrombus arising in these, which extends into the common iliac vein and significantly impedes blood flow, may be suggested by an impaired augmentation response in the femoral veins, or loss of respiratory variation on deep breathing or panting. However, non-occlusive thrombus which is insufficient to produce this effect may be overlooked; transvaginal scanning may be of value in difficult cases. It is important that the proximal extent of any thrombus is defined so that any subsequent extension can be appreciated. In addition, insertion of a caval filter might be considered and it is important to know if access is possible from the groin through the iliac veins and lower IVC. Once a filter has been inserted, the subsequent patency of the cava and iliac veins can be assessed using ultrasound (Fig. 5-25).

Pregnancy. During pregnancy several factors are present which increase the risk of thrombosis. These include changes to the coagulation system and physiological changes to venous flow in the leg veins due to a

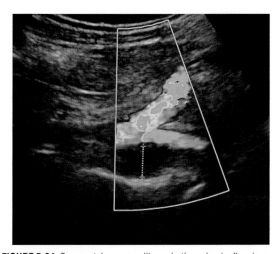

FIGURE 5-24 Segmental common iliac vein thrombosis: flow is seen in the iliac arteries (blue) but no flow is demonstrated in the vein behind them (cursors).

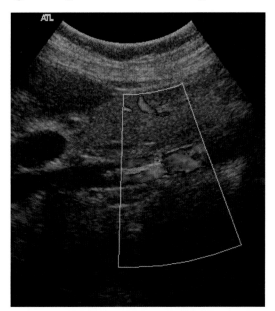

FIGURE 5-25 A caval filter in place. Note the change in colour due to the alteration in direction of flow in relation to the transducer.

combination of hormonal effects and pressure from the enlarging uterus.[30] Some of the technical aspects relating to the ultrasound diagnosis of thrombosis associated with pregnancy have already been discussed. There is also an increased tendency to develop segmental proximal thromboses in the iliac and upper femoral veins. This is more common on the left side,[31,32] perhaps reflecting the additional potential compression from the right common iliac artery, which crosses the left common iliac vein just beyond the aortic bifurcation; in one study[32] only 18% of deep vein thromboses were confined to the right leg. If isolated iliac thrombosis is suspected and the ultrasound examination is less than adequate, then consideration should be given to further imaging with magnetic resonance (MR), or contrast venography.[30] Patients who have undergone caesarean section will have a higher risk of developing a DVT.

OTHER CAUSES OF LEG SWELLING, PAIN OR TENDERNESS

Unlike venography, ultrasound allows examination of other structures in the pelvis and leg. Other pathologies may be seen which account for the patient's symptoms of a swollen, or painful, tender leg; these are given in Box 5-7. It is important to remember that, even if a ruptured popliteal cyst is seen (Fig. 5-26), or a superficial thrombophlebitis is demonstrated (Fig. 5-27), the deep veins must still be examined carefully, as a coexistent DVT may otherwise be overlooked. Labropoulos et al.[33] demonstrated popliteal cysts in 3% of asymptomatic individuals, rising to 10% of patients with symptoms of possible DVT and 20% of patients with painful knees. Langsfeld et al.[34] found popliteal cysts in 3% of patients being examined for possible DVT, 7% of those with cysts had a coexisting DVT.

BOX 5-7 **OTHER CAUSES OF LEG SWELLING, PAIN OR TENDERNESS**

- Popliteal (Baker's) cysts
- Haematoma/muscle injury
- Superficial thrombophlebitis
- Iliac nodes/pelvic masses
- Arteriovenous fistula
- Lymphoedema

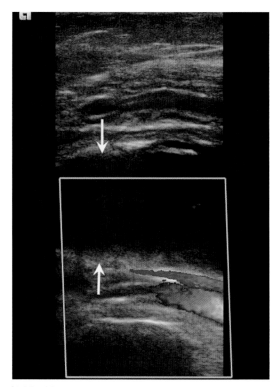

FIGURE 5-26 A popliteal (Baker's) cyst behind the knee joint (arrows) with a patent popliteal vein and artery seen deep to the cyst.

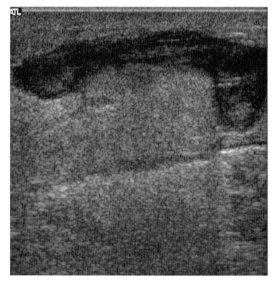

FIGURE 5-27 Thrombosis of the superficial veins is easily recognised but the deep veins should still be examined.

Accuracy in Relation to Other Techniques

Despite these potential problems, ultrasound is a good non-invasive method for the diagnosis of symptomatic DVT, especially between the lower popliteal region and the groin.[3] The key to its value in any given department is that the sonographers must not only be well trained in the technique, but must also be able to recognise an inadequate examination so that appropriate further measures, such as venography or a repeat scan, can be arranged. Should venography be required to clarify areas of doubt, this can be focused on the area of concern identified at the ultrasound examination and only a limited examination may be required.

Many studies have shown that, in comparison to venography, ultrasound is an accurate technique for the diagnosis of symptomatic DVT in the femoropopliteal segments.[3] Used alone, compression is an accurate method for detecting DVT, with sensitivities of 89% and specificity of 100% being reported for proximal thrombosis,[35] and sensitivities of 86–92% and specificities of 96–100% for careful examination of the calf veins.[36] The additional use of colour Doppler allows very accurate diagnosis of DVT, particularly in the femoropopliteal segments. With the development of colour Doppler techniques, further studies have shown the value of ultrasound and that the calf veins can be examined satisfactorily in most cases (Table 5-2).[28,37] The need for an adequate examination must be emphasised. In one study, the initial results in the calf were significantly less accurate than the results for the femoropopliteal segment, but when the examinations were reviewed and only those which were technically adequate were considered, the overall accuracy

improved markedly and reached a similar level to that obtained in the upper part of the limb.[38] In another study,[39] 32% of studies of calf veins were inadequate; if these were excluded then ultrasound showed 93% sensitivity, 98% specificity and 97% accuracy for the diagnosis of lower limb DVT.

In a review of outcomes following negative femoropopliteal ultrasound examinations, Gottlieb and Widjaja[40] showed that only 0.7% of cases developed a subsequent pulmonary embolus, they also reviewed 1797 similar patients reported in the literature and noted that only four (0.2%) of these had developed a pulmonary embolus following a negative ultrasound examination of the thigh area in patients symptomatic for DVT.

It is important to draw a distinction between the accuracy of ultrasound for the diagnosis of symptomatic thrombus and asymptomatic thrombus. The results for the latter are less good as, almost by definition, asymptomatic thrombus will be non-occlusive in many cases and therefore easier to miss. Weinmann et al. noted an overall sensitivity in six reported series of only 59% for proximal thrombus, although the specificity was 98%.[4] In addition, asymptomatic thrombus may be small, or involve one or only a few calf vein segments. A further review by Wells of 17 screening studies in orthopaedic patients showed a sensitivity of 62%, specificity of 97% and a positive predictive value of 66% in those studies which had been carried out with an adequate scientific method.[41]

The continuing developments with MR imaging (MRI) and multislice computed tomography (CT) mean that it is now feasible to consider using these for the diagnosis of DVT. Several authors have

TABLE 5-2	Results of Doppler Ultrasound in the Diagnosis of Deep Vein Thrombosis			
Author	**Sensitivity (%) for all DVT**	**Sensitivity (%) for Proximal DVT**	**Sensitivity (%) for Distal DVT**	**Specificity (%)**
Goodacre et al.[28]				
Duplex (28 studies)	92	96.5	71.2	94
Compression (22 studies)	90.3	93.8	56.8	97.8
Colour Doppler (5 studies)	81.7	95.8	43.5	92.7
Kearon et al.[37]				
Symptomatic (18 studies)	89	97	73	94
Asymptomatic (16 studies)	47	62	53	94

suggested that performing a CT scan of the pelvis and upper legs in patients undergoing CT pulmonary arteriography for pulmonary embolus is a satisfactory way to confirm or exclude the presence of significant proximal thrombus in the leg and pelvic veins.[42,43] However, this technique would not be practical for the assessment of all cases of possible DVT and considerations relating to radiation dose and contrast injection would need to be taken into account. Similarly, MR venography is also of some value[44,45] as it shows not only the thrombus in the lumen of the vein as a filling defect but can also show thrombus directly due to the methaemoglobin present within the thrombus; in addition it also shows the perivascular inflammatory reaction to acute thrombosis.[46] As with CT, MR venography is not practical or suitable for initial assessment of all patients with possible DVT, although incidental findings of DVT in abdominal and pelvic examinations can easily be recognised and research into its role is continuing.

Recurrent Varicose Veins and Chronic Venous Insufficiency

The venous system of the lower limb is relatively fragile and easily damaged by a variety of insults including thrombosis, trauma and inflammation. Previous thrombosis may not clear completely, resulting in chronic obstruction and damage to the valves. In limbs affected by DVT, 50–80% will recanalise months or years after the event; chronic sequelae are most often ascribed to reflux rather than to residual obstruction, although both play a part in the development of chronic problems.[47] This damage results in loss of the protective action of the valves so that a continuous column of blood is present between the heart and the tissues of the calf, ankle and foot. In the erect position this may extend over 1.25 m and the hydrostatic pressure exerted on the tissues interferes with the circulation of blood in the capillaries, the transfer of nutrients and waste matter between blood and the tissues and may also promote local inflammatory responses in the tissues. These changes result in the development of varicose veins, varicose eczema and, ultimately, varicose ulceration. Treatment options include standard varicose vein surgical techniques, pressure stockings, dressings and venous reconstruction techniques. The

pattern of damaged and incompetent veins can be defined using Doppler ultrasound to examine the deep and superficial veins in order to identify thrombosed or partially recanalised veins. Incompetent venous segments, together with incompetent perforating veins, can be mapped out and appropriate surgical or medical techniques applied. Approximately 1% of the population will have venous leg ulceration at some point in their lives,[2] and up to 22% will have evidence of chronic venous insufficiency.[5]

Diagnosis and assessment of primary varicose veins have traditionally been based on clinical assessment in conjunction with hand-held Doppler devices, but it has been shown that a formal colour Doppler assessment prior to surgery will alter the proposed operative procedure in a number of cases and improve the overall results of surgery for primary varicose veins. Blomgren et al.[48] showed that over a 7-year follow-up period, 34% of legs which did not have preoperative duplex required reoperation, compared with 13% of legs on which pre-operative duplex had been carried out. However, applying this principle to all cases of primary varicose veins would result in a heavy workload, so some consideration needs to be given to patient selection and scanning only those in whom there are incomplete, or conflicting clinical findings;[49] or in whom endovascular ablation is to be performed so that an accurate assessment of vessel calibre and anatomy can be made.

Treatment options for varicose veins are no longer restricted to surgical ablation or stripping of the affected vein. Laser or radiofrequency ablation, as well as foam sclerotherapy have been shown to be as effective as surgery.[50] Ultrasound has a major role in the localisation of catheters and ablation devices, as well as monitoring the progress of these treatments.[51]

Recurrence of varicose veins after surgery or sclerotherapy may occur. Three main patterns of recurrence have been described.[52] A patent long saphenous vein may be present, suggesting that it has been missed at the time of the operation. Small collateral veins along the line of the long saphenous vein may enlarge to reconstitute the path of the vein (Fig. 5-28). Finally, drainage can occur through venous collaterals which pass along a variety of courses remote from the normal line of the vein. Colour Doppler is useful to assess the pattern of recurrence, so that appropriate surgical intervention may be planned.[53]

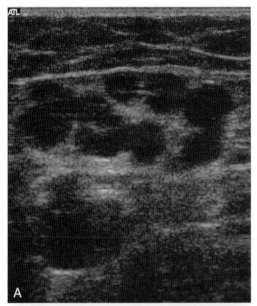

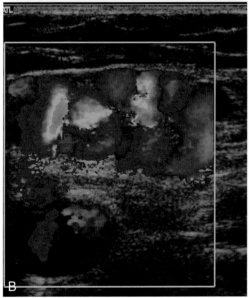

FIGURE 5-28 Collateral channels at the saphenofemoral junction following previous surgery: (A) B-scan image; (B) colour Doppler image.

TECHNIQUE OF EXAMINATION

The patient is best examined standing, or with a large degree of head-up tilt if the couch can be elevated, otherwise inadequate pressure will be exerted on the valves to test their competence and misleading

measurements will be obtained. As the examination may be time-consuming – particularly if both legs are being examined – it is useful if the patients have some means of supporting themselves, such as a handle or rail on the wall; this enables them to stand in reasonable comfort with their weight on the leg that is not being examined and with slight flexion of the leg under examination. Alternatively, they may support themselves by holding the side of the ultrasound machine. It is useful if they are asked to stand on a low plinth, as this makes examination of the popliteal and calf regions less uncomfortable for the examiner.

Various techniques can be used to assess competence or incompetence of a venous segment.[54] The most convenient method for general assessment is to squeeze firmly, then release the patient's calf, or lower thigh, to promote forward flow. Incompetent valves will allow reverse flow back through them after forward flow has ceased (Fig. 5-29), whereas competent valves will stop any reverse flow. Pressure cuffs that can be inflated and deflated rapidly can be used to produce a similar effect and produce a more standardised stimulus than manual compression.[55] They can also be used to compress a segment of leg in order to squeeze out the venous blood and then released suddenly so that any incompetent segments will show up by reversed filling from above. Alternatively, proximal compression may be applied to induce reverse flow. Getting the patient to perform a Valsalva manoeuvre will also show incompetent segments but there are two disadvantages to this technique. First, the effect will only demonstrate reverse flow as far as the first competent valve, so that any incompetent segments below this will not be demonstrated. Second, it is quite difficult to explain to many patients the exact nature and method for performing a Valsalva. Asking the patient to blow into a high-resistance spirometer circuit can produce the desired sudden increase in intra-abdominal pressure and is easier for many patients to understand. In some patients reflux will be seen simply with inspiration.

Reflux can be defined as reverse flow occurring after the cessation of forward flow. It is generally held to be significant if it lasts >0.5 s in the superficial veins, deep femoral and calf veins. For the femoro-popliteal veins, a cut off of 1.0 s is used as their larger diameters and smaller number of valves are thought to contribute to slower valve closure rates.[56] Shorter

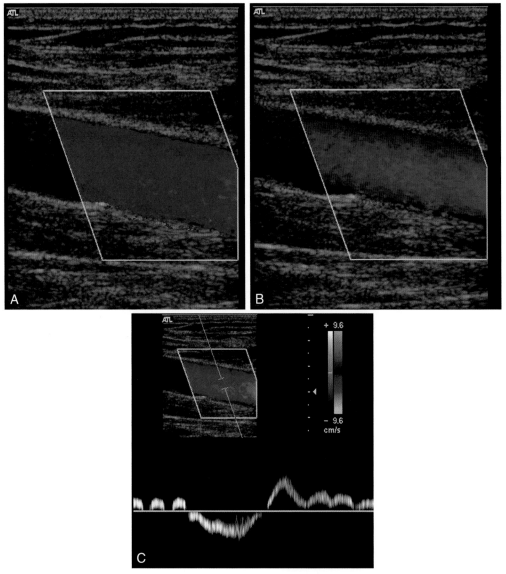

FIGURE 5-29 An incompetent segment of superficial femoral vein showing forward (A, blue) and reverse flow (B, red); (C) the spectral tracing with reverse flow below the baseline lasting for approximately 3 s.

periods of reversed flow may be seen in normal veins and represent the short period as the valve cusps come together and blood in the venous segment settles under the influence of gravity. Reflux should not be confused with the reversed flow which occurs with turbulence, particularly in the common femoral vein and popliteal veins. The difference is usually apparent on colour Doppler, and turbulence is seen on spectral Doppler as reverse flow occurring at the same time as forward flow (Fig. 5-30).

The examination begins in the groin,[57] where the common femoral vein, profunda femoris vein and saphenofemoral junction are identified and assessed. If there is a history of previous venous surgery the details are sometimes uncertain, or even wrong, and the region of the saphenofemoral junction should be

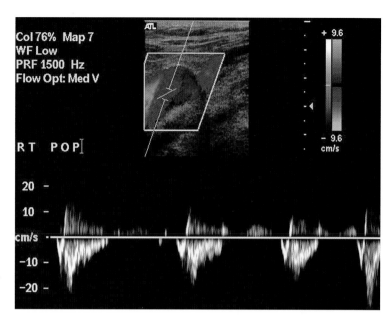

FIGURE 5-30 Turbulence in a vein showing both red and blue signal in the lumen on colour Doppler and simultaneous forward and reversed flow on the spectral display.

examined carefully to assess the type of surgery, whether it was successful and whether there are any significant collaterals, or recanalised segments which are incompetent. The loss of the normal smooth curve of the great saphenous vein as it passes laterally and deeply towards the common femoral vein is suggestive of previous surgery with subsequent recanalisation or collateral formation.

The patency and competence of the deep and superficial veins of the thigh are then assessed down to the level of the knee. Whilst examining the great saphenous vein the presence of incompetent perforators should be sought (Fig. 5-31), especially if the vein becomes incompetent at a level below the sapheno-femoral junction. These can be identified most easily by scanning down the vein transversely whilst

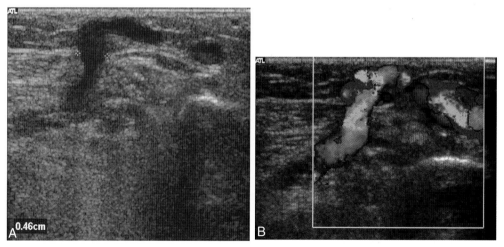

FIGURE 5-31 (A) An incompetent calf perforating vein with a diameter of approximately 5 mm passing through the superficial fascia; (B) colour Doppler shows flow passing from the deep to the superficial veins.

applying recurrent compression to the calf or lower thigh and looking for outward flow with colour Doppler. The commonest of these perforating veins is in the lower thigh at the level of the junction of the middle and lower thirds of the great saphenous vein and is called the mid-thigh perforator vein. The use of tourniquets may help clarify difficult cases but this is not usually required with colour Doppler.

The patient is then turned so that the popliteal region can be examined with the knee partially flexed. The veins in the popliteal fossa are assessed and the saphenopopliteal junction is examined. The level of the saphenopopliteal junction should also be noted, especially if this is not in the expected location. As with the saphenofemoral junction, recurrence after surgery can alter the anatomy and pattern of flow so that care is needed in defining the situation.

Examination of the calf veins may also be performed, although the findings tend to be more variable and their significance more difficult to interpret. Incompetence may be seen in a similar fashion to that demonstrated more proximally. Sometimes the veins appear dilated and it is felt that they should be incompetent, but it is very difficult, or impossible, to induce significant forward flow in the vessels, or any subsequent reflux. Any incompetent calf perforator veins should also be sought using colour Doppler, looking for outward flow from the deep to the superficial systems. The location of any incompetent perforators can be identified in relation to boney landmarks such as the medial malleolus or knee joint. The anatomy and function of the calf veins and the calf perforator veins may have important implications for the development of varicose changes, and this area is the subject of continuing research.

If necessary, varices can be traced proximally in order to identify the point of communication with the deep or superficial segments. This is usually best done with the transducer at right angles to the line of the vein being followed, judicious compression of lower varices will show the course of the veins on colour Doppler and confirm the presence of reflux, where appropriate. Care must be taken not to compress superficial veins with excessive transducer pressure when following the veins.

The findings can be recorded on a diagram of the main lower limb veins where presence of any significant reflux, together with a note of the reflux time, can be indicated on the form (Fig. 5-32).

Saphenous Vein Mapping

The long saphenous vein is the preferred conduit for arterial bypass grafting in the coronary arteries and lower limb. If there is any doubt concerning the suitability of the vein for the procedure, ultrasound can be used to assess the calibre and available length of the vein. Ideally the vein should be more than 3–4 mm wide for much of its length and more than 2 mm at the ankle if a long, femorodistal graft is being considered.[58] The aim of the examination depends on the surgical procedure being contemplated. If the vein is to be removed for a coronary artery or reversed lower limb arterial graft, then the examination can be limited to confirming the presence of the vein and assessing its calibre over the required length. If an in situ lower limb arterial graft is to be performed then a much more detailed examination is required in order to identify perforating veins and superficial branches communicating with the main vein, as these must be ligated during the operation to stop arteriovenous fistulae developing.

TECHNIQUE

The examination is performed with the patient standing, if possible, as this produces distension of the vein, allowing easier location due to dilatation and a better estimation of the calibre of the vessel. If the patient is unable to stand they can be examined sitting with their legs over the side of the couch; if this is not possible then they can be assessed lying supine with a low-pressure tourniquet applied in order to produce distension of the superficial veins.[59] Some operators prefer to mark out the vein with the patient supine as this approximates better to the position during surgery.

One of the problems associated with this examination is that ultrasound gel gums up fibre-tipped markers, making it impossible to mark the course of the vein on the skin, or the location of perforators. In order to avoid this problem the skin should not be covered with gel in the normal manner but the gel should be applied to the transducer and this then placed in the region of the saphenofemoral junction. Once the vein has been located the transducer is aligned along its course, the skin is marked over the

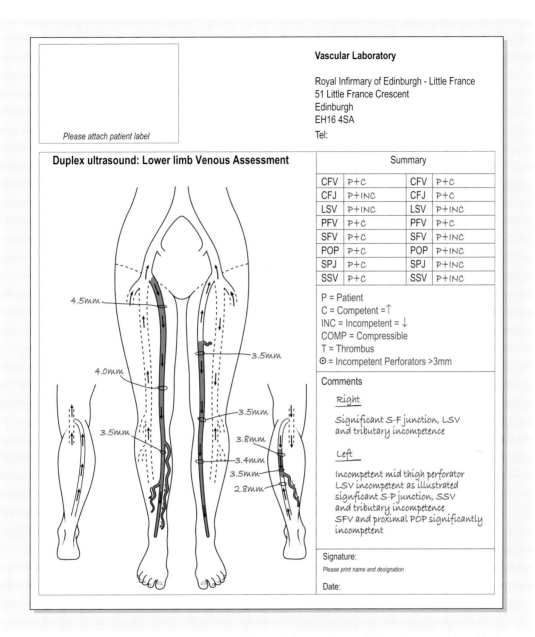

FIGURE 5-32 A sample report form for recording findings of a CVI Doppler examination. Courtesy of S-J Carmichael.

vein at the lower end of the transducer. The transducer is then moved so that its upper end is on the skin mark, aligned along the vein, and a further mark put at the location of the vein at the new position of the lower end of the transducer. The course of the vein is followed down the limb, with skin markings being

made at each transducer length. Care must be taken in the calf, where the long saphenous vein has two main components: the anterior branch usually passes down to the front of the lateral malleolus and is the larger component, with the posterior branch running posteriorly to the posteromedial aspect of the calf.

Once the main marks have been applied, the location of the saphenofemoral junction, together with any other perforator veins, dual segments and tributaries, can be identified and marked. This is usually easier to achieve by scanning transversely along the line of the long saphenous vein with regular augmentation of flow from squeezing the calf. The calibre of the vein is measured in the transverse plane, taking care not to compress the vessel with pressure from the transducer.

Conclusions

Providing care and attention are paid to examination technique then colour Doppler ultrasound is a reliable method for the diagnosis of DVT in symptomatic patients. The technique has become the first-line investigation for DVT in many centres, allowing any subsequent venography to be restricted to the area of doubt or concern on the ultrasound examination. It is important to recognise that the technique has some limitations and that several pitfalls exist.

Ultrasound also provides a non-invasive technique for the investigation of patients with chronic venous disease, or recurrence of varicose veins following surgery, enabling an accurate assessment of the pattern of incompetence or recurrence to be established and allowing an appropriate surgical approach to be developed. It is also of benefit in the assessment of patients with primary varicose veins, especially if there is uncertainty following clinical examination.

The long saphenous vein can be assessed for its suitability as a bypass conduit for arterial or coronary artery bypass procedures. In addition, ultrasound provides a method for examining the central veins prior to central venous line insertion if problems are anticipated in locating a suitable channel for line insertion.

REFERENCES

1. Anderson Jr. FA, Wheeler HB, Goldberg RJ, et al. A population-based perspective of the hospital incidence and case-fatality rates of deep vein thrombosis and pulmonary embolism: the Worcester DVT study. *Arch Intern Med* 1991;**151**:933–8.
2. Callam MJ, Ruckley CV. The epidemiology of chronic venous disease. In: *A textbook of vascular medicine*. London: Arnold; 1996. p. 562–79.
3. Baxter GM. The role of ultrasound in deep vein thrombosis Editorial. *Clin Radiol* 1997;**52**:1–3.
4. Weinmann EE, Salzman EW. Deep vein thrombosis: a review. *New Engl J Med* 1994;**331**:1630–41.
5. Phillips GWL, Paige J, Molan MP. A comparison of colour duplex ultrasound with venography and varicography in the assessment of varicose veins. *Clin Radiol* 1995;**50**:20–5.
6. Da Silva A, Widmer LK, Martin H, et al. Varicose veins and chronic insufficiency: prevalence and risk factors in 4376 subjects of the Basle Study II. *Vasa* 1974;**3**(2):118–25.
7. Caggiatti A, Bergan JJ, Gloviczki P, et al. Nomenclature of the veins of the lower limbs: An international interdisciplinary consensus statement. *J Vasc Surg* 2002;**36**:416–22.
8. Gordon AC, Wright I, Pugh ND. Duplication of the superficial femoral vein: recognition with duplex ultrasonography. *Clin Radiol* 1996;**51**:622–4.
9. Quinlan DJ, Alikhan R, Gishen P, et al. Variations in lower limb venous anatomy: implications for US diagnosis of deep vein thrombosis. *Radiology* 2003;**228**:443–8.
10. Basmajian JV. Distribution of valves in femoral, external iliac and common iliac veins and their relationship to varicose veins. *Surg Gynecol Obstet* 1952;**85**:537–42.
11. Corrales NE, Irvine A, McGuiness CL, et al. Incidence and pattern of long saphenous vein duplication and its possible implications for recurrence after varicose vein surgery. *Br J Surg* 2002;**89**:323–6.
12. Giacomini C. *Osservazioni anatomische per service allo studio della circulazioni venosa delle extremitá inferiori*. Torino: Tip V Vercillino; 1873.
13. Burihan E, Baptista-Silva JCC. Anatomical study of the small saphenous vein (saphena parva): types of termination. *Phlebology* 1995;**10**(Suppl. 1):57–60.
14. Georgiev M, Myers KA, Belcaro G. The thigh extension of the lesser saphenous vein: From Giacomini's observations to ultrasound scan imaging. *J Vasc Surg* 2003;**37**:558–63.
15. Linton RR. The communicating veins of the lower leg and the operative technique for their ligation. *Ann Surg* 1938;**107**:582–93.
16. Wells PS, Anderson DR, Rodger M, et al. Derivation of a simple clinical model to categorize patients' probability of pulmonary embolism: increasing the model's utility with the SimpliRED D-dimer. *Thromb Haemost* 2000;**83**:416–20.
17. Wells PS, Anderson DR, Rodgers M, et al. Evaluation of D-dimer in the diagnosis of suspected deep-vein thrombosis. *NEJM* 2003;**349**:1227–35.
18. Hertzberg BS, Kliewer MA, DeLong DM, et al. Sonographic assessment of lower limb vein diameters: implications for the diagnosis and characterization of deep venous thrombosis. *Am J Roentgenol* 1997;**168**:1253–7.
19. Perlin SJ. Pulmonary embolism during compression US of the lower extremity. *Radiology* 1992;**184**:165–6.
20. Zwiebel WJ, Priest DL. Colour duplex sonography of extremity veins. *Semin Ultrasonogr CT MR* 1990;**11**:136–7.
21. Rosfors S, Eriksson M, Leijd B, et al. A prospective follow-up study of acute deep venous thrombosis using colour duplex ultrasound, phlebography and venous occlusion plethysmography. *Internat Angiol* 1997;**16**:39–44.
22. Franzeck UK, Schalch I, Jager KA, et al. Prospective 12-year follow-up study of clinical and haemodynamic sequelae after deep vein thrombosis in low-risk patients (Zurich study). *Circulation* 1996;**93**:74–9.
23. Baarslag HJ, van Beek EJ, Koopman MM, et al. Prospective study of color duplex ultrasonography compared with contrast venography in patients suspected of having deep venous thrombosis of the upper extremities. *Ann Intern Med* 2002;**136**:865–72.

24. Mustafa S, Stein PD, Patel KC, et al. Upper extremity deep venous thrombosis. *Chest* 2003;**123**:1953–6.

25. Labropoulos N, Webb KM, Kang SS, et al. Patterns and distribution of isolated calf deep vein thrombosis. *J Vasc Surg* 1999;**30**:787–91.

26. Scarvelis D, Wells PS. Diagnosis and treatment of deep-vein thrombosis. *CMAJ* 2006;**175**:1087–92.

27. Davidson BL, Elliot CG, Lensing AWA. Low accuracy of colour Doppler ultrasound in the detection of proximal leg vein thrombosis in asymptomatic high-risk patients. *Ann Intern Med* 1992;**117**:735–8.

28. Goodacre S, Sampson F, Stevenson M, et al. Measurement of the clinical and cost-effectiveness of non-invasive diagnostic testing strategies for deep vein thrombosis. *Health Technol Assess* 2006;**10**:37–42.

29. May R, Thurner J. The cause of the predominantly sinistral occurrence of thrombosis of the pelvic veins. *Angiology* 1957;**8**:419–27.

30. James AH, Jamison MG, Brancaio LR, et al. Venous thromboembolism during pregnancy and the postpartum period: Incidence, risk factor, and mortality. *Am J Obstet Gynecol* 2006;**194**:1311–15.

31. Polak JF, Wilkinson DL. Ultrasonographic diagnosis of symptomatic deep venous thrombosis in pregnancy. *Am J Obstet Gynecol* 1991;**165**:625–9.

32. Ray JG, Chan WS. Deep vein thrombosis during pregnancy and the pueperium: a meta-analysis of the period of risk and leg of presentation. *Obstet Gynecol Surv* 1999;**54**:265–71.

33. Labropoulos N, Shifrin DA, Paxinos O, et al. New insights into the development of popliteal cysts. *Br J Surg* 2004;**91**:1313–18.

34. Langsfeld M, Matteson B, Johnson W, et al. Baker's cysts mimicking the symptoms of deep vein thrombosis: diagnosis with venous duplex scanning. *J Vasc Surg* 1997;**25**:658–62.

35. Cronan JJ, Dorfman GS, Scola FH, et al. Deep venous thrombosis: US assessment using vein compression. *Radiology* 1987;**162**:191–4.

36. Atri M, Herba MJ, Reinhold C, et al. Accuracy of sonography in the evaluation of calf deep vein thrombosis in both postoperative surveillance and symptomatic patients. *Am J Radiol* 1996;**166**:1361–7.

37. Kearon C, Julian JA, Newman TE, et al. Non-invasive diagnosis of deep vein thrombosis. *Annals Int Med* 1998;**128**:663–7.

38. Rose SC, Zweibel WJ, Nelson BD, et al. Symptomatic lower limb venous thrombosis: accuracy, limitations and role of colour duplex flow imaging in the diagnosis. *Radiology* 1990;**175**:639–44.

39. Theodorou SJ, Theodorou DJ, Kakitsubata Y. Sonography and venography of the lower extremities for diagnosing deep vein thrombosis in symptomatic patients. *Clin Imaging* 2003;**27**:180–3.

40. Gottlieb RH, Widjaja J. Clinical outcomes of untreated symptomatic patients with negative findings on sonography of the thigh for deep vein thrombosis: our experience and a review of the literature. *AJR Am J Roentgenol* 1999;**172**:1601–4.

41. Wells PS, Lensing AW, Davidson BL, et al. Accuracy of ultrasound for the diagnosis of deep vein thrombosis in asymptomatic patients after orthopaedic surgery: A meta-analysis. *Ann Intern Med* 1995;**122**:47–53.

42. Thomas SM, Goodacre SW, Sampson FC, et al. Diagnostic value of CT for deep vein thrombosis: results of a systematic review and meta-analysis. *Clin Radiol* 2008;**63**:299–304.

43. Lim KE, Hsu WC, Hsu YY, et al. Deep venous thrombosis: comparison of indirect multidetector CT venography and sonography of lower extremities in 26 patients. *Clin Imaging* 2004;**28**:439–44.

44. Fraser DG, Moody AR, Davidson IR, et al. Deep venous thrombosis: diagnosis by using venous enhanced subtracted peak arterial MR venography versus conventional venography. *Radiology* 2003;**226**:812–20.

45. Sampson FC, Goodacre SW, Thomas SM, et al. Accuracy of MRI in diagnosis of suspected deep vein thrombosis: systematic review and meta-analysis. *Eur Radiol* 2007;**17**:175–81.

46. Froehlich JB, Prince MR, Greenfield LJ, et al. 'Bull's-eye' sign on gadolinium-enhanced magnetic resonance venography determines thrombus presence and age: a preliminary study. *J Vasc Surg* 1997;**26**:809–16.

47. Nicolaides AN. Investigation of chronic insufficiency: a consensus statement. *Circulation* 2000;**102**:e126–63.

48. Blomgren L, Johansson G, Emanuelson L, et al. Late follow up of a randomized trial of routine duplex imaging before varicose vein surgery. *Br J Surg* 2011;**98**:1112–16.

49. Kent PJ, Weston MJ. Duplex scanning may be used selectively in patients with primary varicose veins. *Ann R Coll Surg Engl* 1998;**80**:388–93.

50. Rasmussen LH, Lawaertz M, Bjoern B, et al. Randomized clinical trial comparing endovenous laser ablation, radiofrequency ablation, foam sclerotherapy and surgical stripping for great saphenous varicose veins. *Br J Surg* 2011;**98**:1079–87.

51. Mowatt-Larssen E, Shortell CK. Treatment of primary varicose veins has changed with the introduction of new techniques. *Semin Vasc Surg* 2012;**25**:18–24.

52. Stonebridge PA, Chalmers N, Beggs I, et al. Recurrent varicose veins: a varicographic analysis leading to a new, practical classification. *Br J Surg* 1995;**82**:60–2.

53. Bradbury AW, Stonebridge PA, Callam MJ, et al. Recurrent varicose veins: assessment of the saphenofemoral junction. *Br J Surg* 1994;**81**:373–5.

54. Allan PL. The role of ultrasound in the assessment of chronic venous insufficiency. *Ultrasound Q* 2001;**17**:3–10.

55. Markel A, Meissner MH, Manzo RA, et al. A comparison of the cuff deflation method with Valsalva's maneuver and limb compression in detecting venous valvular reflux. *Arch Surg* 1994;**129**:701–5.

56. Labropoulos N, Tiongson J, Pryor L, et al. Definition of venous reflux in lower-extremity veins. *J Vasc Surg* 2003;**38**:793–8.

57. Coleridge-Smith P, Labropoulos N, Partsch H, et al. Duplex ultrasound of the veins in chronic venous disease of the lower limbs – UIP consensus document. Part 1: Basic Principles. *Eur J Vasc Endovasc Surg* 2006;**31**:83–92.

58. Leopold PW, Shandall A, Kupinski AM, et al. Role of B-mode venous mapping in infrainguinal in situ vein arterial bypasses. *Br J Surg* 1989;**76**:305–7.

59. Hoballah J, Corry DC, Rossley N, et al. Duplex saphenous vein mapping: venous occlusion and dependent position facilitate imaging. *Vasc Endovasc Surg* 2002;**36**:377–80.

Chapter 6

The Aorta and Inferior Vena Cava

Paul L. Allan

Doppler examination in the abdomen is associated with specific problems which are not encountered in peripheral vascular examinations and these are particularly relevant to examinations of the aorta, inferior vena cava and their associated vessels.

Respiratory motion and cardiac pulsation impair the examination, but getting the patient to suspend respiration for any length of time results in relative hypoxia and subsequently increased respiratory movement. It is therefore better to scan as much as possible during quiet respiration, asking the patient to hold their breath only for short periods in order to obtain a spectral trace. In most cases only two or three cardiac cycles are needed for assessment.

Many vessels will always seem to be orientated at right angles to the scan plane, especially with sector or curved linear transducers. Different angles of approach and repositioning of both the transducer and the patient may be required in an attempt to improve the Doppler angle.

Bowel gas is also a problem as it can obscure a vessel, or produce distracting motion artefacts as it bubbles past; scanning after an overnight fast may improve the situation, as may an injection of hyoscine. It has been suggested that patients should receive bowel preparation as for an enema, but this author feels that this is not usually justified for the small advantage it may occasionally confer.

Abdominal Doppler examinations are performed on vessels which lie more deeply than the peripheral vessels and this has several consequences. First, lower-frequency transducers are used and this limits the size of Doppler shift which will be obtained for a given velocity. Second, longer-pulse repetition intervals are required to allow the sound to travel the greater distances; this also limits the size of Doppler shift which can be measured as a result of the Nyquist

limit (see Chapter 1). Operators should therefore seek to minimise the scan depth and use the highest-frequency transducer compatible with adequate visualisation.

The Aorta

ANATOMY

The aorta enters the abdomen at the level of T12 and runs down the posterior abdominal wall to the left of the midline, with the inferior vena cava to its right side. It divides into the common iliac arteries at the level of L4, which is about the level of the iliac crests. Para-aortic nodes are distributed anteriorly and on both sides of the vessel.

The abdominal aorta gives branches to the abdominal organs and to the abdominal wall. The parietal branches to the abdominal wall are not usually large enough to be seen regularly using colour Doppler and will not be considered further. The visceral branches (Fig. 6-1) supply the liver, kidneys, adrenal glands, gonads, spleen, bowel and pancreas. The vessels to the adrenals and gonads are also usually too small to be seen reliably on ultrasound; the renal, hepatic and iliac arteries are covered elsewhere in greater detail.

The splanchnic arteries supply the bowel and associated organs. The coeliac trunk (Fig. 6-2) arises from the anterior aspect of the aorta just after it has entered the abdomen. The trunk is only about 1 cm long and divides into three branches: the common hepatic artery, the splenic artery and the left gastric artery. The common hepatic artery passes to the right over the head of the pancreas, where it gives off the gastroduodenal artery which can be seen passing inferiorly between the head of the pancreas

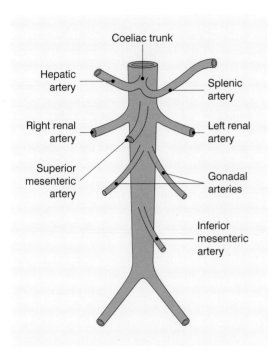

FIGURE 6-1 The abdominal aorta and its major branches.

to the porta of the liver, where it divides into right and left hepatic arteries. The splenic artery passes to the left and runs along the superior margin of the body of the pancreas to the hilum of the spleen. It has a tortuous course and an arterial loop may be mistaken for a small cyst in the pancreas if the situation is not recognised; colour Doppler allows quick identification of the true nature of the 'cyst'. The right gastric artery arises from the splenic artery but is not usually seen on ultrasound.

The superior mesenteric artery (Fig. 6-3) arises 1–2 cm below the coeliac trunk and supplies the small bowel and colon to the distal transverse colon. The superior mesenteric vein is seen on the right side of the upper portion of the artery and can be followed to its confluence with the splenic vein, forming the portal vein. The individual branches of the superior mesenteric artery are not usually seen clearly on ultrasound. The inferior mesenteric artery (Fig. 6-4) arises from the anterior aorta about 3–4 cm above the bifurcation and runs inferiorly to the left side of the aorta. The inferior mesenteric vein may be seen

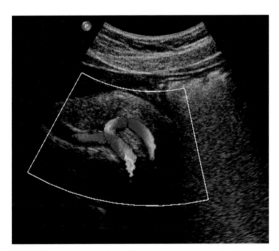

FIGURE 6-2 Transverse view of the coeliac axis showing the splenic artery on the right and the hepatic artery on the left.

and the margin of the duodenum; the other branches from this segment of the hepatic artery are not usually apparent on ultrasound. The artery ascends in the lesser omentum as the proper hepatic artery, in company with the portal vein and common bile duct,

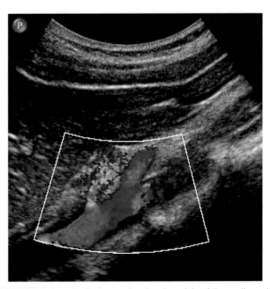

FIGURE 6-3 Longitudinal scan showing the origin of the coeliac axis superiorly and the superior mesenteric artery just below this. Colour Doppler shows aliasing and a tissue bruit around a stenotic coeliac axis origin.

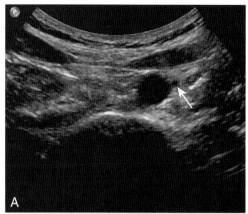

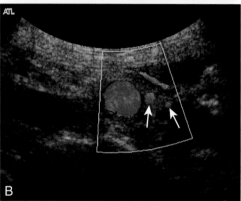

FIGURE 6-4 (A) Transverse scan showing the inferior mesenteric artery lying adjacent to the aorta (arrow); (B) colour Doppler image showing the inferior mesenteric artery and vein (arrows).

on the left of the artery but diverges as it passes up to join the splenic vein.

Several variations in the anatomy of the splanchnic arteries are well recognised. The most important one in relation to ultrasound is the origin of the right hepatic artery from the superior mesenteric artery. Occasionally the coeliac trunk is absent with its branches arising separately from the aorta; the left hepatic artery may arise from the left gastric artery and accessory hepatic arteries may arise from the superior mesenteric artery or other arteries in the region.

SCANNING TECHNIQUE
Aorta

The upper abdominal aorta can nearly always be examined through the left lobe of the liver; the coeliac

trunk and superior mesenteric arteries are also visible from this approach. A 3 or 5 MHz transducer is used depending on the build of the patient. The patient should fast for 8 h prior to the examination, for two reasons: first, fasting will improve visualisation of the aorta and its branches; second, splanchnic blood flow will be in the basal fasting state, rather than the dynamic postprandial state.

If the aorta is the main object of the investigation it is followed distally to its bifurcation. The vessel should be scanned both longitudinally and transversely, taking note of the overall diameter, the presence of any aneurysmal dilatation and any para-aortic masses or pathology. If visualisation from an anterior approach is impaired, then scanning in a coronal plane through the right lobe of the liver will allow the upper aorta to be visualised; scanning in a coronal oblique plane from a left posterolateral approach can provide a view of the mid- and lower aorta, together with the bifurcation. The calibre of the vessel used to be measured from the outer aspect of the vessel wall, ideally during systolic expansion. However, it has been shown that measurement of the systolic diameter between the inner aspects of the vessel wall is a more repeatable measurement to make and this is therefore used for follow-up of aneurysm patients. It is important to ensure that the true anteroposterior diameter is measured, particularly in ectatic, tortuous arteries, as oblique measurements will result in falsely high measurements. Colour Doppler and spectral Doppler are used to assess any potential disturbances of flow which may result from atheroma or dissection.

Splanchnic Arteries

The coeliac trunk and its main branches are examined using colour and spectral Doppler. The main trunk is short but it is directed towards the transducer so that an excellent Doppler angle is achieved. The proximal hepatic and splenic arteries, together with the superior mesenteric artery, are often orientated almost at right angles to the transducer with an anterior approach (Fig. 6-2), so that some experimentation with points of access is required to get acceptable Doppler angles. The hepatic artery is followed to the right and the gastroduodenal artery can be identified beside the head of the pancreas. The proper hepatic artery is traced towards the porta where it divides into the right and left hepatic arteries. The origin of the superior mesenteric artery is examined (Fig. 6-3) and the vessel traced as far distally as it remains visible. Firm pressure with the transducer may help in displacing bowel gas from in front of the vessel, but care must be taken not to compress the artery and produce a spuriously high Doppler shift. Colour Doppler is used to identify any abnormal areas of flow, including 'visible bruits', or tissue vibrations, which may be seen in cases of severe stenosis (Fig. 6-3). Power Doppler is of less value in the abdomen than in peripheral vessels as arterial pulsation, respiratory movement and bowel gas motion can all cause marked motion artefacts which obscure the signal from the vessel.

The inferior mesenteric artery is sometimes difficult to locate. It can be found by scanning transversely up from the bifurcation and it may be identified just to the left of the aorta, 2–4 cm above the bifurcation (Fig. 6-4).

NORMAL AND ABNORMAL FINDINGS
Aorta

The calibre of the normal aorta varies with the age, sex and build of the patient, being larger in men, older patients and tall patients. The calibre also varies with the level in the abdomen. Goldberg et al. found an average diameter of 22 mm above the renal arteries, 18 mm just below the renal arteries and 15 mm above the bifurcation.[1] The normal Doppler waveform in the aorta also varies with location. In the upper aorta there is a narrow, well-defined systolic complex with forward flow during diastole; below the renal arteries the diastolic flow is much reduced and above the bifurcation it is absent, or reversed diastolic flow may occur, with a waveform similar to that seen in the lower limb arteries (Fig. 6-5).[2]

The main abnormalities affecting the aorta are atheroma, aneurysm, dissection and para-aortic masses. Atheroma can affect the aorta and produce stenosis (Fig. 6-6), or occlusion; aortic disease, unless severe is usually overshadowed clinically by symptoms arising from the peripheral or the coronary arteries. Sometimes there is uncertainty as to whether aortic

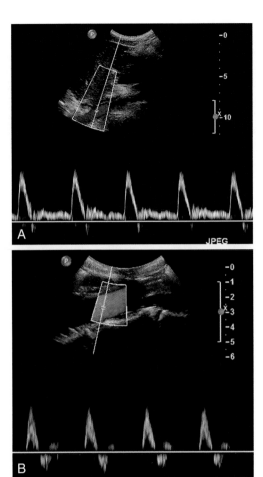

FIGURE 6-5 (A) The aortic waveform in the upper abdomen showing diastolic flow. (B) The aortic waveform above the bifurcation with absent diastolic flow and a waveform similar to that seen in the lower limb arteries.

disease seen on arteriography is clinically significant. In these cases velocity ratios taken from above and at the stenosis can be used to assess the degree of haemodynamic compromise. However, accurate criteria are not as fully developed for aortic stenosis, unlike the situation for carotid and peripheral Doppler examinations; however, in one study[3] a peak systolic velocity ratio of 2.8 correlated (86% sensitivity, 84% specificity) with aortoiliac stenoses of >50% diameter reduction and a ratio of 5.0 showed some correlation (65% sensitivity, 91% specificity) with stenoses >75%. If the stenotic area is clearly seen, a direct measurement

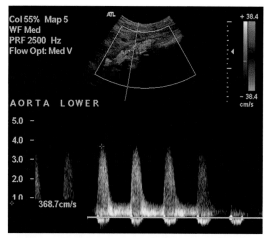

FIGURE 6-6 Colour Doppler image of a stenosis in the middle aortic segment showing significant turbulence and a peak systolic velocity of 3.7 m/s.

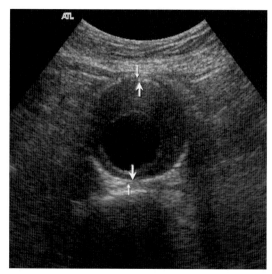

FIGURE 6-7 Transverse view of an aneurysm. The smaller arrows show the outer to outer measuring points. The larger arrows show the inner to inner (ITI) measurement used by screening programmes.

of diameter or area stenosis may be obtained; colour or power Doppler is of value in defining the margins of the residual lumen.

An aneurysm of the abdominal aorta can be defined as an increase of the anteroposterior diameter over 3 cm, or a localised increase of 1.5 times the diameter of the adjacent normal aorta. Aneurysms may extend into the abdomen from the thoracic aorta, or may arise within the abdominal aorta, usually affecting the infrarenal segment. Aneurysms are nearly always true aneurysms secondary to degeneration of the connective tissue in the vessel wall. Occasionally mycotic aneurysms secondary to infection, or pseudoaneurysms secondary to trauma, may be seen. Ultrasound diagnosis is normally straightforward; the cardinal measurement is the anteroposterior (AP) diameter, which is best obtained by scanning transversely with the ultrasound beam at right angles to the long axis of the vessel, in order to ensure a true anteroposterior measurement. The technique of diameter measurement has been amended since the advent of screening programmes so that the AP diameter of the aneurysm is measured between the inner aspects of the aneurysm wall in the antero-posterior dimension (the inner to inner method, ITI) (Fig. 6-7); and not the previous measurement using the outer aspects of the wall. In terms of a screening programme, the ITI method has been shown to be more reproducible and it is therefore preferred.[4] It is also important to locate the upper and

lower margins of the aneurysmal segment, particularly in relation to the renal arteries. If these cannot be identified with certainty it should be remembered that the main renal arteries usually arise from the aorta 1–2 cm below the superior mesenteric artery, and this vessel can therefore be used as an approximate marker for the renal vessels. The proximal common iliac arteries should also be checked.

Colour and spectral Doppler may show turbulent flow within the aneurysm, or indeed very slow flow with very little forward movement of the blood. However, examination of normal-calibre vessels below the aneurysm will show rapid reconstitution of the waveform as the pressure wave is constrained by the narrower-calibre vessels. Doppler can also be used to confirm renal blood flow, particularly after surgery, if there is any question that this has been cut off.

The main complications from aneurysms are leakage or rupture; occasionally an aortocaval or aortoduodenal fistula may develop (Fig. 6-8); high-volume pulsatile flow is seen in the inferior vena cava on Doppler in cases of caval fistula. Ultrasound does not have a major role in the diagnosis of these conditions as CT or angiography provide more comprehensive information if the patient's condition allows time for imaging before surgery. FAST (Focused Assessment with Sonography in Trauma) scanning in the

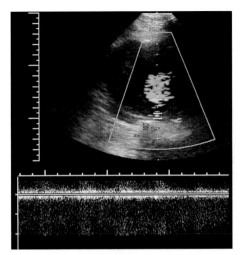

FIGURE 6-8 Colour Doppler image of an aortocaval fistula in a patient with an aneurysm. The spectral Doppler gate is on the fistula and the spectral display shows a turbulent signal which is largely off the spectral range at these settings.

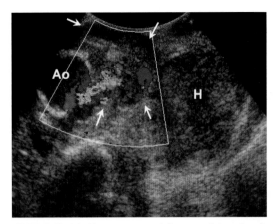

FIGURE 6-10 A leaking aneurysm of the aorta. Colour Doppler shows the leak from the aorta (Ao) into a partly thrombosed pseudo-aneurysm (arrows), with a further, large haematoma (H) seen lateral to this.

Emergency Department may be used for initial identification of an aneurysm in a patient with abdominal symptoms which may be related to a leaking aneurysm. If an aneurysm is seen, the patient can then be transferred directly for emergency surgery or appropriate imaging if the clinical status allows time for this.

Occasionally ultrasound may show a para-aortic haematoma in a patient if an aneurysm has not been suspected (Fig. 6-9); and rarely, a leaking, ruptured aneurysm may be seen on ultrasound (Fig. 6-10).

Screening for aortic aneurysms in men over 60–65 is beneficial in terms of reducing mortality;[5,6]

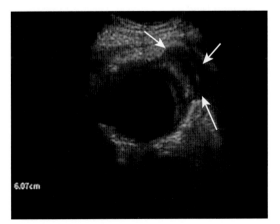

6.07cm

FIGURE 6-9 Transverse image of a leaking aortic aneurysm with a haematoma visible (arrows).

approximately 4% of men and 1% of women over 65 have been shown to have an aorta more than 3 cm in diameter. The NHS Abdominal Aortic Aneurysm Screening Programme offers ultrasound scans to men over 65; if a diameter greater than 3 cm is found then a follow-up scan is offered at 1 year if the diameter is 3–4.4 cm and in 3 months if the diameter is 4.5–5.4 cm. If the diameter is more than 5.5 cm the patient is referred for vascular surgery assessment. Growth of a smaller aneurysm by >1 cm in a year, or the development of tenderness in patients with smaller aneurysms also leads to vascular surgery referral.

Ultrasound can also be used in the follow up of patients who have had endovascular aneurysm repair (EVAR). Although contrast-enhanced CT is considered the gold standard technique for demonstrating leaks,[7] Doppler ultrasound with echo-enhancing agents has been shown to be a useful method for assessment and may show leaks that have not been apparent on CT.[8,9] Ultrasound can be used to monitor the size of the aneurysmal sac: following a successful EVAR the sac may or may not shrink but an increase in size of more than 0.5 cm indicates an endoleak. Ultrasound is also useful for identifying graft limb occlusions or stenoses. However, ultrasound is less good for detecting structural problems with the stent graft, such as stent distortion or fracture.[10] Unenhanced colour Doppler is less reliable when compared with CT angiography and digital subtraction arteriography. One suggested strategy is to alternate CT and ultrasound in the follow-up of stent graft patients[10] as this could result in substantial cost reduction, reduced radiation exposure and reduction in the risk of contrast-induced nephrotoxicity.

Dissection of the abdominal aorta nearly always results from the extension of a dissection of the thoracic aorta extending into the abdomen (Fig. 6-11). Rarely, it may originate in the abdominal aorta, or result from trauma. The aorta is usually dilated to some extent but dissection can occur in the presence of a normal-calibre aorta. The flap may be visible depending on its orientation in relation to the ultrasound beam, and if a dissection is suspected the aorta should be examined from several different approaches in an effort to show the flap. Spectral and colour Doppler will show the presence and character of any flow in the true and false lumens and, even if a flap is not visible, the different flows in the two channels may be apparent on Doppler; reversed flow may be seen in the non-dominant channel due to compression in systole; if one of the channels is thrombosed then the appearances can be a little confusing. Doppler can also be used to assess blood flow in the major branches supplying the bowel, liver, kidneys and lower limbs.[11] Clevert et al.[12] reported on the role of ultrasound in the assessment of a series of 68 dissections, 25 of which involved the aortic and iliac segments. For the 13 aortic dissections the sensitivity for colour Doppler was 85%, power Doppler 85% and B-flow 98%; for the 12 iliac dissections, the sensitivity for colour Doppler was 67%, power Doppler 75% and 98% for B-flow when compared with the reference techniques (a mix of CT, magnetic resonance angiography and digital subtraction angiography).

Splanchnic Arteries

Blood flow in the superior and inferior mesenteric arteries varies depending on whether the patient is fasting, or has recently eaten. In the fasting state the flow is consistent with a relatively high-resistance vascular bed with low diastolic flow. Following the ingestion of food there is a reduction in the peripheral resistance of the mesenteric vessels, resulting in increased diastolic flow, together with an increase in peak systolic velocity (Fig. 6-12).

The main indication for examination of blood flow in the splanchnic arteries is the investigation of possible intestinal ischaemia. One population study[13] showed a prevalence of 17.4% for mesenteric artery stenosis in a population with a mean age of 77 years. Of the patients with mesenteric artery stenosis, 86% had isolated coeliac artery stenosis (Fig. 6-3), 7% had combined coeliac and superior mesenteric artery stenosis, 5% had isolated superior mesenteric artery stenosis and 2% had coeliac axis occlusion; however none of those affected had symptoms of intestinal ischaemia. The usual indication for ultrasound examination is possible subacute or chronic ischaemia; significant acute ischaemia presents as an acute abdomen and is managed accordingly. The splanchnic circulation is capable

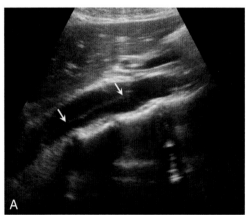

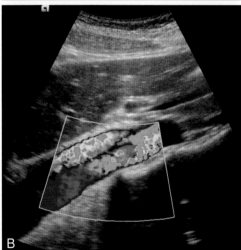

FIGURE 6-11 Longitudinal view of the abdominal aorta showing a dissection flap (A); colour Doppler (B) shows flow in different directions in the two compartments.

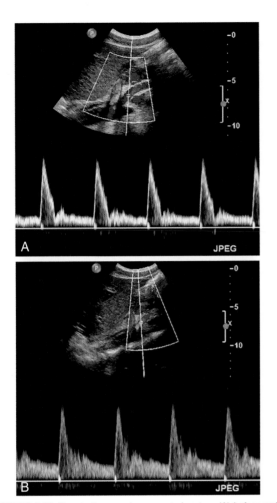

FIGURE 6-12 Flow in the superior mesenteric artery (A) before and (B) after food.

the ultrasound beam. In addition, colour Doppler may show a visible tissue bruit if there is a significant stenosis. The proximal 2–3 cm of the vessels is the most common site for disease and a peak velocity of more than 2.8 m/s in the superior mesenteric artery correlates well with a stenosis of more than 70% diameter reduction with a sensitivity of 92% and a specificity of 96%; whereas the equivalent peak systolic velocity for the coeliac axis is 2 m/s (87% sensitivity, 80% specificity).[14] Indirect signs of intestinal ischaemia include oedema of the mucosa and bowel wall and also reduced peristalsis. In severe cases gas bubbles may be seen in the portal vein flow; these produce a characteristic popping sound on spectral Doppler (Fig. 6-13).

The problems associated with the diagnosis of mesenteric ischaemia are illustrated by the fact that 18% of patients over 60 years without symptoms of mesenteric ischaemia have been shown to have significant disease on Doppler.[13,15] This emphasises the need to assess the findings in the light of the clinical situation.

Aneurysms of the hepatic and splenic arteries may occur. Splenic artery aneurysms are associated with acute pancreatitis and trauma; hepatic artery aneurysms can be associated with these conditions but may also arise following liver transplantation.

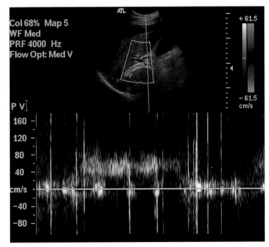

FIGURE 6-13 The spectral display from the portal vein of a patient with severe ischaemia and a transjugular intrahepatic portosystemic shunt (TIPS) showing the characteristic high-intensity echoes from bubbles of gas in the blood.

of developing multiple collateral channels and this makes the assessment of possible gut ischaemia difficult. The demonstration of stenosis of two of the three splanchnic arteries is strongly suggestive of the diagnosis and, in the appropriate clinical situation, the demonstration of severe stenosis in one vessel with occlusion of another is also supportive of the diagnosis. Colour Doppler is of value in identifying the abnormal segment (Fig. 6-3), although care must be taken not to mistake a high shift resulting from disease with the high shift from normal velocity flow, which is seen due to the low Doppler angle resulting from the orientation of the coeliac trunk and proximal superior mesenteric artery to

OTHER APPLICATIONS

The nature of para-aortic masses can be clarified using colour Doppler and masses can be distinguished from aneurysms.

An aorta which is prominent but of normal calibre in a thin patient, or the aorta in a patient with a marked lumbar lordosis, may be mistaken clinically for a mass or an aneurysm. Ultrasound can confirm the normal calibre of the vessel and the lack of pathology in these patients.

Blood flow in the coeliac and mesenteric arteries is also responsive to a variety of pharmacological agents such as glucagon and somatostatin, or pathological states such as cirrhosis and Crohn's disease.[16] Doppler ultrasound can show flow changes associated with these situations and may hold some promise for the future in the assessment of disease activity, or response to treatment.

The Inferior Vena Cava

ANATOMY

The inferior vena cava is formed by the confluence of the common iliac veins at the level of the 5th lumbar vertebra and runs cranially to the right of the midline. It passes through the diaphragm at the level of the 8th thoracic vertebra and enters the right atrium. In the embryo there is a complex arrangement of venous sinuses which form during embryogenesis, and several of these contribute to the inferior vena cava; this means that there are many variations of anatomy which may be seen. The most common variation is that the common iliac veins continue cranially as paired 'venae cavae' (Fig. 6-14), with the left component crossing to join the right side at the level of the left renal vein. Many other variations have been recorded; these are more easily assessed using contrast-enhanced CT than ultrasound, but may cause some confusion if they are seen during an ultrasound examination and not recognised.

TECHNIQUE

The inferior vena cava can be examined using the techniques described for the abdominal aorta. However, in the supine position the vessel may be narrow in the anteroposterior plane and difficult to define. Scanning transversely with colour Doppler and using the aorta

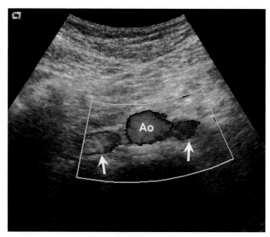

FIGURE 6-14 Transverse scan of the lower abdominal aorta (Ao) showing paired venae cavae (arrows) running on either side in front of the vertebral body.

as a guide may allow localisation of the vein in these circumstances; or elevation of the leg(s) by an assistant will increase flow and the calibre of the vein, thus making it more visible. The calibre of the cava will vary with the state of hydration of the patient. In a well-hydrated patient it will be distended, whereas in a dehydrated patient it will be collapsed, narrow and more difficult to visualise. Excessive transducer pressure applied in an effort to disperse bowel gas will also compress the cava, therefore a balance must be sought in order to visualise segments of the vessel in some patients.

NORMAL AND ABNORMAL FINDINGS

Flow in the inferior vena cava is slow and varies with both respiration and cardiac pulsation (Fig. 6-15). On inspiration the diaphragm descends. This results in negative pressure in the chest and increased pressure in the abdomen, and blood therefore flows from the abdomen to the chest; the reverse occurs on expiration. Superimposed on this is the more rapid periodicity resulting from cardiac activity; this is seen particularly in the upper abdomen. The prominence of the caval waveform also depends on the degree of hydration of the patient. A dehydrated patient's cava will be narrow and difficult to see below the renal veins, whereas in fluid overload the cava is dilated and there is cardiac periodicity detectable down into the iliac veins.

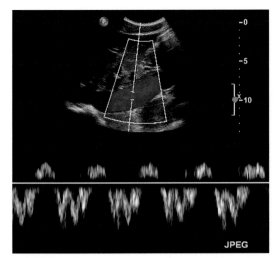

FIGURE 6-15 The inferior vena cava in the upper abdomen showing the variations in flow which occur with respiration and cardiac activity; the various components of the waveform in the inferior vena cava and hepatic veins are described in detail in Chapter 8 and Figure 8-12.

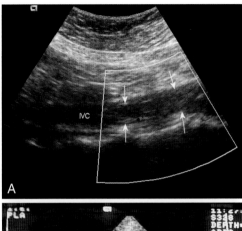

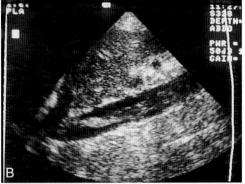

FIGURE 6-16 (A) Thrombus from an iliac DVT extending into the lower IVC (arrows) (B) A tongue of thrombus extending into the upper inferior vena cava in a patient with deep vein thrombosis.

One of the most common indications for specific examination of the inferior vena cava is to assess whether thrombus from a pelvic or lower limb deep vein thrombosis has extended up into the cava. Thrombus may fill the lumen of the cava and even produce some expansion of the vessel; alternatively, a tongue of thrombus may be seen lying free in the lumen, extending up towards the right atrium (Fig. 6-16).

Caval filters are inserted in some patients who are at risk of pulmonary embolus from more distal thrombus. There are several types but all are inserted in the mid- or lower cava, below the renal veins. Identifying a metallic, echogenic structure within the inferior vena cava above the level of the renal veins may indicate migration of the filter. There is a small risk that thrombus may extend past the filter, or develop at the site of the filter. Colour Doppler is a quick and easy method for confirming patency of the cava around and above the filter.[17] The metal struts of the filter can be recognised within the lumen of the cava and colour Doppler, or power Doppler, will show blood flow past the level of the filter (Fig. 6-17).

Renal tumours and hepatocellular carcinoma are two tumours which have a tendency to invade venous channels and, as a result, tumour thrombus may extend into the cava (Fig. 6-18) from the renal or hepatic vein.[18] Compromise of the venous drainage of the liver or kidneys is shown by loss of the normal cardiac and respiratory periodicity of the venous waveform and the tumour thrombus may be clearly seen as it extends into the caval lumen. Some tumours in the retroperitoneum may compress or directly invade the inferior vena cava causing obstruction to the venous return from the lower abdomen and legs. Although the caudal segments of the inferior vena cava and the iliac veins usually remain patent, they will often be dilated, flow will be sluggish or reversed, the flow profile will be flat, and there will be an absence of the normal Valsalva response. Rarely, intrinsic tumours, usually mesenchymal in origin such as fibrosarcomas or leiomyosarcomas, may develop in the caval wall; lipomas have also been reported.[19]

Following liver transplantation the cava should be assessed to ensure satisfactory flow. The appearances

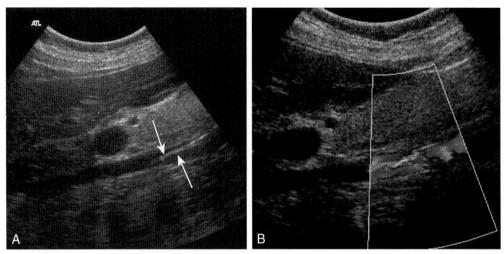

FIGURE 6-17 (A) Real time image of an IVC containing a filter in the lower segment; (B) colour Doppler image of the same patient with a caval filter. The change in colour reflects the changing Doppler angle as the blood flows through the sector scan.

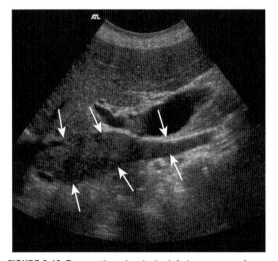

FIGURE 6-18 Tumour thrombus in the inferior vena cava from a renal carcinoma (arrows).

will depend on the type of anastomosis performed. In the past, the segment of donor cava attached to the new liver replaced the equivalent segment of native cava, which had been removed with the diseased liver. Many surgeons now perform a 'piggyback' technique, where the native cava is left in place, the inferior end of the donor caval segment is oversewn and the upper end anastomosed to the native cava.

This results in a postoperative appearance which can be confusing if it is not recognised, as there will appear to be two cavae associated with the transplanted liver (Fig. 6-19).

Other postoperative problems which may occur in relation to the cava following transplantation include compression, if the new liver is relatively large; distortion of the cava may also occur if there is relative twisting of the caval channel as a result of fitting the donor liver into the native abdomen. In the longer term stenosis may develop at the sites of anastomosis. Liver transplantation is covered further in Chapter 7.

Retroperitoneal and other abdominal masses may compress or occlude the inferior vena cava. The situation is usually apparent, especially with colour Doppler, which shows the cava entering the mass and becoming narrowed or occluded with absent flow. Congenital webs can occur, particularly at the upper end of the cava. These may produce a variable degree of caval narrowing and in some cases may predispose to hepatic vein thrombosis and a Budd–Chiari syndrome.

Fistulae involving the cava may rarely occur spontaneously, often secondary to an aortic aneurysm (Fig. 6-8), or they may be surgically created as is the case with portocaval shunts. In the case of aortocaval fistulae, colour Doppler may show a visible tissue bruit with pulsatile flow in the cava above the level of the fistula; sometimes the fistula itself is difficult to

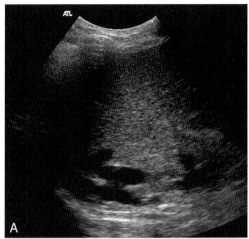

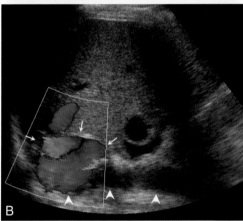

FIGURE 6-19 (A) A real time image of the upper caval region in a liver transplant patient with a 'piggyback' caval anastomosis, showing the native cava posteriorly and the donor cava just anterior to it; (B) colour Doppler image showing the donor cava (arrows) and native cava (arrowheads).

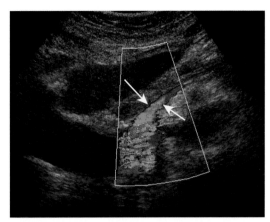

FIGURE 6-20 Colour Doppler image of a portocaval shunt. The portal vein (arrows) has been surgically anastomosed to the inferior vena cava.

Conclusions

The aorta and inferior vena cava, together with their major branches and tributaries, can be examined in most patients, provided that care and attention is spent in finding the best scan plane and ensuring that the system is set appropriately for the specific examination concerned, both in terms of imaging and Doppler settings. CT and three-dimensional reconstruction is the technique of choice for imaging the aorta, particularly if percutaneous stent/grafts are contemplated but ultrasound can contribute significant information to guide management of patients with disorders of the aorta and its major branches. Similarly, ultrasound continues to have a significant role in relation to both initial diagnosis and follow-up of patients with abnormalities relating to the inferior vena cava and its tributaries.

identify. Surgical portocaval shunts are usually side-to-side shunts in the upper abdomen at the level where the proximal main portal vein passes close in front of the cava (Fig. 6-20). A tissue bruit may be apparent and the shunt is more easily identified if the liver can be used as a window through to the point of anastomosis; turning the patient up onto the left side may facilitate visualisation. However, these are rarely performed now, having been replaced by transjugular intrahepatic portosystemic shunts (TIPS) (see Chapter 7).

REFERENCES

1. Goldberg BB, Ostrum BJ, Isard HJ. Ultrasonographic aortography. *J Am Med Assoc* 1996;**198**:353–8.
2. Taylor KJW, Burns PN, Woodcock JP, et al. Blood flow in deep abdominal and pelvic vessels: ultrasonic pulsed Doppler analysis. *Radiology* 1985;**154**:487–93.
3. De Smet AA, Kitslaar PJ. A duplex criterion for aortoiliac stenosis. *Eur J Vasc Surg* 1990;**4**:275–8.
4. Hartshorne TC, McCollum CN, Earnshaw JJ, et al. Ultrasound measurement of aortic diameter in a national screening programme. *Eur J Vasc Endovasc Surg* 2011;**42**:195–9.

5. US Preventive Services Task Force. Screening for abdominal aortic aneurysm: recommendation statement. *Ann Intern Med* 2005;**142**:198–202.

6. Cosford PA, Leng GC, Thomas J. Screening for abdominal aortic aneurysm. *Cochrane Database Syst Rev* 2007;(Issue 2). Art. No.: CD002945http://dx.doi.org/10.1002/14651858.CD002945.pub2.

7. Raman KG, Missig-Carroll N, Richardson T, et al. Color-flow duplex ultrasound scan versus computed tomographic scan in the surveillance of endovascular aneurysm repair. *J Vasc Surg* 2003;**38**:645–51.

8. Napoli V, Bargellini I, Sardella SG, et al. Abdominal aortic aneurysm: contrast-enhanced US for missed endoleaks after endoluminal repair. *Radiology* 2004;**233**:217–25.

9. Bendick PJ, Bove PG, Long GW, et al. Efficacy of ultrasound contrast agents in the noninvasive follow-up of aortic stent grafts. *J Vasc Surg* 2003;**37**:381–5.

10. Thurnher S, Cejna M. Imaging of aortic stent-grafts and endoleaks. *Radiol Clin North Am* 2002;**40**:799–833.

11. Thomas EA, Dubbins PA. Duplex ultrasound of the abdominal aorta – a neglected tool in aortic dissection. *Clin Radiol* 1990;**42**:330–4.

12. Clevert DA, Rupp N, Reiser M, et al. Improved diagnosis of vascular dissection by ultrasound B-flow: a comparison with color-coded Doppler and power Doppler sonography. *Eur Radiol* 2005;**15**:342–7.

13. Hansen KJ, Wilson DB, Craven TE, et al. Mesenteric artery disease in the elderly. *J Vasc Surg* 2004;**40**:45–52.

14. Moneta GL. Screening for mesenteric vascular insufficiency and follow-up of mesenteric artery bypass procedures. *Semin Vasc Surg* 2001;**14**:186–92.

15. Roobottom CA, Dubbins PA. Significant disease of the coeliac and superior mesenteric arteries in asymptomatic patients: predictive value of Doppler sonography. *Am J Radiol* 1993;**161**:985–8.

16. Perko MJ. Duplex ultrasound for assessment of superior mesenteric artery blood flow. *Eur J Vasc Endovasc Surg* 2001;**21**:106–17.

17. Smart LM, Redhead DN, Allan PL, et al. Follow-up study of Gunther and LGM inferior vena caval filters. *J Intervent Radiol* 1992;**7**:115–18.

18. Bissada NK, Yakout HH, Babanouri A, et al. Long-term experience with management of renal cell carcinoma involving the inferior vena cava. *Urology* 2003;**61**:89–92.

19. Grassi R, Di Mizio R, Barberi A, et al. Case report. Ultrasound and CT findings in lipoma of the inferior vena cava. *Br J Radiol* 2002;**75**:69–71.

Chapter 7

Haemodialysis Access

Heidi R. Umphrey, Lauren F. Alexander, Michelle L. Robbin
and Mark E. Lockhart

Arteriovenous Fistulas and Synthetic Arteriovenous Grafts

At the end of 2009, there were 571,414 patients being treated for end-stage renal disease in the United States with 116,395 new cases in that year[1]; approximately 65% of these patients received haemodialysis.[1] Complications associated with vascular access procedures are a major cause of morbidity and increasing healthcare costs in patients undergoing haemodialysis.[2] For patients with end-stage real disease (ESRD) requiring haemodialysis, there are two options for vascular access, either the surgical creation of an arteriovenous fistula (AVF) or implantation of a synthetic arteriovenous graft (graft). Due to the lower rates of infection and thrombosis, mature AVFs are the preferred access when possible.[3,4] Preoperative ultrasound evaluation of the upper extremity arteries and veins has been shown by several studies to increase the success rate of AVF creation by influencing surgical planning.[5–7] While sonographic postoperative haemodialysis access evaluation may be beneficial in assessing AVF maturation,[8,9] the role of postoperative ultrasound monitoring for early detection of access pathology allowing prompt intervention to increase the longevity of an access is still evolving.[10–15]

When clinically feasible and anatomically possible, the surgical creation of an AVF is preferred over a graft. Access placement in the non-dominant arm allows activities of daily living to continue as the non-dominant arm recovers; however, it is preferential to place a dominant arm AVF as opposed to a non-dominant arm graft in most patients. Potential haemodialysis access sites in decreasing order of preference are as follows: (1) forearm AVF (radiocephalic AVF or transposed forearm basilic vein to radial artery AVF); (2) upper arm brachiocephalic AVF or transposed brachiobasilic AVF; (3) forearm loop graft; (4) upper arm straight graft (brachial artery to upper basilic/axillary vein); (5) upper arm axillary artery to axillary vein loop graft; and (6) thigh graft. Other less common access configurations may also be utilised based on surgical experience.[16] Cephalic vein use is preferred over a basilic vein transposition for fistula formation because the cephalic vein procedure involves less dissection and venous handling.

Preoperative Evaluation

Ultrasound exam optimisation has been previously reported.[9,17–19] For evaluation of upper extremity arteries and veins, the patient should preferably be sitting upright. Following arterial assessment, a tourniquet is placed for evaluation of the veins[20] (Fig. 7-1). The tourniquet should be repositioned on the arm above each level of examination, so those veins are maximally distended. Assessment of the internal jugular and subclavian veins should be performed with the patient supine for improved distension.

The vascular structures are generally superficial and a high-frequency linear array transducer, at 12–15 MHz or higher, can provide good spatial resolution with adequate penetration. A light touch and plenty of coupling gel are recommended, so as to not deform the circular shape of the vessels. Preoperative criteria suggested by the literature include a minimum intraluminal arterial diameter of 2.0 mm (Fig. 7-2) and a minimal intraluminal venous diameter of 2.5 mm (Fig. 7-3) to allow successful AVF creation.[5,9]

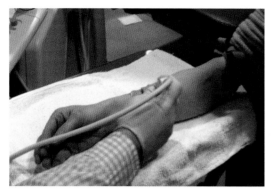

FIGURE 7-1 Photograph shows optimal patient positioning for preoperative upper extremity sonographic evaluation and tourniquet placement for evaluation of forearm veins. Sonographer is using a high-frequency 17 MHz transducer for best vascular visualisation.

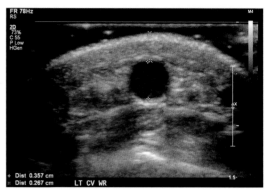

FIGURE 7-3 Greyscale transverse image of the forearm cephalic vein at the wrist demonstrates with (+) caliper placement an intraluminal diameter of 3.6 mm and with (×) caliper placement a distance of 2.7 mm from skin surface to anterior venous wall.

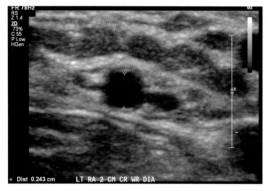

FIGURE 7-2 Greyscale transverse image of the left radial artery at the wrist demonstrates with caliper placement an intraluminal diameter of 2.4 mm satisfactory for access placement. Note use of high-frequency transducer and optimised technique.

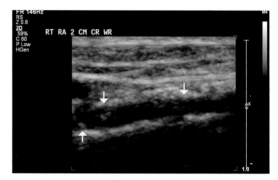

FIGURE 7-4 Greyscale longitudinal image shows calcifications in the caudal third of this right radial artery (arrows).

Suggested criteria for graft creation include a minimum intraluminal venous diameter of 4.0 mm and a minimum arterial diameter threshold of 2.0 mm.[5] In addition to diameter measurements, the caudal third of the brachial and radial arteries are evaluated for intimal thickening, calcification, stenosis or occlusion. Severity of arterial calcification may be categorised, depending on surgeon preference (Fig. 7-4). Evaluation for a normal triphasic or biphasic arterial waveform is performed, and peak systolic velocity (PSV) is measured in the region of artery planned for use (Fig. 7-5). If two arteries with paired veins are seen in the upper arm, a high radial artery take-off from the brachial artery should be suspected (Fig. 7-6). These arteries should be followed into the forearm to confirm high radial artery take-off and to exclude a prominent arterial branch supplying the elbow.

Venous assessment is performed with a tourniquet in place, and each vein should be visually inspected and compressed along the entire venous length to exclude thrombus. Internal transverse diameters of the cephalic vein are measured in the forearm at multiple levels. Internal diameters of the cephalic and basilic veins are measured in the upper arm at multiple levels in a similar fashion. The axillary vein, subclavian vein, and internal jugular vein should be assessed for compressibility and/or normal waveforms (Fig. 7-7).

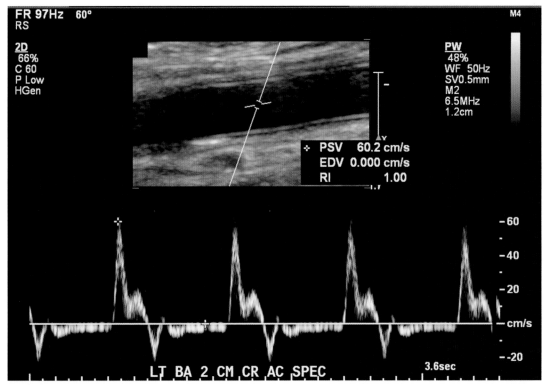

FIGURE 7-5 Spectral Doppler image shows a normal biphasic arterial waveform of this left brachial artery just above the antecubital fossa. PSV 60.2 cm/s.

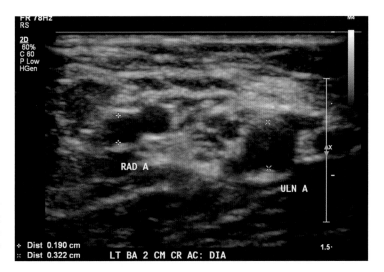

FIGURE 7-6 High bifurcation of the brachial artery should be suspected when two arteries are present near the antecubital fossa. Calipers (+) denote the radial artery (RAD A) and calipers (×) denote the ulnar artery (ULN A).

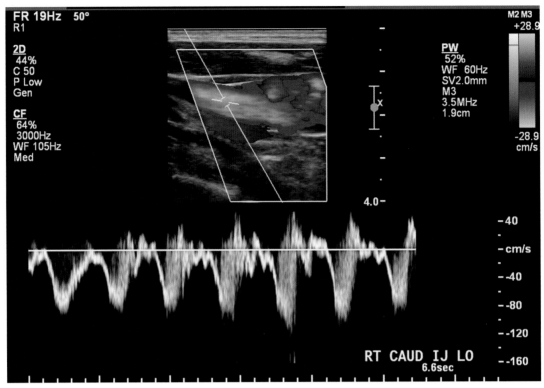

FIGURE 7-7 Spectral Doppler image shows both cardiac periodicity and respiratory phasicity in the right internal jugular vein.

Postoperative Ultrasound Evaluation

A surgically created dialysis access can have a variety of complications, and most of these can be identified and evaluated by ultrasound. Prior to the sonographic evaluation of a haemodialysis access, pertinent patient history and surgical notes are reviewed. An initial cursory ultrasound scan is performed to obtain an overview of the haemodialysis access. Once the general layout is understood, sonographic assessment is performed with greyscale and Doppler. The caudal third of the feeding artery is assessed for possible stenosis, and the intraluminal diameter is measured in the transverse plane. Colour and spectral Doppler assessment of the feeding artery is performed in the longitudinal plane to confirm the presence of normal low-resistance flow (Fig. 7-8). The anastomosis(es) are evaluated with both colour and spectral Doppler to assess for stenosis. The draining vein of the AVF or graft is inspected for wall thickening, stenosis, and thrombosis along its entire length. For a fistula, the intraluminal draining vein diameter and the vein depth from skin surface are measured at several points cranial to the arteriovenous anastomosis. A depth greater than 5 mm may suggest the need for superficialisation to improve accessibility. The draining vein is evaluated for accessory vein branches (Fig. 7-9). Internal diameter and distance from anastomosis are recorded for each identified accessory vein branch within 10–15 cm of the anastomosis. Flow volume measurements are obtained within the mid draining vein of an AVF or within the graft. This measurement is obtained in an area with parallel vessel walls, minimal vessel tortuosity and no stenosis (Fig. 7-10).

If intraluminal thrombus is identified within an access or draining vein, a longitudinal greyscale image is obtained for documentation. Colour and spectral Doppler should be performed when access occlusion is suspected to confirm and document absent flow.

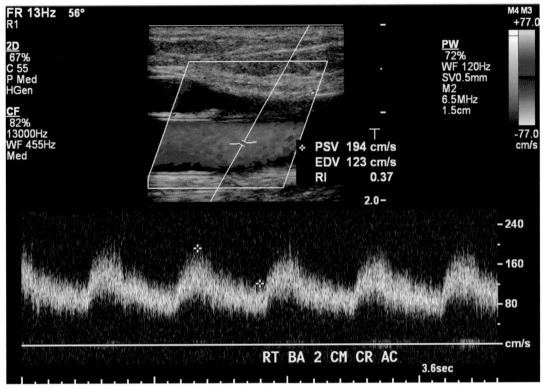

FR 13Hz 56°
R1

2D
67%
C 55
P Med
HGen

CF
82%
13000Hz
WF 455Hz
Med

PW
72%
WF 120Hz
SV0.5mm
M2
6.5MHz
1.5cm

M4 M3
+77.0

-77.0
cm/s

PSV 194 cm/s
EDV 123 cm/s
RI   0.37

2.0-

240

160

80

cm/s

RT BA 2 CM CR AC

3.6sec

FIGURE 7-8 Spectral Doppler waveform in the right brachial artery 2 cm cranial to the antecubital fossa shows a normal low-resistance waveform seen in an AVF feeding artery. PSV 194 cm/s. EDV 123 cm/s.

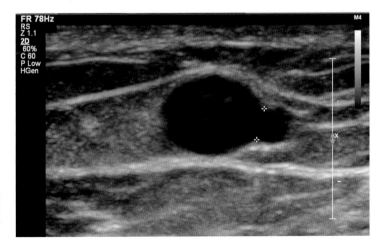

FIGURE 7-9 Greyscale image shows a venous branch from a left upper arm fistula draining vein measuring 2.0 mm located 10 cm cranial to the anastomosis.

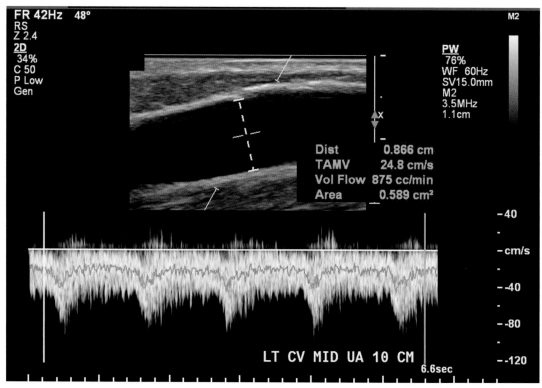

FIGURE 7-10 Volume flow measurement in the draining vein of an AVF 10 cm cranial to the anastomosis is 875 cc/min.

If there is any uncertainty, power Doppler should be utilised since it is more sensitive for detection of residual slow flow. If fluid collections are present, they should be measured and inspected for echogenic foci or gas. Subcutaneous air within a collection or adjacent to the access can be the result of recent access cannulation. Echogenic foci associated with a fluid collection, however, can represent a developing infection or an abscess.

The artery downstream from the arterial anastomosis is routinely evaluated for flow reversal, which may be asymptomatic. If there are clinical symptoms suspicious for arterial steal, such as hand pain, the arterial flow to the hand should be carefully evaluated. In severe cases, revision or sacrifice of the access may be necessary.

In the setting of upper extremity swelling, the subclavian and internal jugular veins should be included in the postoperative sonographic evaluation. Doppler imaging of the internal jugular and subclavian veins provides indirect assessment of the brachiocephalic veins. In a patient

with an AVF, spectral Doppler evaluation of normal central veins shows respiratory phasicity and/or transmitted cardiac periodicity (Fig. 7-7). Monophasic subclavian and internal jugular venous waveforms are suggestive of central venous stenosis or occlusion, especially if these veins are distended (Fig. 7-11). MR venography may be useful to exclude critical stenosis in this setting.

A normal AVF has antegrade flow through both the arterial and venous limbs without visible narrowing, thrombus, or flow disturbance. Potential signs of stenosis include areas of visible narrowing, aliasing, or focal increased velocity, and are further described in the following pathology section. A functioning AVF has flow volume of at least 300 to 800 mL/min (Fig. 7-10).[8,21] When an AVF has a minimum draining vein diameter of ≥ 4 mm or a blood flow rate of ≥ 500 mL/min, approximately 70% can be successfully used for haemodialysis.[8] When both criteria are present, the likelihood of fistula maturation is 95%.[8] If neither of these are met, only 33% of fistulas are adequate for haemodialysis.[8] The National Kidney

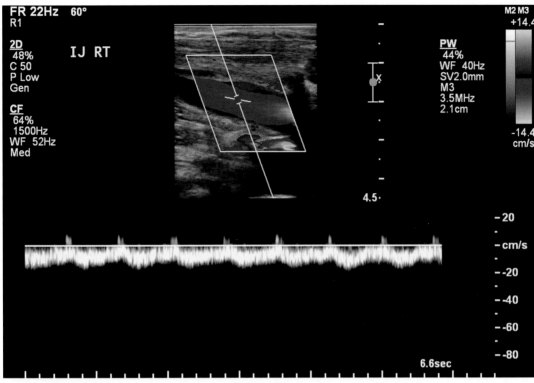

FIGURE 7-11 Spectral Doppler image of the right internal jugular vein shows relatively monophasic flow suggestive of central obstruction such as thrombosis or stenosis.

Foundation Kidney Disease Outcomes Quality Initiative published sonographic criteria suggestive of maturation that included the following: draining vein greater than 6 mm diameter, blood flow rate greater than 600 cc/min, and less than 6 mm skin depth.[3] However, these criteria exclude many fistulas that can still be successfully used for haemodialysis.

A normal haemodialysis graft is seen as two echogenic lines that represent strong specular reflection from the polytetrafluoroethylene (PTFE) material. Flow within the graft should be antegrade demonstrating low resistance, arterialised flow on spectral Doppler. Findings suggestive of stenosis include visible narrowing, focal turbulence, or focally elevated velocity. Antegrade flow without focal turbulence or aliasing is seen in the draining vein of a normal graft. Because of the larger blood flow volume within grafts, the lack of phasicity or periodicity in the central veins is less specific for central occlusion in patients with a graft than in patients with an AVF.

Diagnosis of Pathology

Pathology associated with AVFs includes stenosis, thrombosis/occlusion, pseudoaneurysm, peri-fistula fluid collections, and arterial steal. Two features characterise AVF stenosis; visual narrowing as assessed on greyscale imaging and an increased ratio of the PSV at the stenosis as compared to the PSV measured 2 cm upstream from the stenosis. The diagnostic criteria vary in accordance with the location of the stenosis. A juxta-anastomotic stenosis is defined by the following criteria: (1) location within 2 cm of the anastomosis, encompassing the feeding artery and the draining vein;[22-23] (2) visible narrowing; and (3) a PSV ratio of greater than or equal to 3:1 (Fig. 7-12). A draining vein stenosis is defined by visible narrowing and by a PSV ratio of 2:1. Stenoses of the feeding artery are rare but can occur and are characterised by visible narrowing and a PSV ratio of 2:1. Poststenotic waveforms with a delayed systolic upstroke (tardus parvus) may

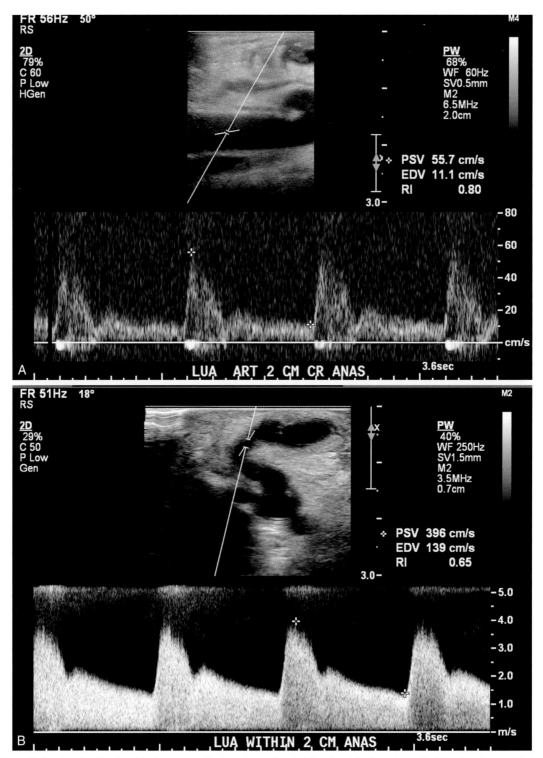

FIGURE 7-12 Spectral Doppler of AVF juxta-anastomotic stenosis. (A) Spectral Doppler of feeding artery with PSV of 55.7 cm/s. (B) Spectral Doppler of juxta-anastomotic area of narrowing 1 cm downstream to the anastomosis with PSV of 396 cm/s. Given PSV in (A) this yields a PSV ratio of 7.1:1.

suggest proximal arterial stenosis and prompt further direct evaluation.

Stenoses associated with an AVF are listed in order of decreasing frequency by location as follows: the juxta-anastomotic region, the draining vein, the feeding artery, and central veins. Stenoses are clinically relevant since they can be associated with subsequent thrombosis. If thrombosis occurs, it is usually visualised within the vessel lumen on greyscale imaging (Fig. 7-13) and confirmed when no colour or spectral Doppler flow is identified within the affected portion of the AVF or draining vein. If the thrombus is

nonocclusive, slow flow or a trickle of flow may be identified with power Doppler.

Pseudoaneurysms may develop anywhere along the course of a fistula secondary to suboptimal compression after cannulation. Colour Doppler of a pseudoaneurysm shows a typical 'yin/yang' circular flow pattern (Fig. 7-14). There may be 'to-and-fro' flow in the pseudoaneurysm neck. If the pseudoaneurysm thromboses, there may be clot partially filling the space or total lack of flow on Doppler. Avascular, hypoechoic lesions usually represent post access or post procedure haematomas and can be seen

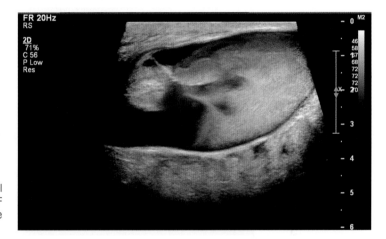

FIGURE 7-13 Occluded AVF. Greyscale longitudinal image of the draining vein of a left upper arm AVF 4 cm cranial to the anastomosis reveals occlusive echogenic thrombus filling a dilated vein lumen.

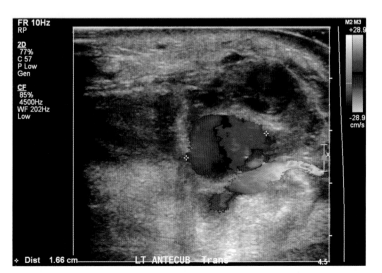

FIGURE 7-14 Colour Doppler image of a pseudoaneurysm reveals the typical bidirectional blue and red 'yin-yang' flow.

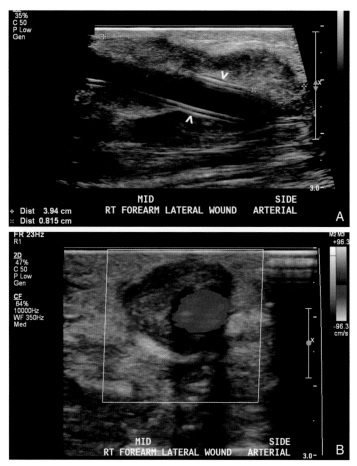

FIGURE 7-15 Peri-access haematoma. (A) Greyscale longitudinal image reveals a 39 × 8 mm complex collection denoted by calipers adjacent to the arterial end of a graft (arrowheads). (B) Colour Doppler image shows patent graft with avascular surrounding material consistent with peri-access haematoma.

associated with fistulas or grafts (Fig. 7-15). Fluid collections complicated by echogenic foci with 'dirty' shadowing suspicious for gas may represent abscess in the appropriate clinical setting.

Graft abnormalities are similar to those described above for AVFs, with slight variations and differences in the diagnostic thresholds and criteria. Studies have shown that grafts with decreased blood flow are at increased risk for thrombosis.[24–26] The four sonographic criteria utilised to characterise graft stenosis are as follows: (1) visual luminal narrowing on greyscale imaging; (2) a high-velocity jet on colour Doppler; (3) a PSV ratio greater than 2:1 for the venous anastomosis[17] or draining vein; and (4) a PSV ratio greater than 3:1 for the arterial anastomosis. The most common sites of graft stenosis are in decreasing order of frequency as follows: the venous anastomosis, draining vein, intragraft, arterial anastomosis, and the central veins.[27] Graft thrombosis is characterised by echogenic material identified within the graft lumen and by lack of flow within the graft (Fig. 7-16); power Doppler should be utilised to exclude slow flow.

The formation of pseudoaneurysms along grafts is relatively common with typical 'yin/yang' flow pattern

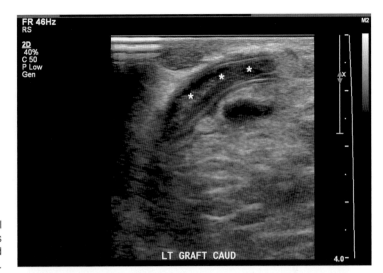

FIGURE 7-16 Occluded graft. Greyscale longitudinal image through the caudal aspect of a graft reveals luminal echogenic material (***). Colour and spectral Doppler (not shown) confirm the occlusion.

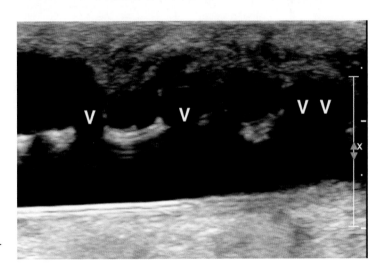

FIGURE 7-17 Greyscale image demonstrates irregularity (arrowheads) of the graft wall.

seen with colour Doppler within the cavity or 'to-and-fro' flow at the neck. Degeneration of graft synthetic material is unique to grafts. At ultrasound, irregularity of the graft wall can be seen and may be associated with numerous pseudoaneurysms along the length of the graft wall (Fig. 7-17). Arterial steal is defined as flow reversal in the native artery caudal to the anastomosis and may be associated with hand pain and paraesthesias that may worsen during dialysis. If severe, ischaemia or tissue necrosis of the fingers can occur. However, not all flow reversal is symptomatic. Sonographic evaluation demonstrates reversal of

flow in the distal artery and rarely shows an arterial occlusion (Fig. 7-18). Brief manual compression of the graft will usually demonstrate a change in the reversed arterial flow, yielding an antegrade high-resistance flow pattern toward the hand.[28]

Conclusions

The sonographic evaluation of the haemodialysis access has become a mainstream diagnostic technique, and it continues to gain importance as the number of patients with renal failure progressively increases.

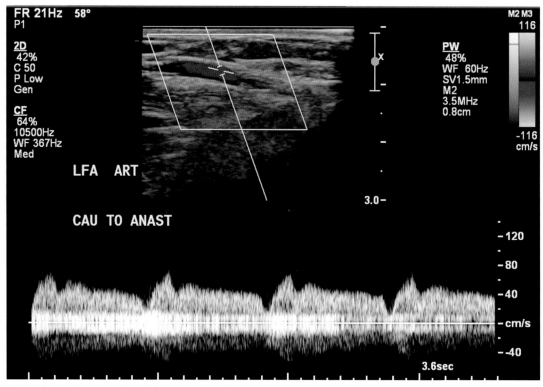

FIGURE 7-18 Spectral Doppler of the radial artery caudal to the anastomosis shows reversal of flow consistent with arterial steal (flow is directed toward head, away from hand).

Doppler can aid in the selection of the optimal access type and location for fistula or graft creation in these patients. Once an access is surgically created, sonography is useful to determine maturation of the access for successful use in haemodialysis. Furthermore, it can identify the common complications associated with these accesses.

REFERENCES

1. U.S. Renal Data System, USRDS 2011 . *Annual Data Report: Atlas of Chronic Kidney Disease and End-Stage Renal Disease in the United States*. Bethesda, MD: National Institutes of Health, National Institute of Diabetes and Digestive and Kidney Diseases; 2011.
2. Feldman HI, Kobrin S, Wasserstein A. Hemodialysis vascular access morbidity. *J Am Soc Nephrol* 1996;**7**:523–35.
3. KDOQI clinical practice guidelines and clinical practice recommendations for vascular access 2006. *Am J Kidney Dis* 2006;**48** (Suppl. 1):S176–S322.
4. Hodges TC, Fillinger MF, Zwolak RM, et al. Longitudinal comparison of dialysis access methods: risk factors for failure. *J Vasc Surg* 1997;**26**:1009–19.
5. Silva Jr MB, Hobson 2nd RW, Pappas PJ, et al. A strategy for increasing use of autogenous hemodialysis access procedures: impact of preoperative noninvasive evaluation. *J Vasc Surg* 1998;**27**:302–7.
6. Gibson KD, Caps MT, Kohler TR, et al. Assessment of a policy to reduce placement of prosthetic hemodialysis access. *Kidney Int* 2001;**59**:2335–45.
7. Allon M, Lockhart ME, Lilly RZ, et al. Effect of preoperative sonographic mapping on vascular access outcomes in hemodialysis patients. *Kidney Int* 2001;**60**:2013–20.
8. Robbin ML, Chamberlain NE, Lockhart ME, et al. Hemodialysis arteriovenous fistula maturity: US evaluation. *Radiology* 2002;**225**:59–64.
9. Robbin ML, Gallichio MH, Deierhoi MH, et al. US vascular mapping before hemodialysis access placement. *Radiology* 2000;**217**:83–8.
10. Allon M, Bailey R, Ballard R, et al. A multidisciplinary approach to hemodialysis access: Prospective evaluation. *Kidney Int* 1998;**53**:473–9.
11. Robbin ML, Oser RF, Lee JY, et al. Randomized comparison of ultrasound surveillance and clinical monitoring on arteriovenous graft outcomes. *Kidney Int* 2006;**69**:730–5.
12. Lumsden AB, MacDonald MJ, Kikeri D, et al. Prophylactic balloon angioplasty fails to prolong the patency of expanded polytetrafluoroethylene arteriovenous grafts: Results of a prospective randomized study. *J Vasc Surg* 1997;**26**:382–92.

13. Ram SJ, Work J, Caldito GC, et al. A randomized controlled trial of blood flow and stenosis surveillance of hemodialysis grafts. *Kidney Int* 2003;**64**:272–80.
14. Malik J, Slavikova M, Svobodova J, et al. Regular ultrasound screening significantly prolongs patency of grafts. *Kidney Int* 2005;**67**:1554–8.
15. Dember LM, Holmberg EF, Kaufman JS. Randomized controlled trial of prophylactic repair of hemodialysis arteriovenous graft stenosis. *Kidney Int* 2004;**66**:390–8.
16. Jennings WC, Sideman MJ, Taubman KE, et al. Brachial vein transposition arteriovenous fistulas for hemodialysis access. *J Vasc Surg* 2009;**50**:1121–5.
17. Robbin ML, Osler RF, Allon M, et al. Hemodialysis access graft stenosis: US detection. *Radiology* 1998;**208**:655–61.
18. Lockhart ME, Robbin ML. Hemodialysis ultrasound. *Ultrasound Q* 2001;**17**:157–67.
19. Umphrey HR, Lockhart ME, Abts CA, et al. Dialysis grafts and fistulae: planning and assessment. *Ultrasound Clin* 2011;**6**:477–89.
20. Lockhart ME, Robbin ML, Fineberg NS, et al. Cephalic vein measurement before forearm fistula creation: does use of a tourniquet to meet venous diameter threshold increase the number of useable fistulas? *J Ultrasound Med* 2006;**25**:1541–5.
21. Falk A. Maintenance and salvage of arteriovenous fistulas. *J Vasc Interv Radiol* 2006;**17**:807–13.
22. Clark TW, Hirsch DA, Jindal KJ, et al. Outcome and prognostic factors of restenosis after percutaneous treatment of native hemodialysis fistulas. *J Vasc Interv Radiol* 2002;**13**:51–9.
23. Beathard GA, Arnold P, Jackson J, et al. Aggressive treatment of early fistula failure. Physician Operators Forum of RMS Lifeline. *Kidney Int* 2003;**64**:1487–94.
24. May RE, Himmelfarb J, Yenicesu M, et al. Predictive measures of vascular access thrombosis: a prospective study. *Kidney Int* 1997;**52**:1656–62.
25. Shackleton CR, Taylor DC, Buckely AR, et al. Predicting failure in polytetrafluoroethylene vascular access grafts for hemodialysis: a pilot study. *Can J Surg* 1987;**30**:442–4.
26. Robbin ML, Oser RF, Allon M, et al. Hemodialysis access graft stenosis: US detection. *Radiology* 1998;**205**:655–61.
27. Beuter JJG, Lezana AH, Calvo JH, et al. Early detection and treatment of hemodialysis access dysfunction. *Cardiovasc Intervent Radiol* 2000;**23**:40–6.
28. Valji K, Hye RJ, Roberts Ac, et al. Hand ischemia in patients with hemodialysis access grafts: angiographic diagnosis and treatment. *Radiology* 1995;**196**:697–701.

Chapter 8

The Liver

Myron A. Pozniak

Introduction

There have been impressive advances recently in the application of ultrasound contrast medium to liver imaging; but these agents are not universally available. Researchers have shown the benefits of microbubble-enhanced lesion detection and characterisation.[1] Unfortunately governing agencies across the world have not uniformly endorsed these agents and there is limited ability and/or interest to apply them in many centres. This chapter is, therefore, written for those ultrasound practitioners who do not have access to or routinely use intravenous ultrasound contrast. For discussion of hepatic applications of sonographic contrast please refer to Chapter 17.

The standard hepatic US examination should include a brief survey with spectral and colour Doppler (Box 8-1). This serves a two-fold purpose: first, it adds valuable haemodynamic information to the evaluation of the liver, in most cases reinforcing normality, but occasionally revealing an unexpected finding. Second, by consistently integrating Doppler into the routine hepatic examination, sonologists will continually refine their Doppler skills so that when presented with significant haemodynamic abnormalities, they can be identified quickly and evaluated accurately. Although a cursory Doppler survey of the hepatic vasculature may add 2–3 min to an abdominal examination, regular practice enables the examiner to become more adept at perceiving abnormalities, dialling in the settings to optimise the display, and more expert in analysing the results. Not infrequently altered blood flow may be the only abnormal finding to suggest the presence of pathology. The Doppler survey may reveal distortion of vascularity around a subtle lesion of which the examiner was otherwise unaware. It may display hypervascularity of an observed lesion and this awareness may increase diagnostic certainty. The use of colour Doppler in the hepatic examination also helps to differentiate vascular from non-vascular structures. Care must be taken, however, to ensure that equipment settings are appropriate: if gain, pulse repetition frequency, and filtration are not optimised, slow flow can be missed in vascular structures or artifactual colour can be painted into non-vascular structures.[2]

Executing the Liver Doppler Study

SCAN TECHNIQUE

The patient is scanned in a supine or left lateral decubitus position. Depending on vessel orientation and body habitus, the portal vein and hepatic artery are best interrogated by either a subcostal approach pointing posterocephalad, or a right intercostal approach pointing medially. Since the portal vein and hepatic artery travel together in

---

BOX 8-1 **PRINCIPLES OF THE LIVER DOPPLER EXAMINATION**

- General examination of liver parenchyma and abdomen
- Colour and spectral Doppler assessment of the portal vein, superior mesenteric and splenic veins, together with main intrahepatic portal branches
- Colour and spectral Doppler assessment of the hepatic artery from the coeliac axis to the porta, together with main intrahepatic branches
- Colour and spectral Doppler assessment of the main hepatic veins and the upper inferior vena cava
- Assessment of flow to any observed intrahepatic mass or abnormality

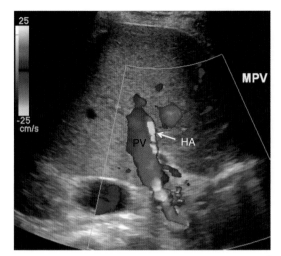

FIGURE 8-1 Oblique colour Doppler image of the porta hepatis. The hepatic artery (HA) accompanies the portal vein (PV) and bile ducts. With the colour scale appropriately set for the slow flow within the portal vein, hepatic arterial flow projects as colour aliasing.

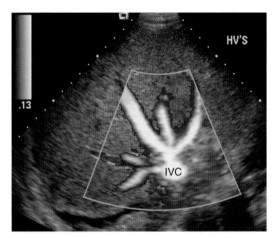

FIGURE 8-2 Power Doppler transverse view of the liver with a subcostal approach. This crow's foot appearance of the hepatic veins shows the convergence of five hepatic veins onto the IVC. The presence of accessory branches is very common.

the portal triad, along with the common duct, these approaches should satisfactorily interrogate both vessels (Fig. 8-1).

Scanning the left hepatic and middle hepatic veins is best accomplished from a substernal approach. The transducer should be oriented transversely, pointing posterocephalad, and swept up and down across the liver. For the right hepatic vein, a right lateral intercostal approach is used with the transducer pointed cephalad. If the patient's liver extends below the costal margin during inspiration, a subcostal transverse view, angled cephalad, is useful for the confluence of the hepatic veins (Fig. 8-2).

There is no specific acoustic window that is ideal for all patients and the operator must determine the best approach on an individual basis. This usually requires trying multiple windows at varying degrees of inspiration. During respiration, the upper abdominal organs move back and forth under the US transducer. When patients are able to cooperate, the operator should ask them to intermittently hold their breath during the Doppler examination or at least to breathe gently. This improves the colour Doppler image and allows acquisition of longer spectral Doppler tracings. Patients who are unable to hold their breath can pose a significant problem and the operator may have to carefully 'ride' the vessel in real time as it moves with

respiration. An experienced sonologist may be able to 'rock' the transducer back and forth in synchrony with the patient's respiration, thus maintaining the sample volume over the area of interest and obtaining a longer tracing. If the patient is short of breath or unable to cooperate, short segments of spectral tracings are all that may be possible.

Some patients, when asked to hold their breath perform a vigorous Valsalva manoeuvre. This results in increased intrathoracic pressure which will impede venous return, affecting flow profiles and velocities, particularly in the hepatic veins and inferior vena cava (IVC). This will often alter the hepatic vein profile, creating the perception of hepatic venous outflow obstruction (HVOO). Scanning must be performed in neutral breath-hold to avoid producing a misleading Doppler tracing.[3]

Varying the width of the sample volume can be advantageous when examining the porta hepatis. If the examiner is screening for vascular patency or trying to locate a specific vessel, a large sample volume is appropriate for rapid interrogation of a broad area; for example, when ruling out hepatic artery thrombosis in a liver transplant recipient. If, however, the examiner wants to precisely characterise flow within a vessel and evaluate waveform detail, then the sample volume must be small and placed near the centre of the vessel, thereby interrogating the highest velocity lamina

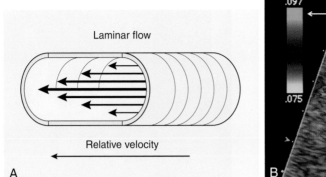
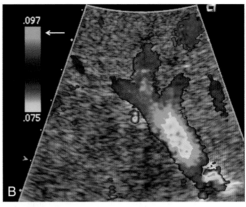

FIGURE 8-3 (A) Schematic representation of normal laminar flow. The velocity of fluid along the wall of a vessel is slowed because of frictional forces causing drag; therefore its relative velocity is less than that at the centre of the vessel. The travelling wave assumes a parabolic form. (B) Colour Doppler image of portal vein flow with a green tag assigned to high velocities towards the transducer. Additionally the pulse repetition frequency (velocity scale) is set low to cause aliasing. This distortion of the colour-encoding thus permits a display of several velocity lamina. Note the transition from the slowest velocities, red through orange, green and blue from the periphery to the centre of the vessel. The actual velocity displayed on a spectral Doppler tracing is, therefore, dependent on sample volume placement relative to these various velocity lamina. A small, centrally placed sample volume will display a higher measured velocity than a peripherally placed sample volume.

(Fig. 8-3). A wide sample volume, by incorporating the slower lamina along the wall together with the faster central lamina, will broaden the spectral Doppler tracing and mimic turbulence.[4]

The presence of bowel gas is also an obvious impediment to a successful examination. Having the patient fast for 4–6 hours prior to an abdominal examination helps minimise the amount of gas, thereby increasing the likelihood that an appropriate sonographic window will be available for any particular vessel of interest. In addition, consistently scanning fasting patients decreases the risk of misinterpreting flow dynamics altered by a nutrient load.

Patient obesity is a well-known limiting factor for an adequate Doppler examination. Delineation of anatomical detail is impaired when the examination is conducted at lower frequencies. During US imaging, the operator may need to press firmly to displace some of the overlying adipose tissue and position the transducer closer to the area of interest. Such a manoeuvre, however, is not appropriate during a Doppler examination as pressure from the transducer compresses the underlying organ and its vasculature, thereby altering flow profiles and velocities. Compression of an organ or vessel with the transducer causes increased

resistance to diastolic blood flow, thereby elevating the measured resistive index.

Some sonologists place considerable emphasis on the measurement of flow velocity, but too great a dependence on a number may lead to diagnostic errors. Numerous systemic factors affect blood flow in the hepatic vasculature. These include the patient's state of hydration, cardiac output, blood pressure, vascular compliance, the interval since the previous meal, and haemodynamic effects of medications. These factors affect measured velocities in a variety of ways and to varying degrees. Therefore, although the measured velocity may be above or below the diagnostic threshold for disease in any individual vessel; that specific velocity may not necessarily be a reflection of focally disordered haemodynamics due to underlying pathology. Furthermore, defining flow within a vessel as normal or abnormal by simply comparing the measured velocity to a predetermined normal range is a poor method of establishing a diagnosis, as a few degrees difference in the angle of insonation or improper angle correction can markedly change the measured velocity. Assigning the proper degree of angle correction may be difficult if the vessel is poorly visualised, curved, or visualised only over a short segment.

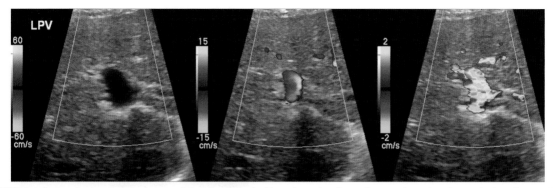

FIGURE 8-4 Series of colour Doppler images of the left portal vein. The only setting changed among these three images is the pulse repetition frequency (colour Doppler scale). On the first image with scale set high (60 cm/s), no colour is displayed within the portal vein which therefore could be interpreted as thrombosed. The second image with scale set appropriately (15 cm/s), relative to normal portal velocity, reveals appropriate colour saturation and confirms patency. On the final image with scale set too low (02 cm/s), colour aliasing distorts the image.

Differentiating a patent from a thrombosed vessel is critically dependent on Doppler settings and transducer frequency. Gain, filtration, and pulse repetition frequency settings must be adjusted throughout the study. The settings must be carefully reviewed if one is about to make a diagnosis of thrombosis (Fig. 8-4).

TERMINOLOGY

When performing Doppler ultrasound of the liver, it is important to be consistent in the use of terms relating to blood flow: the term 'pulsatility' should be reserved for velocity variations in arterial flow. 'Phasicity' should be reserved for changes in velocities secondary to respiration. The term 'periodicity' is recommended when referring to velocity variation in the SVC, IVC, hepatic and portal veins secondary to cardiac activity. Normal flow in the portal vein towards the liver is properly termed 'hepatopetal' (as in centripetal force, not 'hepatopedal'). Reversed portal vein flow is referred to as 'hepatofugal' (as in centrifugal force).

Indications

Patients referred for right upper quadrant (RUQ) US typically have elevated liver enzymes of unknown aetiology incidentally detected on screening blood tests. Although sonographic imaging of the liver may reveal diffuse abnormality or focal disease, the majority of these examinations are normal (Box 8-2). Doppler US, however, may reveal flow alterations caused by inflammatory disease, neoplasm, or other disorders which are too subtle or too small to cause perceptible imaging irregularities. Being able to differentiate flow profile and velocity alterations in the hepatic vasculature between those caused by hepatic versus cardiac disease will help identify those patients needing additional cardiac evaluation versus those who would benefit from liver biopsy. Additionally, the identification of a Doppler abnormality can define those patients who would benefit from further hepatic imaging with computed tomography (CT), magnetic resonance imaging (MRI), or angiography.

When portal hypertension is suspected, Doppler US characterises changes in portal haemodynamics and identifies pathways of portosystemic collateralisation.[5] Doppler can confirm the patency of surgical or percutaneous shunts which have been performed

---

BOX 8-2 INDICATIONS FOR DOPPLER ULTRASOUND OF THE LIVER

- Part of the routine examination of the liver and right upper quadrant
- Assessment of portal hypertension
- Pre- and post-procedural assessment of transjugular portosystemic shunt (TIPS) procedures
- Postoperative follow-up of liver transplants
- Assessment of focal liver disease

in patients with bleeding oesophageal varices. Identification and differentiation of bland thrombus from tumour thrombus within the hepatic or portal veins by Doppler has significant implications for medical, surgical or ablation treatment planning. Doppler US plays a key role in the postoperative monitoring of liver transplant recipients, confirming vascular patency.

The role of Doppler in the characterisation of parenchymal liver disease and screening for hepatocellular carcinoma (HCC) is controversial. Marked alterations in flow profiles and velocities can be seen and have been described in the literature.[6–9] It is rare, though, to be able to precisely pinpoint a specific diagnosis based on Doppler findings since there is considerable overlap in velocity and waveform alterations among various disease states.

Vascular Anatomy and Normal Flow Profiles

PORTAL VEIN

The portal vein is formed by the confluence of the splenic and superior mesenteric veins. It supplies around 70% of incoming blood volume to the liver. It is accompanied by the hepatic artery and common bile duct which together make up the portal triad (Fig. 8-1). The triad has echogenic margins as it enters the liver, due to the intrahepatic extension of Glisson's capsule and presence of perivascular fat. After forming the right and left branches, these vessels progressively branch to supply the liver segments as defined by Couinaud whose US appearance was described by La Fortune.[10] The Couinaud system divides the liver vertically along the planes of the hepatic veins, and horizontally along the planes of the left and right portal veins. A thorough understanding of this anatomy is critical for surgical planning in liver resection and living related donation. Anatomic variations of the portal vein are rare.

The portal vein Doppler flow profile in a fasting patient has a relatively constant velocity of approximately 18 cm/s (± 5 cm/s) towards the liver (hepatopetal) (Fig. 8-5A). The flow velocity is uniform because cardiac pulsation is damped by the splenic parenchyma and the capillaries of the gut at one end of the portal system and by the liver sinusoids at the

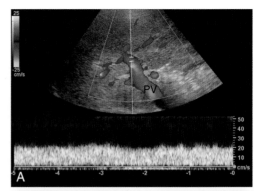

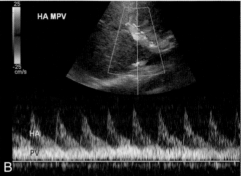

FIGURE 8-5 (A) Spectral Doppler tracing of normal portal vein flow. The flow velocity of 20 cm/s is relatively uniform and in a hepatopetal direction. (B) Spectral Doppler tracing of normal portal vein and hepatic artery flow. Slight periodicity is present in this patient's portal vein tracing. The dip in antegrade velocity coincides with hepatic arterial systole. The comparison of the two flow profiles is achieved by interrogating with a wide sample volume that encompasses both the artery and the vein in one tracing. Velocity variation may also occur due to pressure change with the hepatic vein A-wave but those are harder to compare since the vessels are separated and cannot be simultaneously interrogated.

other. Slight phasicity may be seen on the portal spectral tracing due to respiration and a mild degree of periodicity may be present, due either to retrograde pulsation transmitted from the right heart via the hepatic vein (A-wave) or to the hepatic artery systolic pressure wave. Because these brief pressure surges into the liver transiently elevate intracapsular pressure, they increase resistance to portal venous inflow and, thereby, effect a momentary slowing of antegrade flow in the portal vein (Fig. 8-5B).[11] Although some periodicity may be expected in portal vein flow, marked velocity variation or reversal of flow, even if brief, should be considered an abnormal finding.[12] The blood in the portal vein is relatively deoxygenated since it comes to the liver after perfusing the intestine and spleen. It is rich in nutrients after a meal, and arrives at the liver to be processed by the cells of the hepatic sinusoids.

HEPATIC ARTERY

The hepatic arterial blood supply arises solely from the celiac axis in approximately 75% of individuals. The celiac trifurcates into the splenic artery, left gastric artery and common hepatic artery. After the take-off of the gastroduodenal artery, the common hepatic is then called the proper hepatic artery. It enters the liver alongside the portal vein (Fig. 8-1) where it divides into left and right hepatic arteries and from there branches into the Couinaud segments. There are, however, numerous variants of hepatic artery anatomy. These include accessory vessels which exist in conjunction with normal branches of the hepatic artery and replaced arteries which make up the sole supply of a segment or lobe. For example, a replaced right hepatic artery arising from the superior mesenteric artery (SMA) is the sole blood supply to the entire right lobe of the liver in 15% of the population.[13] In a slender patient, colour Doppler US may be able to identify the replaced right hepatic artery behind the main portal vein as it courses towards the right lobe from the SMA (Fig. 8-6). A branch of the left gastric artery may supply the left lobe of the liver. This occurs less frequently and is more difficult to identify by Doppler US because of its small size.

The normal proper hepatic artery in a fasting patient has a low-resistance Doppler flow profile, [about 60–70% resistive index (RI)] (Fig. 8-7). During systole, the velocity is approximately 30–60 cm/s; while during diastole, it normally slows to approximately 10–20 cm/s. Normal systolic acceleration time of the hepatic artery is brisk – less than 0.07 seconds.

Diastolic arterial velocity approximates the velocity of the portal vein. A comparison between hepatic artery diastolic velocity and the portal vein velocity is called the liver (or hepatic) vascular index. To acquire this comparison one can increase the sample volume size so that both vessels are incorporated into the same tracing (Fig. 8-5B) or swing the sample volume from one vessel to the other in the same tracing (Fig. 8-8).[12,14]

HEPATIC VEINS

The hepatic veins are relatively straight, tubular structures that converge on the IVC approximately 1 cm below its confluence with the right atrium. The walls of the hepatic veins are relatively hypoechoic which helps to differentiate them from the portal veins in the more echogenic portal triads. There are no valves

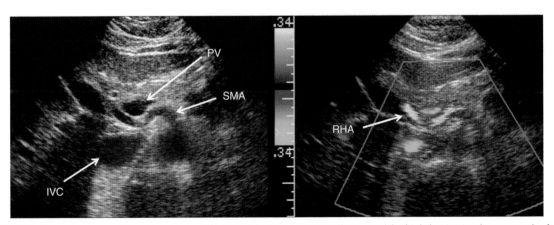

FIGURE 8-6 Transverse image of the mid-abdomen at the level of the superior mesenteric artery origin. A tubular structure is seen coursing from the superior mesenteric artery (SMA) to the right lobe of the liver, between portal vein (PV) and the inferior vena cava (IVC). The addition of colour Doppler identifies this tubular structure as a vessel. An arterial signal on spectral Doppler, identification of its SMA origin and a course towards the right lobe of the liver confirm this to be a replaced right hepatic artery.

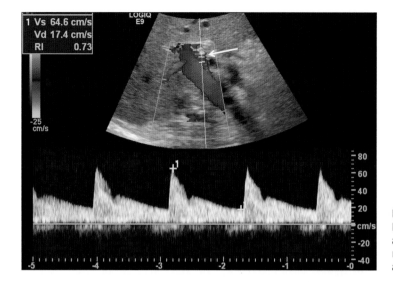

FIGURE 8-7 Spectral Doppler tracing of a normal hepatic artery. Systolic upstroke is brisk with acceleration time <0.07 s. Resistive index measures 73%. Velocity at end diastole approximates 17 cm/s.

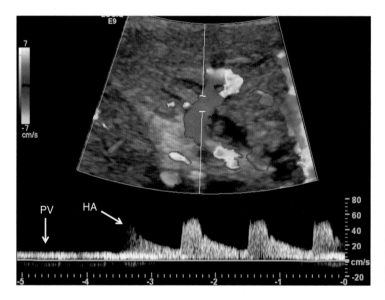

FIGURE 8-8 Colour image and spectral Doppler tracing of the porta hepatis. A comparison of hepatic artery and portal vein velocities is achieved on a single tracing by gently rocking the transducer from one vessel to the other.

in the hepatic veins so cardiac periodicity can be expected to extend into the liver.

The right, middle, and left hepatic veins enter the IVC in a 'crow's foot' configuration when viewed in the transverse plane (Fig. 8-2). The left and middle hepatic veins usually enter as a common trunk along the left anteromedial aspect of the IVC. Over 50% of individuals have additional hepatic veins that are seen with colour Doppler; a right superior anterior segmental vein may be seen draining into the middle hepatic

vein, marginal hepatic veins may drain into the right and left hepatic veins, and a large accessory right hepatic vein may be seen entering the IVC several centimetres inferior to the junction of the three main hepatic veins in 6–10% of people (Fig. 8-9). The venous drainage from the central liver, and the caudate lobe, empties directly into the IVC and is not normally detected by colour Doppler since these veins are small and deep (Fig. 8-10). This separate drainage pathway is responsible for the unique behaviour of the caudate

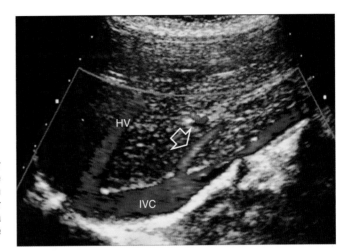

FIGURE 8-9 Longitudinal colour Doppler image of the liver and inferior vena cava (IVC) through the right flank. There is a prominent accessory hepatic vein (open arrow) from the inferior posterior segment of the right lobe of the liver (Couinaud segment 6). This vein joins the inferior vena cava approximately 4 cm inferior to the junction of the main three hepatic veins (HV).

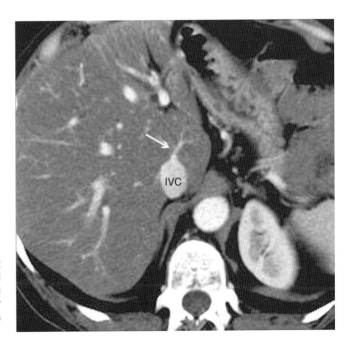

FIGURE 8-10 CT scan at the level of the mid-liver in a patient with steatosis. Because of the fatty background, small central hepatic veins (arrow) can be seen draining directly into the inferior vena cava. This unique drainage of the central liver is the underlying cause for caudate hypertrophy in patients with main hepatic vein thrombosis or cirrhosis.

lobe in diffuse liver disease, and for the distinctive enhancement pattern seen on contrast-enhanced CT scans of patients with hepatic vein thrombosis.

The normal hepatic vein waveform is referred to as triphasic and is a result of pressure waves emanating from the right heart (Fig. 8-11A). It is similar to the jugular vein waveform. There are four components to this waveform and occasionally a fifth may be perceived. Since hepatic vein flow courses toward the centrally located IVC, the hepatic vein flow is towards the heart and away from the transducer. Therefore, the majority of flow registers below the baseline. During right atrial contraction blood is forced back into the liver and is therefore displayed above the baseline. These directions are best described as being 'antegrade' (towards the heart) and 'retrograde' (away from the heart).

This complex hepatic vein tracing and associated velocities have been described by Abu-Yousef.[15] Figure 8.11B shows the hepatic vein waveform in relationship with an electrocardiogram (ECG) tracing, tricuspid M-mode scan, and atrial and ventricular status. The following stages can be identified:

1. The most distinctive feature is the retrograde A-wave, which is the result of right atrial contraction triggered by the P-wave on the ECG. Since there is no valve between the right atrium and the IVC, a burst of reversed flow travels down the IVC and into the hepatic veins, which has a mean velocity of approximately 18 cm/s.

2. At the end of right atrial contraction, flow returns to the antegrade direction as the atrium relaxes. However, as the right ventricular contracts, the tricuspid valve is slammed shut and bulges back into the right atrium, creating its own pressure wave: the C-wave. This is a subtle brief pause in the steadily increasing antegrade flow. It is infrequently detected. The C-wave coincides with the beginning of ventricular systole and occurs with the QRS complex on the ECG.

3. The right atrium continues to dilate and antegrade flow builds to a relatively high velocity of approximately 30 cm/s. Eventually atrial filling approaches completion and antegrade flow starts to slow. This transition from accelerating to decelerating flow is known as the S-wave and occurs during ventricular systole within 0.15 s of the QRS complex.

4. At the end of atrial filling, antegrade velocity decelerates, or may even briefly reverse. The tricuspid valve then opens and velocities accelerate in the antegrade direction. This is known as the V-wave and has a mean velocity of approximately −1 cm/s. In relation to the ECG, this occurs following the T-wave.

5. As the right ventricle relaxes flow in the hepatic veins again accelerates in the antegrade direction, as both the right atrium and right ventricle

fill. Velocity builds to a mean of approximately 22 cm/s. Eventually, the right heart chambers become filled passively and antegrade flow decelerates. This change from accelerating to decelerating velocity is referred to as the D-wave, and occurs during ventricular diastole. We then return to the A-wave as the atrium again contracts to begin another cardiac cycle.

This waveform is seen in the hepatic veins and upper IVC in the vast majority of patients. However, not all individuals have a similar degree of periodicity within the hepatic veins. The percentage of patients that manifest an identifiable C-wave is relatively small (Fig. 8-12). The degree of flow reversal of the A-wave and V-wave may vary depending on the patient's cardiac status, state of hydration, heart rate, and the distance of Doppler interrogation from the heart. In a survey of a population of normal volunteers, a 9% incidence of a flattened hepatic vein flow profile has been reported.[12,16]

Because the heart is located within the thorax, pressure changes caused by respiration affect the hepatic vein flow profile. When the patient forcefully exhales or bears down against a closed glottis, the elevated intrathoracic pressure resists antegrade flow, causing the S- and D-waves to be less prominent. The reversed component of flow increases so the A- and V-waves become more pronounced (Fig. 8-13). Conversely, during forced inspiration with increasing negative intrathoracic pressure, the S- and D-waves become more prominent, while the A- and V-waves are less pronounced and may actually not manifest as reversed flow.[17]

Assessment of Disease

PORTAL VEIN

Portal Hypertension

In hepatocellular disease, the sinusoids are damaged, destroyed or replaced. As the volume of normally functioning liver parenchyma decreases, the resistance to portal venous flow increases, the portal vein dilates, and portal flow decreases and with increasing severity, reverses.[18–20] An elevation of pressure in the portal system above 6 mmHg is considered portal hypertension. Above 12 mmHg pressure, portal hypertension becomes clinically evident.

Use of the 'congestive index' has been recommended to help diagnose portal hypertension. This index is the

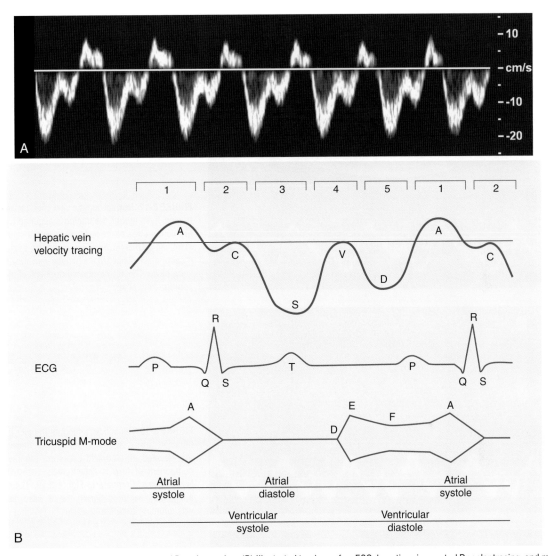

FIGURE 8-11 (A) Normal hepatic vein spectral Doppler tracing. (B) Illustrated tracings of an ECG, hepatic vein spectral Doppler tracing, and mitral valve M-mode tracing with correlation to atrial and ventricular systole and diastole. The divisions at the top of these tracing 1–5 correspond to the discussion in the text.

ratio of the portal vein cross-sectional area (cm^2) divided by the mean portal flow velocity (cm/s). This takes into account portal vein dilatation and decreased flow velocity, the two physiological changes associated with portal hypertension. In normal subjects, this ratio is less than 0.7. Although there is theoretical value in this index, the interobserver variability in portal vein area measurements and velocity measurements is relatively high, and error is further compounded when the parameters

are combined in a ratio. Therefore, few centres now rely on this index.[21,22]

As liver disease worsens, the periodicity in the portal vein may become more pronounced, usually coinciding with hepatic arterial systole (Fig. 8-14).[19,23] Finally, with end-stage liver disease, continuous hepatofugal flow is observed, usually with increased periodicity. Blood entering the liver in the hepatic artery normally passes through the hepatic sinusoids to the hepatic

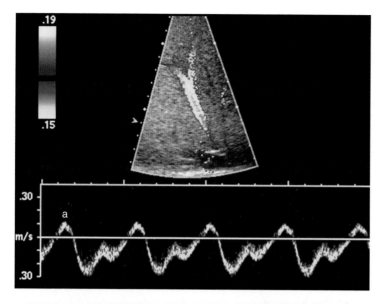

FIGURE 8-12 Normal hepatic vein spectral Doppler tracing. Even though the tracing is acquired within a few centimetres of the heart, the C-wave cannot be identified on this tracing. This is, indeed, the tracing most often visualised in the hepatic vein and inferior vena cava. The retrograde component of flow is appropriately small.

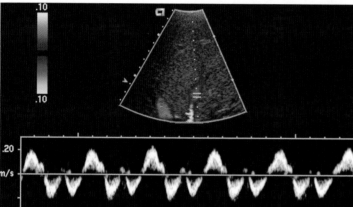

FIGURE 8-13 Hepatic vein spectral Doppler tracing obtained during Valsalva manoeuvre. Because of the elevated intrathoracic pressure, the reversed component of flow is accentuated. Forward flow is decreased. Compare to Figure 8.12. The colour image was captured during the 'a wave' as flow was coursing back into the liver.

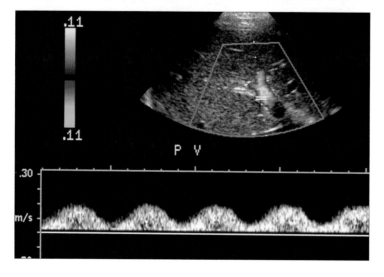

FIGURE 8-14 Spectral hepatic vein Doppler tracing in a patient with alcoholic cirrhosis. Portal vein flow profile has become more sinusoidal although the flow direction does remain hepatopetal throughout the cardiac cycle. This degree of periodicity is beyond what we would expect in a normal portal vein. The dip in antegrade velocity coincides with hepatic arterial systole.

veins, but with increasing hepatocellular disease, scarring, fibrosis, and capillary leak the pathway of least resistance for the arterial inflow becomes the portal vein. Arterial blood shunts to the portal vein via vasa-vasorum, or via direct arteriovenous shunting at the level of the sinusoids. Thus, the origin of hepatofugal flow leaving the liver in the portal vein is blood shunted from the hepatic artery[24] (Fig. 8-15).

Pronounced periodicity may be seen in the portal vein, which does not coincide with hepatic arterial systole. This is usually due to cardiac disease, such as right ventricular dysfunction or tricuspid regurgitation, and is caused by a prominent reversed component of flow in the hepatic veins, either a 'cannon' A-wave or a reversed S-wave[25,26] (Fig. 8-16).

Varices

As portal hypertension progresses and pressure rises to 15 or 20 mmHg, sufficient pressure exists to cause the development of varices. These collateral pathways shunt blood from the portal to the systemic circulation.[27] The more common channels are the short gastric, left gastric

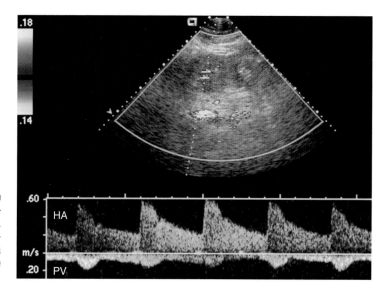

FIGURE 8-15 Portal vein spectral Doppler tracing in a patient with severe hepatocellular injury secondary to paracetamol (acetaminophen) overdose. Portal vein flow is hepatofugal throughout the cardiac cycle. We again see increased periodicity with a velocity surge concurrent with arterial systole secondary to capillary leak.

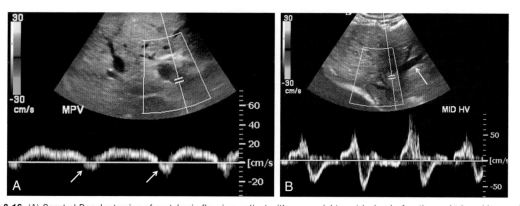

FIGURE 8-16 (A) Spectral Doppler tracing of portal vein flow in a patient with severe right ventricular dysfunction and tricuspid regurgitation. There is marked periodicity in the portal vein waveform. Hepatopetal flow decreases, and briefly reverses, coinciding with the large regurgitant component of hepatic vein flow during tricuspid regurgitation. (B) Colour image and spectral Doppler tracing of the middle hepatic vein. Note the veins are distended. There is complete distortion of the triphasic hepatic vein waveform with a large regurgitant component of flow. This large reversed pressure wave impedes portal vein inflow.

and coronary veins; recanalised umbilical or paraumbilical vein; and splenorenal-mesenteric collaterals (Fig. 8-17). Other, less typical, pathways include pericholecystic, iliolumbar, gonadal, haemorrhoidal, and ascending retrosternal veins. Indeed, any vein in the abdomen may serve as a potential collateral to the systemic circulation and may be incorporated in a very convoluted shunt.[28,29]

Short gastric varices coursing between the spleen and the greater curvature of the stomach are best

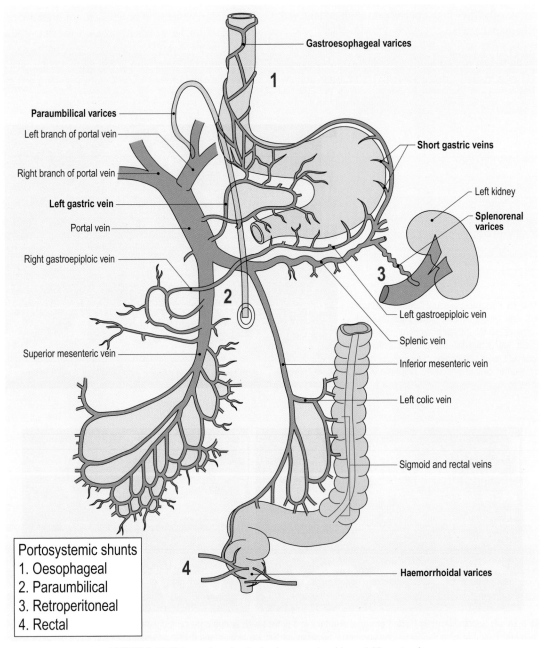

FIGURE 8-17 Major portosystemic shunts encountered in portal hypertension.

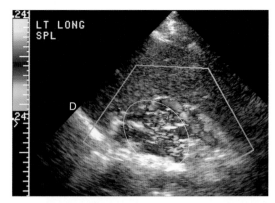

FIGURE 8-18 Longitudinal colour Doppler view of the left flank in a patient with portal hypertension and splenomegaly. A tangled web of veins (arrows) is seen coursing cephalad from the splenic vascular pedicle and extends towards the diaphragm (D). These are short gastric varices coursing from the splenic vein, along the greater curvature of the stomach and from there to the systemic circulation via oesophageal varices.

imaged via the left flank, using the enlarged spleen as a window (Fig. 8-18). Left gastric or coronary vein varices course from the splenic or portal veins along the lesser curvature of the stomach and are best imaged through the left lobe of the liver (Fig. 8-19). Both sets of varices then converge on the gastro-oesophageal junction (Fig. 8-20A). From there, blood flow proceeds upwards through oesophageal varices to eventually communicate with the azygous vein and the systemic circulation (Fig. 8-20B). Because of the potential lethal

risk from spontaneous, brisk haemorrhage from oesophageal varices, a variety of endoscopic, surgical, or percutaneous procedures have been developed to divert blood away from them.

In utero, oxygenated blood flows from the placenta up the umbilical vein to the left portal vein and then through the ductus venosus into the IVC and right atrium. After birth, this pathway involutes and the umbilical vein remnant becomes the ligamentum teres in the falciform ligament. In portal hypertension, paraumbilical veins in this ligament or the umbilical vein itself can dilate and carry blood from the left portal vein along the anterior abdominal wall to the umbilical region (Fig. 8-21). From the umbilicus, the blood may pass to the superior or inferior epigastric veins, or through subcutaneous veins in the anterior abdominal wall, known as the 'Caput Medusa', to reach the systemic circulation. Because inferior epigastric varices run just deep to the rectus muscles, they are not apparent on clinical examination but are easily identified by colour Doppler (Fig. 8-22). Patients with known portal hypertension, who present with an umbilical hernia, should undergo imaging evaluation prior to surgery as the hernia may contain a dilated varix, rather than bowel. This pathway has less risk of life-threatening variceal bleeding.[30]

Splenorenal-mesenteric collaterals are typically quite large, elongated and very tortuous. Spontaneous

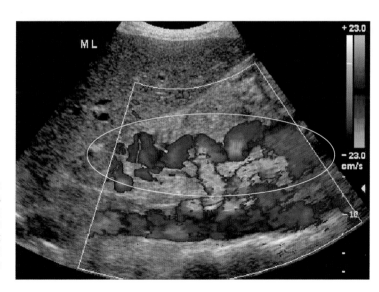

FIGURE 8-19 Longitudinal colour Doppler image in the midline of a patient with portal hypertension. A large tortuous left gastric varix is seen coursing from the region of the coeliac axis towards the gastro-oesophageal junction. Whereas short gastric varices tend to be a plexus of small vessels, the left gastric varix is typically a single large tortuous vessel. (Image courtesy of a friend.)

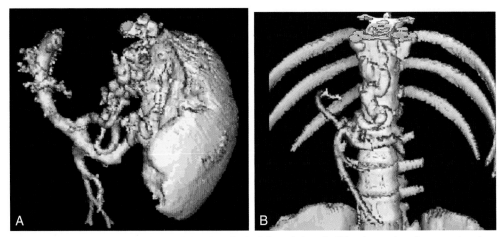

FIGURE 8-20 (A) Anterior view of a colour-coded shaded surface display 3-D rendering of a CT angiogram/portal venous phase in a patient with portal hypertension and splenomegaly. Short gastric varices (green) are best imaged from the left flank using the spleen as a sonographic window. The left gastric varix (red) is best imaged through the left lobe of the liver. (B) Anterior view of a colour-coded shaded surface display 3-D rendering of the portal vasculature in a patient with portal hypertension. The portal venous system is coloured red. The vessel coded blue is a large left gastric varix. Note the serpiginous course of this vessel as it courses cephalad, eventually branching into multiple oesophageal varices.

splenorenal varices are almost never a direct communication between splenic and renal veins. They are seen in the left flank taking an extremely convoluted course, often extending between diaphragm and pelvis (Fig. 8-23). Very often this pathway arrives at the renal vein via the left gonadal vein.

Pericholecystic varices can occur in the gallbladder wall and are associated with portal vein thrombosis. It is common to find pericholecystic varices associated with cavernous transformation of the portal vein. US imaging may reveal cystic or tubular structures in the gallbladder wall. These should not be confused with the Rokitansky Aschoff sinuses of hyperplastic cholecystosis. Colour Doppler is useful to show flow within these vessels; with the spectral tracing showing portal venous flow profile (Fig. 8-24). From the gallbladder, subhepatic collaterals communicate with the abdominal wall and subcostal veins.

Haemorrhoidal collaterals are not routinely studied by Doppler, but can be seen on endoscopic examination.

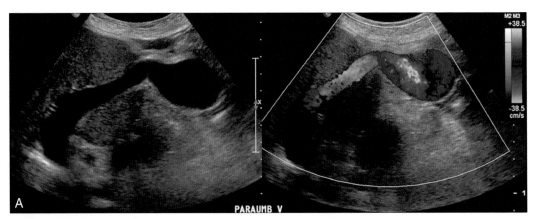

FIGURE 8-21 (A) Longitudinal colour Doppler image of a patient with portal hypertension. A large vein carries flow from the left portal vein towards the transducer. It courses along the falciform ligament and then turns caudad along the abdominal wall passing towards the umbilicus, deep to the rectus muscles.

Continued

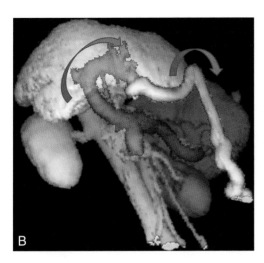

FIGURE 8-21—CONT'D (B) Shaded surface display three-dimensional reformat of the upper abdominal solid organs and portal venous system. Flow in the main portal vein courses towards the liver but immediately channels into a large left portal vein (open arrow). Flow then continues anteriorly towards the anterior abdominal wall and down towards the umbilicus in a large recanalised umbilical vein (pink).

Portal Vein Thrombosis

Portal vein thrombosis may be completely asymptomatic in patients with cirrhosis; however, more than half of cases present with life-threatening complications, such as gastrointestinal haemorrhage or intestinal infarction.[31,32] Portal vein thrombosis must be considered when no Doppler signal is detected within the portal vein. It may be due to blood clot, or to tumour invasion. However, the examiner should first review the scanner set-up and re-evaluate scale, gain, and filtration settings (Fig. 8-3). If these are found to be set appropriately and there is still no perceptible flow, the patient should be asked to perform a Valsalva manoeuvre. This elevates intrathoracic and right atrial pressure, transmitting higher pressure to the IVC, hepatic veins and subsequently into the liver parenchyma. This increased pressure causes even greater resistance to portal venous inflow and may convert stagnant portal flow to hepatofugal flow (Fig. 8-25) thereby decreasing the risk of misdiagnosis of thrombosis. If available, one may also consider the use of intravenous US contrast to enhance perception of very slow flow.[33]

Early thrombosis of the intrahepatic portal vein branches may be difficult to visualise with US imaging alone as fresh clot can be of similar echogenicity to the

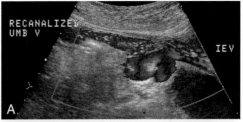

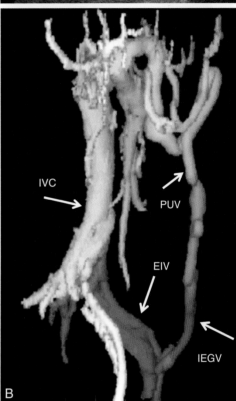

FIGURE 8-22 (A) Longitudinal colour Doppler image directly over the umbilicus. A recanalised umbilical vein carries blood towards the umbilicus. No caput medusa was present in this patient since flow drains from the umbilical region via the inferior epigastric vein (IEV). (B) Right lateral view of a colour-coded shaded surface display 3-D rendering of the portal vasculature in a patient with a large recanalised umbilical vein. The umbilical vein (UV) courses towards the umbilicus. From there flow continues back to the systemic circulation via the left inferior epigastric vein (IEGV) to the left external iliac vein (EIV) and eventually the inferior vena cava (IVC).

adjacent liver (Fig. 8-26). As clot matures, it becomes more echogenic and retracts, allowing partial recanalisation of the portal vein (Fig. 8-27). Patients with longstanding portal vein thrombosis may develop collateral flow into the liver via a lace-like network of veins. This

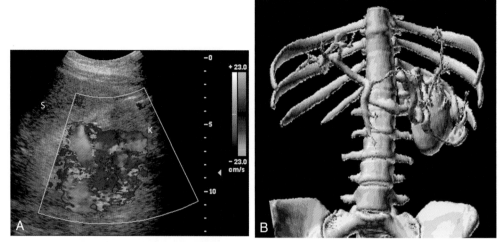

FIGURE 8-23 (A) Longitudinal colour Doppler image of the left flank. A large varix occupies the space between the splenic hilum (S) and the left kidney (K). This represents a convoluted splenorenal varix. (B) Anterior view of a colour-coded shaded surface display 3-D rendering of the portal vasculature in a patient with portal hypertension. The portal venous system is shaded pink. The red vessel represents a large serpiginous splenorenal varix. The kidney and its renal vein are illustrated in yellow. (The spleen has been removed for ease of visualisation of this varix.)

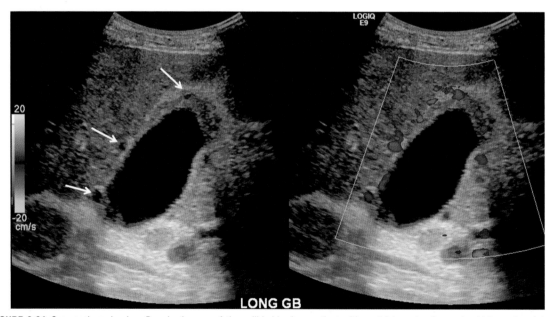

FIGURE 8-24 Grey scale and colour Doppler images of the gallbladder in a patient with portal hypertension and a history of portal vein thrombosis. Several cystic areas are seen in the gall bladder wall. Colour Doppler reveals that these are blood vessels and not sinuses from chronic cholecystitis. Spectral Doppler revealed a portal vein waveform as would be expected in varices and not an arterial waveform as would be seen in the cystic artery. Gallbladder wall varices are seldom seen without portal vein thrombosis.

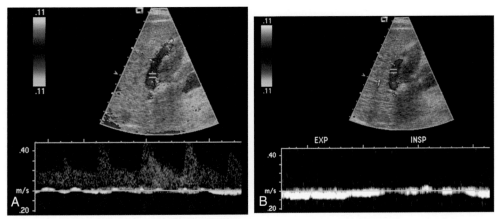

FIGURE 8-25 (A) Spectral Doppler tracing of a patient with end-stage liver disease being considered for liver transplantation. With neutral breath-hold, flow in this portal vein is barely perceptible. It oscillates between hepatofugal during arterial systole and hepatopetal during arterial diastole. (B) When instructed to forcefully breathe in and out, this patient's portal flow became more dynamic. During forced expiration with elevated intrathoracic pressure there is increasing resistance to hepatic venous outflow forcing portal vein flow to become hepatofugal. During inspiration with negative intrathoracic pressure, this decreases the resistance to hepatic venous outflow, thereby causing flow to become almost stagnant. Note also that colour Doppler flow in the portal vein is reversed from the prior image, simply by the change in intrathoracic pressure.

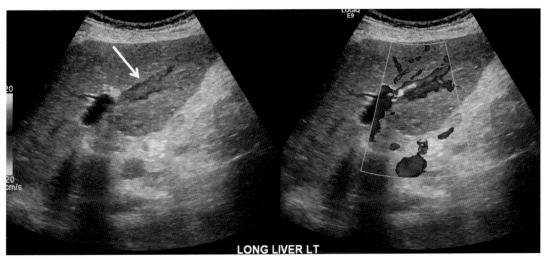

FIGURE 8-26 Oblique colour Doppler image of the left portal vein. The pulse repetition frequency is appropriately set at a low level. A tubular echogenic plug of thrombus is seen within the left portal vein (arrow). Its echogenicity is very similar to that of the adjacent liver parenchyma. The colour image shows a small trickle of flow between the vessel wall and the clot.

is known as cavernous transformation of the portal vein or cavernoma.[34] The absence of a clearly definable portal vein is the notable finding on greyscale imaging alone. Colour Doppler reveals a web of numerous serpiginous small veins which typically involve a fairly wide area of the liver hilum (Fig. 8-28). Spectral Doppler shows portal flow in the branches of the cavernoma.

Neoplastic Invasion

HCC has a propensity to invade the portal and hepatic veins. Intravascular tumour is classified as stage IV disease and is considered unresectable. Involvement of the portal vein by tumour may cause an increase in its cross-sectional area and a decrease in portal vein flow. Tumour in the portal vein receives its blood supply from

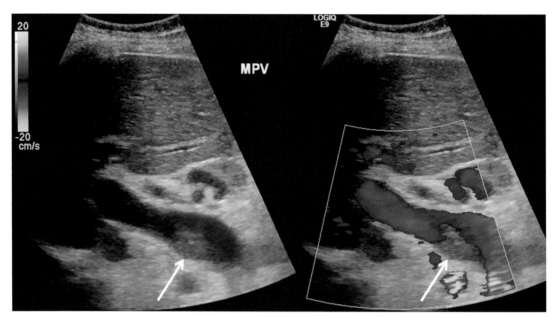

FIGURE 8-27 Oblique colour Doppler along the porta hepatis. An echogenic clot is adherent to the posterior wall of this enlarged portal vein. Colour Doppler shows flow coursing around it. This patient with a long-standing history of hypercoagulability has been successfully managed with anti-coagulant therapy.

the hepatic artery and spectral Doppler of the 'thrombus' will show an arterial waveform. Arterial velocities usually project in a hepatofugal direction, supplying the tumour as it grows out of the liver. Bland thrombus will not manifest such a tracing on Doppler, so that invasive tumour can be differentiated from bland thrombus and the diagnosis of stage IV HCC with vascular invasion confirmed (Fig. 8-29).[35,36]

Portal Vein Aneurysm

Aneurysm of the portal vein has been reported, but it is extremely rare. The vein may enlarge to a diameter of 3 cm or larger. Spectral Doppler should be applied to confirm a portal vein waveform and rule out hepatic artery aneurysm since the latter carries a much higher incidence of complications and rupture.[37]

Portal Vein Gas

Air bubbles may be seen in the portal vein and its branches in a variety of gastrointestinal disorders, such as sepsis, obstruction with distension, necrotising enterocolitis, infarction or ulceration. Numerous tiny hyperechoic foci can be seen in the portal vein, flowing into the liver. Since these bubbles are moving fairly

rapidly, their perception is best with high temporal resolution. This is accomplished by limiting the field of view to the area of the portal vein, scanning with a single focal zone and minimising, or turning off, frame averaging. The spectral Doppler tracing reveals sharp bidirectional spikes superimposed on the Doppler tracing of the portal vein. These spikes do not reflect a higher velocity of the air bubbles but are due to artefact resulting from the system being set to the strength of reflected signal from red blood cells. Since air bubbles are much more intense reflectors, their echoes register as spikes of noise on the tracing (Fig. 8-30).[38]

HEPATIC ARTERY

A comparison of hepatic arterial velocities with those of the portal vein may be used as an indicator of liver disease. The normal portal vein velocity in a fasting patient is about 18 cm/s, the normal systolic velocity in the hepatic artery is 25–40 cm/s and 10–15 cm/s in diastole. If the waveforms of the hepatic artery and portal vein can be captured simultaneously on a Doppler tracing, the normal hepatic arterial diastolic velocity will therefore be seen to dip just below that of the portal vein (Fig. 8-5).

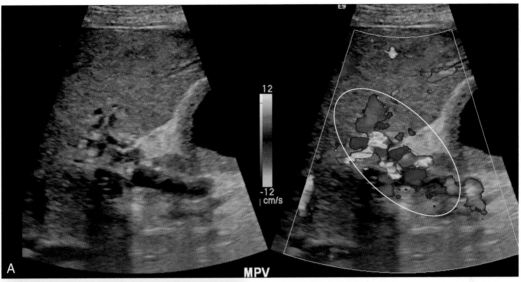

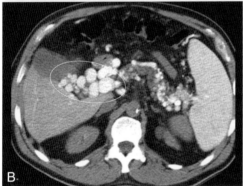

FIGURE 8-28 (A) Oblique greyscale and colour Doppler image of the porta hepatis. A normal portal vein could not be visualised. Instead there is a plexus of small vessels with tortuous, but mostly hepatopetal flow (circled). After portal vein thrombosis this web of vessels reconstitutes portal flow to the liver and is known as cavernous transformation of the portal vein. (B) Axial contrast-enhanced CT scan at the level of the porta hepatis. Note the numerous tributaries of this portal cavernoma after portal vein thrombosis.

Almost all liver disease processes receive their blood supply primarily from the hepatic artery. As the process becomes more severe, or involves a larger area of liver, hepatic artery velocities increase. As liver disease worsens, portal venous inflow encounters progressively increasing resistance. This results in decreased hepatopetal portal velocity. Therefore, if the Doppler examination shows hepatic arterial diastolic velocities twice or more than that of the portal vein, the liver parenchyma should be carefully evaluated to identify possible focal lesions or diffuse distortion of echotexture.[18] This finding, however, is non-specific and can be seen with neoplasm (both primary and metastatic), infection (viral, bacterial, parasitic or fungal), severe steatosis or ingestion of toxins

(acetaminophen overdose) (Fig. 8-31).[39] Benign conditions such as haemangioma or focal, geographic steatosis do not perceptibly affect main hepatic artery or portal vein flow (Fig. 8-32).

Hepatic artery resistance has been studied in several disease states. Alterations in resistance may be observed but, to date, have not been shown to be sufficiently specific or sensitive in the diagnosis of any one particular condition.[40,41] Rapid onset of oedema or inflammation of the liver may produce a substantial amount of congestion, leading to higher resistance to hepatic arterial inflow and elevation of the RI. Elevated RI in the hepatic artery has been reported as a predictor of fulminant and severe acute liver failure.[42] Hypervascular disorders, especially those with arterial

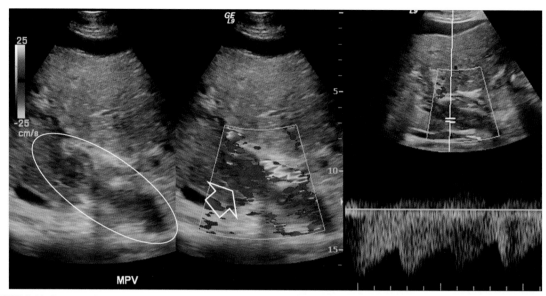

FIGURE 8-29 Greyscale imaging, colour Doppler and spectral Doppler tracing over the portal vein in a patient with known advanced hepatocellular carcinoma (HCC). Echogenic material fills the portal vein. Colour Doppler shows numerous small vessels with flow but in a hepatofugal direction. Spectral Doppler tracing over these vessels shows a very low-resistance arterial waveform. This is vascular invasion of the portal vein by hepatocellular carcinoma. The tumour originates in the liver and grows outward; therefore, the arterial supply runs in a hepatofugal direction. This is tumour neovascularity, therefore, resistance is low.

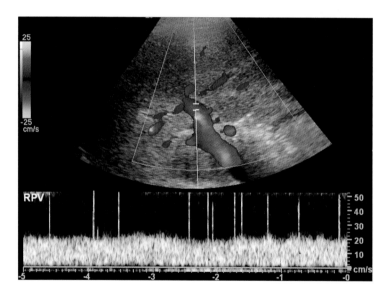

FIGURE 8-30 Spectral Doppler tracing of the portal vein in a patient with pneumatosis intestinalis. The spikes present in this spectral Doppler tracing are caused by air bubbles in the portal vein. These bubbles are travelling at the same velocity as the rest of the blood in the portal vein, but with the spectral gain set for blood, the intense sound reflection caused by the passing air bubbles creates spikes of noise.

venous shunting, such as neoplasm, can lower the arterial resistance. A tardus-parvus waveform and low-resistance flow may also be perceived downstream from hepatic arterial inflow obstruction such as with hepatic artery stenosis, or a diaphragmatic crus defect of the celiac axis. This is also known as arcuate ligament syndrome and is most often seen in slender females. The hepatic artery tracing can change from normal to tardus-parvus between inspiration and expiration. This waveform variation is diagnostic of this condition and is caused by a changing degree of compression of the celiac axis as the patient breathes. It is further reinforced by the identification of aliasing and a high-velocity jet in the celiac artery (Fig. 8-33).

Hepatic Artery Aneurysm/Arteriovenous Fistula

Most hepatic artery aneurysms are extrahepatic and may be congenital or acquired. Pancreatitis, trauma, or liver biopsy are the most common aetiologies. Mycotic aneurysms can be seen in immune-compromised patients, those with bacterial endocarditis or those abusing intravenous drugs. Sonography demonstrates a rounded area with swirling flow on colour. The spectral tracing is usually quite distorted

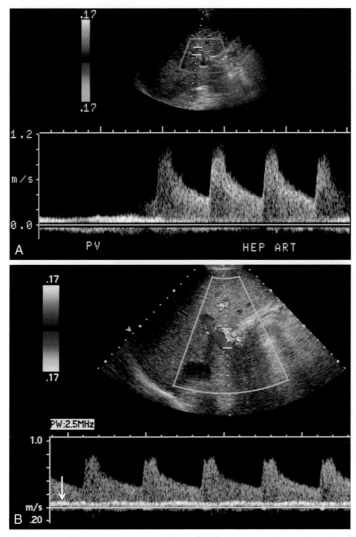

FIGURE 8-31 (A) Spectral Doppler tracing of the porta hepatis in a patient with biopsy-proven chemical hepatitis. This tracing was obtained by a slight change in orientation of the transducer during the scan, traversing from portal vein to the hepatic artery. Hepatic arterial velocities are markedly increased with low resistive index and high diastolic flow. Portal vein flow has decreased to the point where it is barely perceptible. (B) Combined hepatic artery and portal vein tracing at the porta hepatis in a patient with HIV. In contrast to (A) this tracing was obtained with a sample volume opened wide, including the flow profiles of both the hepatic artery and portal vein in the same tracing. Similar alteration in velocities is again perceived with bounding arterial flow and markedly diminished portal vein inflow.

Continued

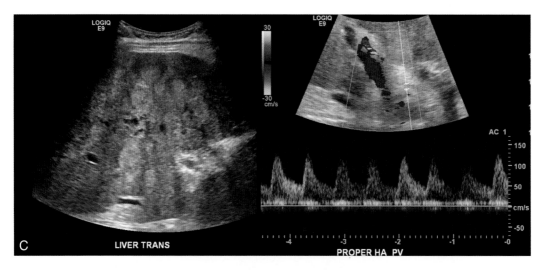

FIGURE 8-31—CONT'D (C) Ultrasound image of the liver and combined Doppler tracing of the porta hepatis in a patient with metastatic lung cancer. The bounding arterial flow is supplying the rapidly growing tumour metastases. Portal venous flow is decreased as the liver sinusoids are being replaced by tumour.

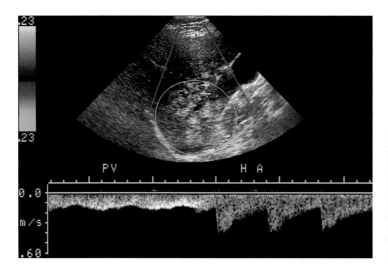

FIGURE 8-32 Transverse image of the right lobe of the liver. A geographic echogenic area is perceived in the inferior aspect of the right lobe (circle). The postero-inferior branch of the right hepatic artery and vein are interrogated by spectral Doppler. The hepatic artery and portal vein supplying this mass reveal normal flow profiles and velocities. The ratio of flow is not altered between the two vessels. Biopsy proved this mass to be focal fatty infiltration.

due to turbulence. A clot may eventually develop within the aneurysm or pseudoaneurysm (Fig. 8-34).

In this era of percutaneous intervention for diagnosis, if biopsies are performed closer to the centre or hilum of an organ, there is greater risk of an arteriovenous fistula developing. Hepatic arterial inflow can fistulise to either the hepatic veins (Fig. 8-35) or portal vein (Fig. 8-36A). Colour Doppler findings depend upon the scale settings. With a relatively low PRF, the vibration of adjacent tissues induced by the fistula causes a flash of colour artefact. With a higher PRF, the feeding artery and draining vein may be more easily identified along with the nidus of the fistula. Spectral Doppler flow profiles show low-resistance arterial inflow with high velocities, and arterialisation of the venous outflow vein (Fig. 8-36B).[43,44]

Hereditary Haemorrhagic Telangiectasia (Osler–Rendu–Weber Disease)

This disease is characterised by multiple small aneurysmal telangiectases distributed over the skin, mucous membranes, alimentary tract, liver, brain and spleen. These patients have a tendency for frequent haemorrhages requiring transfusion. Vascular lesions in the liver can evolve into arterial venous fistulas and aneurysms. Ultrasound may reveal large hepatic arteries feeding large, ectatic, serpiginous arteriovenous malformations, which in turn feed large draining veins.[45,46]

Hepatic Venous Outflow Obstruction

When most of us hear the term Budd–Chiari syndrome we assume hepatic vein thrombosis. Budd–Chiari syndrome, however, refers to liver dysfunction caused by a wide array of conditions that compromise hepatic vein outflow, both thrombotic and non-thrombotic. The term hepatic venous outflow obstruction (HVOO) is now preferred over Budd–Chiari syndrome. Spectral and colour Doppler are capable of identifying numerous non-thrombotic causes of HVOO and differentiating them from hepatic vein thrombosis. Aetiology may be related to pregnancy, tumour, hypercoagulable state or IVC membranes, but the majority of cases are idiopathic. The clinical presentation of HVOO will vary, depending upon how rapidly it develops and the degree of obstruction. Approximately 50% of patients first present with RUQ pain and hepatomegaly. Almost all develop ascites, while a few progress to mild jaundice. Patients with chronic, partial obstruction may

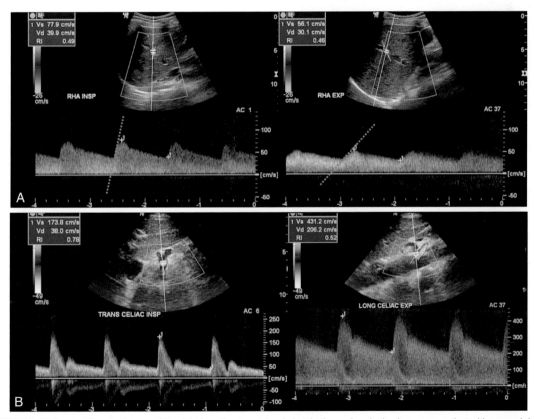

FIGURE 8-33 (A) Spectral Doppler tracing of the right hepatic artery taken in inspiration and expiration in a young patient with upper abdominal pain. The waveform, in inspiration, shows a moderate tardus-parvus configuration. Upon expiration however, it significantly worsened. There is a slow upstroke in systole and a very low resistive index. This indicates inflow compromise which varies with breathing. (B) Spectral Doppler tracing of the celiac artery also in inspiration and expiration. The waveform in inspiration appears completely normal. In expiration, however, it becomes very turbulent with a velocity greater than 4 m/s.

Continued

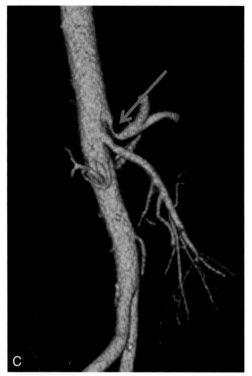

FIGURE 8-33—CONT'D (C) CT angiography confirms celiac artery compression by the arcuate ligament of the diaphragm. The origin of the celiac artery is markedly narrowed and pinched against the aorta.

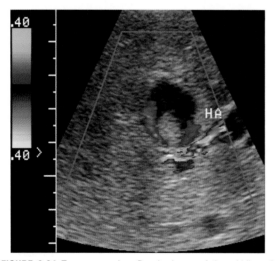

FIGURE 8-34 Transverse colour Doppler image of the mid-liver. A rounded lesion is present with some internal debris. Flow is perceived around this debris. A turbulent arterial spectral Doppler waveform was identified at the neck. Angiography confirmed that this was a partially thrombosed intrahepatic hepatic artery aneurysm.

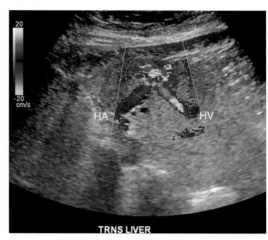

FIGURE 8-35 Transverse colour Doppler image of the mid-liver. The patient had undergone a liver biopsy two months prior. A prominent area of marked turbulent disordered colour flow represents the nidus of the arteriovenous fistula. A large feeding hepatic artery enters from one side. An enlarged draining hepatic vein with turbulent flow is seen coursing away from the lesion.

develop cirrhosis and portal hypertension. If the obstruction progresses to complete occlusion, then shock, hepatic coma and death may ensue.[9,47]

Sonographic imaging features of HVOO may include echogenic intraluminal material (either thrombus or tumour), diffuse narrowing and compression of the veins from generalised liver swelling, or focal vascular compromise by a mass. Doppler findings include complete absence of hepatic vein flow (Fig. 8-37) or localised flow disturbances due to focal partial obstruction. With a more proximal obstruction, the central portions of the hepatic veins (distant from the IVC) that remain patent will become distended and display low-velocity continuous flow, rather than the periodicity seen when the venous flow continues unimpeded to the right atrium. Finally, liver congestion due to HVOO will also cause flow abnormalities in portal vein flow, such as diminished hepatopetal, bidirectional or hepatofugal (reversed) flow. The diagnosis of complete thrombosis by US imaging is difficult since the echogenicity of the clot is often similar to that of the adjacent liver parenchyma. Because the identification of absent blood flow by Doppler is an exclusionary diagnosis, it is difficult to determine with absolute certainty that the cause is thrombosis.

For our discussion we will divide HVOO into four categories: hepatic vein thrombosis, non-thrombotic

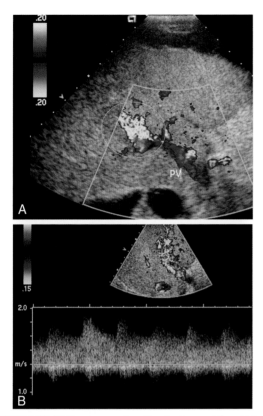

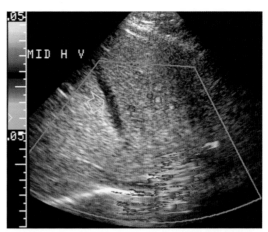

FIGURE 8-37 Transverse colour Doppler image of the upper liver. Even with maximised Doppler sensitivity, no flow was perceived in the middle hepatic vein of this patient (arrow). The hepatic vein had become thrombosed when a central line was inadvertently advanced through the heart into the inferior vena cava and up into the middle hepatic vein. This relatively acute thrombus is hypoechoic compared to the surrounding liver parenchyma. As thrombus matures, however, the echogenicity tends to become isoechoic with the adjacent liver and the thrombus becomes harder to perceive.

FIGURE 8-36 (A) Transverse colour Doppler image of the mid-liver. Flash artefact is seen in the mid-liver. This is due to tissue vibration adjacent to a large arteriovenous fistula. Flow in the portal vein is hepatofugal. This is due to a combination of the underlying liver disease and shunting of blood at the fistula. (B) Spectral Doppler tracing just proximal to the fistula. Very high-velocity, turbulent, low-resistance arterial flow pours into the fistula. The venous outflow is arterialised.

predispose to thrombosis, but in two-thirds of cases, the cause is unknown. The caudate lobe has a separate venous drainage to the IVC. The smaller veins are usually spared from thrombosis, resulting in caudate enlargement and a more normal appearance on contrast-enhanced CT (Fig. 8-38). Occasionally, thrombosis is limited to only one or two of the hepatic veins,

focal compromise of hepatic vein drainage (e.g. stricture, web or neoplasm), reduced compliance of liver parenchyma (e.g. hepatitis, cirrhosis or transplant rejection) or cardiopulmonary resistance to outflow. The first three categories result in decreased or absent hepatic vein periodicity. Cardiopulmonary causes will result in disordered hepatic vein waveforms, with increased accentuated periodicity, especially the reversed components.

Hepatic vein thrombosis most commonly occurs in patients with a hypercoagulation disorder. For instance, females using oral contraceptives have a two and a half time's increased risk of hepatic vein thrombosis. Hepatic vein injury and phlebitis may also

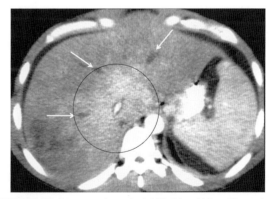

FIGURE 8-38 Contrast-enhanced axial CT of the mid-liver. The caudate lobe and central portion of the liver are uniformly enhancing (encircled), but peripherally the enhancement is decreased and irregular. No contrast is seen within the three hepatic veins because they are thrombosed (arrows).

resulting in intrahepatic shunting of blood from the affected lobe to the unaffected side through hepatic venous collaterals (Fig. 8-39).

A strategically located mass (either benign or malignant) may expand and press upon the ostia of the hepatic veins, resulting in impaired venous drainage. Renal cell carcinoma extending from the renal vein into the IVC can extend up to the right atrium and obstruct hepatic vein outflow. Renal cell carcinoma metastases to the liver maintain this same propensity for vascular invasion.

Membranous obstruction (fibrous web) of the IVC has been reported as one of the major causes of HVOO in South Africa and Asia. The aetiology of these is probably acquired since chronic hepatitis B infection is common in these patients, and up to 50% develop HCC. The hypothesis of congenital membranous obstruction of the IVC has faded and the membrane is now considered to be a sequela of thrombosis. The web is usually at, or just above, the level of the hepatic vein ostia; with resultant damping of cardiac periodicity into the IVC and the hepatic veins and flattening of the Doppler waveform.[48]

Diffuse hepatic parenchymal disease resulting in a reduction of liver compliance can easily compromise hepatic venous drainage as it is a low-pressure system (basically the same as the right atrium; i.e. $-2/+7$ mmHg). Both oedema from acute inflammation and fibrosis from chronic parenchymal disease can narrow the hepatic veins, producing HVOO. Some periodicity may be perceived in close proximity to the junction of the hepatic veins with the IVC, but it quickly fades as the sample volume is moved further away from the heart (Fig. 8-40).[49–51]

Non-thrombotic occlusion of small hepatic veins (hepatic veno-occlusive disease) can occur in bone

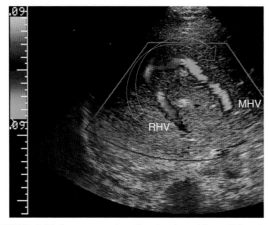

FIGURE 8-39 Transverse colour Doppler view of the mid-liver in a patient with catheter-related inferior vena cava thrombus that obstructed the ostium of the right hepatic vein. Flow in the right hepatic vein (RHV) is reversed and coursing towards the transducer. A prominent collateral vein (arrow) then carries flow to the middle hepatic vein (MHV) and back towards the heart. Intrahepatic venovenous collateralisation develops quickly in response to focal hepatic venous outflow obstruction of a single branch.

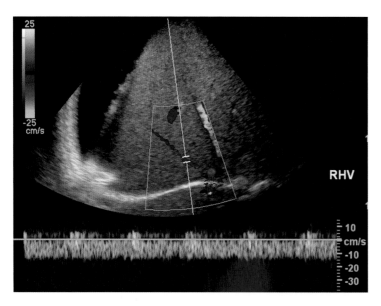

FIGURE 8-40 Transverse image of the liver in a patient with severe cirrhosis and ascites. The liver is small, nodular and very echogenic. The spectral Doppler tracing of the right hepatic within the liver confirms patency but flow is markedly compromised by compression of this vessel. There is complete absence of periodicity and a relatively slow velocity.

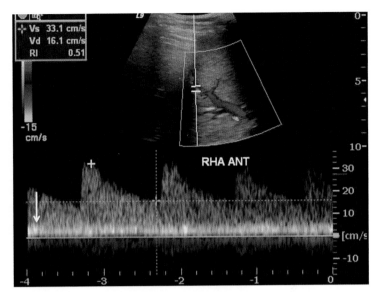

FIGURE 8-41 Transverse image of the liver in a recent bone marrow transplant recipient with worsening liver function tests. This spectral tracing incorporates both artery and portal vein. Note the alteration of the liver vascular index. Portal vein inflow is very slow. Hepatic arterial velocities, however, are still appropriate. This was biopsy-proven venoocclusive disease.

marrow transplant recipients, secondary to chemo-therapy or radiation therapy or with alkaloid toxicity. The obstruction of terminal hepatic venules presents as jaundice, hepatomegaly, pain, ascites and altered liver functions. If the associated coagulopathy is severe, it may preclude biopsy for diagnosis. Spectral Doppler of the hepatic veins typically shows a normal flow profile. Portal vein inflow velocities, however, decrease and may actually reverse. Hepatic artery flow develops increased resistance when the process becomes severe (Fig. 8-41).[52,53]

Near the heart, the normal spectral Doppler tracing of the hepatic vein has a small retrograde component of flow above the baseline, the A-wave (Fig. 8-12). It is relatively small when compared to the antegrade components below the baseline: the S- and D-waves. The ratio of retrograde to antegrade flow decreases during inspiration (which lowers intrathoracic pressure) or when the Doppler sample volume is moved further from the heart (Fig. 8-42). A consistently large component of retrograde flow is an abnormal finding, and if identified, the examiner should consider the presence

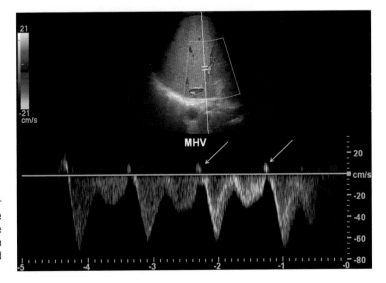

FIGURE 8-42 Transverse spectral and colour Doppler view of the middle hepatic vein. The sample volume is more centrally positioned in the liver. At this distance from the heart, although there is still robust periodicity, the reversed component of flow is actually quite small.

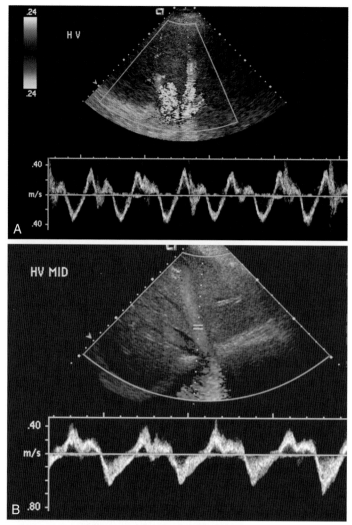

FIGURE 8-43 (A) Transverse spectral and colour Doppler view of the hepatic veins. The hepatic veins are markedly engorged as would be expected with chronic cardiac congestion. Spectral Doppler waveform shows appropriate periodicity within these vessels. The overall amount of retrograde flow, however, is disproportionately large. When summating the area of flow above and below the baseline it becomes apparent that there is relatively little total antegrade flow as would be expected with cardiac congestion. (B) Spectral Doppler tracing in another patient with cardiac congestion. Although periodicity is identified in the tracing it is more disordered than the standard triphasic waveform. Flow away from the heart (above the baseline) is only slightly less than flow towards the heart (below the baseline). This decreased total antegrade flow is a manifestation of cardiac congestion.

of cardiac or pulmonary disease (Fig. 8-43). Distortion of the triphasic hepatic vein waveform can occur with many different cardiac disorders including cardiomyopathy, constrictive pericarditis, tamponade, tricuspid or pulmonary valve disease, atrioventricular dissociation, atrial fibrillation and right ventricular dysfunction. Pulmonary hypertension and massive pulmonary

embolism may also distort the hepatic vein waveform. Basically, any condition restricting cardiac inflow will compromise hepatic outflow.

Specific patterns of hepatic vein velocity profile distortion have been described in restrictive ventricular cardiomyopathy, tricuspid stenosis, pericardial constriction and tamponade. The common property of these conditions is that they prevent right ventricular filling. With right atrial contraction, since flow is restricted from entering the ventricle, there is accentuated reversal of the A-wave.

Tricuspid regurgitation (TR) results in a large volume of blood pushed back through a diseased/incompetent tricuspid valve by the forceful contraction of the right ventricle. In mild TR, the hepatic vein flow profile is characterised by attenuation of the S-wave and a relative increase in V-wave amplitude. In severe TR, systolic reversal of the S-wave and fusion of the S- and V-waves is seen. Instead of forward flow filling the atrium during atrial diastole, the high right ventricular systolic pressure forces blood back through the tricuspid valve into the IVC and the hepatic veins[54,55] (Fig. 8-44).

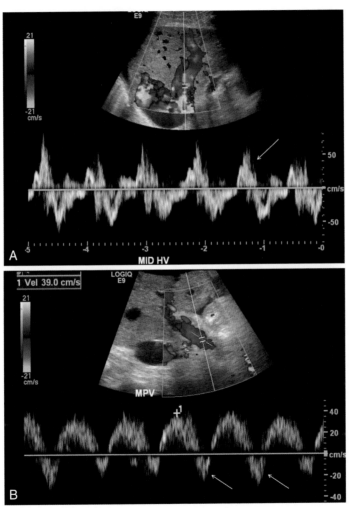

FIGURE 8-44 (A) Spectral Doppler tracing of the hepatic vein in a patient with severe tricuspid regurgitation. The hepatic vein waveform is distorted and basically biphasic. The reversed component of flow is disproportionately large. In the absence of an ECG tracing it is impossible to determine whether this is a reversed S-wave due to tricuspid regurgitation versus a Canon A-wave due to right ventricular dysfunction. Recognition of an inappropriately large retrograde component of flow in conjunction with a disordered waveform and large distended hepatic veins, however, should be enough to channel a patient such as this for a cardiac workup. (B) Spectral Doppler tracing of the portal vein. Instead of uniform flow this waveform is sinusoidal with a brief component of reversed flow. This finding further reinforces the need for a cardiac workup since the retrograde pressure wave of the hepatic vein flow profile is able to resist and actually reverse portal vein inflow.

In atrioventricular dissociation, the atrial and ventricular electromechanical events occur independently of each other. With complete heart block, atrial contraction against the closed tricuspid valve can result in a markedly accentuated A-wave, as the entire atrial volume regurgitates back into the SVC and IVC. Clinically, the palpable increased jugular vein pulsations are described as 'cannon A-waves'. The same phenomenon can occur in patients with premature ventricular ectopic beats which follow atrial contraction.

With atrial arrhythmias, the A-wave may have a varying relationship to the S-wave due to premature atrial contraction or a variable PR interval as seen in Mobitz I heart block. In atrial flutter, multiple small-amplitude A-waves may be present. The lack of organised atrial activity in atrial fibrillation leads to the loss of rhythmic A-waves in the hepatic vein tracing (Fig. 8-45).

In patients with moderate to severe right ventricular (RV) dysfunction, hepatic vein Doppler flow profiles fall into three basic patterns. The first Doppler indication of RV dysfunction is accentuation of the atrial A-wave, due to reduced RV compliance which cannot accommodate all of the right atrial output. Further deterioration of RV function results in attenuated systolic forward flow (S-wave) due to a decrease in the descent of the base of the right ventricle. There is increased early diastolic forward flow (D-wave), because of increased early diastolic filling of the right ventricle and increased A-wave amplitude. Patients with severe RV dysfunction usually have associated tricuspid insufficiency. This results in S-wave reversal. S-wave amplitude changes may also reflect reduced right atrial compliance, reduced RV systolic function or tricuspid insufficiency.

The precise diagnosis of HVOO caused by cardiopulmonary dysfunction requires correlation of the hepatic vein waveform with the ECG tracing (further refined by correlating with the tricuspid M-mode tracing). The average ultrasound department does not have routine access to these tools. Nevertheless, recognition of hepatic vein waveform distortion, especially with accentuated reversed components of flow should identify the patient who would benefit from further work-up in a cardiac echo lab (Fig. 8-46).

Arterialised Hepatic Vein Flow

An arterial waveform within the hepatic veins is an extremely rare finding. It may be seen with a fistula from the hepatic artery to the hepatic vein following biopsy or surgery (Fig. 10-31). Rarely, erosion of a hepatic artery aneurysm into the hepatic vein will result in pulsatile arterial flow in the veins.

FOCAL LIVER LESIONS – MALIGNANT

Hepatocellular carcinoma (HCC) is the most common primary malignant neoplasm of the liver. It occurs primarily in patients with underlying chronic liver disease, such as hepatitis B or C infection, or alcoholic cirrhosis. US is part of screening for hepatocellular carcinoma in high-risk countries where screening programmes exist. Non-contrast enhanced US, however has difficulty detecting HCC on a background of nodular cirrhosis, with a sensitivity of only 50%. Specificity is even worse. The distorted, nodular echo-texture of the cirrhotic liver parenchyma, together with the tumour's variable sonographic appearance, makes it difficult to distinguish HCC with confidence.[56–58]

HCC is typically a hypervascular neoplasm and several authors have promoted the use of spectral and colour Doppler in helping with its diagnosis. Tumour neovascularity with intratumoral arterio-venous shunting, results in decreased vascular impedance and a low-resistance Doppler waveform. A basket pattern of flow within the lesion on colour Doppler has been described in HCC; the internal branching vessels within the tumour, combined with the network of surrounding vessels being responsible for this appearance. However, these findings can occur in other conditions and so the specificity is low. A low-RI, high-velocity flow with systolic frequency shifts approximating 3 m/s may be seen in the feeding arteries; but there is too much overlap with other conditions, so again specificity is low.[59]

Vascular invasion is a hallmark of advanced HCC. Any echogenic plug of tissue within the portal vein should be interrogated with spectral and colour Doppler. The presence of an arterial signal, usually hepatofugal, within the plug makes the diagnosis.[35] HCC invades portal veins (Fig. 8-29) more frequently than hepatic veins.

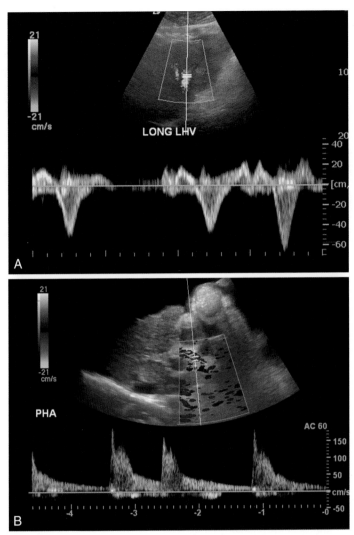

FIGURE 8-45 (A) Spectral Doppler tracing of the left hepatic vein. There is complete distortion of the triphasic waveform. Surges of antegrade flow are not rhythmic. There are reversed components of flow but nothing that resembles an A-wave. (B) Spectral Doppler tracing of the hepatic artery. Arrhythmia is clearly evident by temporal distortion of the systolic spikes.

Metastasis

Metastatic liver lesions occur with a frequency 20 times greater than primary hepatic neoplasms. The sonographic appearance is markedly variable, but most often has a target pattern or halo sign. The hypoechoic rim surrounding the lesion is caused by compressed liver parenchyma, or by proliferating tumour at the edge of the lesion. Colour Doppler may reveal displacement of normal liver vasculature by the expanding metastatic lesion. Little if any flow is seen in the metastasis itself. Spectral Doppler can reveal low-resistance, high-velocity flow in the hepatic artery (Fig. 8-31C). However, this is not consistent enough to obviate the need for biopsy. Power Doppler imaging can assess vascularity in the majority of small liver nodules, but the pattern distribution of tumoral vascular signals does not provide reliable differential diagnostic criteria.[60]

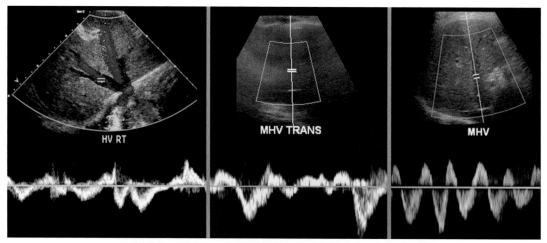

FIGURE 8-46 Spectral Doppler tracing of a hepatic vein in three different patients. None of them is normal. Without an ECG tracing, the precise diagnosis cannot be made. Nevertheless, recognition of a functional hepatic venous outflow obstruction is sufficient to identify the heart as the potential cause of disordered liver function tests and channel the patient's workup towards cardiology.

FOCAL LIVER LESIONS – BENIGN

Hepatic Steatosis (Fatty Liver)

The liver can accumulate triglycerides within the hepatocytes in response to hepatocellular disease. This reversible cellular response may be seen with obesity, alcoholic liver disease, diabetes, parenteral nutrition, and numerous other disorders. Ultrasound commonly reveals a bright echogenic liver with poor through transmission. The central vasculature is often poorly visualised due to compression of these vessels by surrounding fat-laden parenchyma. Fatty infiltration can be patchy and irregular (geographic), with geometric margins or wedge-shaped sub-segmental distribution. Doppler ultrasound shows little change in the hepatic haemodynamics, or vascular distribution in focal steatosis or mild to moderate diffuse steatosis. Absence of velocity alterations is helpful in reinforcing the impression of mild benign fatty infiltration in cases where the imaging appearance is confusing (Fig. 8-32). If significant doubt exists, CT or MR can clinch the diagnosis. With severe steatosis, however, vascular compression will result in inflow resistance and loss of hepatic vein periodicity (Fig. 8-47).[61]

Haemangiomas

Haemangiomas are the most common solid benign neoplasms of the liver. On US, small haemangiomas (<3 cm) are well-defined, homogeneous and hyperechoic. Echotexture becomes distorted with larger haemangiomas due to haemorrhage, fibrosis, or calcification. Doppler (without contrast) adds nothing to the diagnosis of haemangioma as the flow is typically too slow to register, even at the most sensitive settings (Fig. 8-48).

Focal Nodular Hyperplasia

Focal nodular hyperplasia (FNH) is the second most common benign solid tumour of the liver and makes up approximately 8% of all primary hepatic tumours, typically seen in young to middle-aged women. It is believed to be a hormone-dependent non-neoplastic, hyperplastic response to a congenital vascular malformation. Ultrasound reveals a solitary, small lesion, often at the periphery of the liver. The echogenicity is varied with hypo-, hyper-, and isoechoic FNH reported with equal frequency. A central scar has been reported as a dominant feature of FNH, however, it is seldom seen sonographically but, even if seen, it does not help clinch a benign diagnosis since fibrolamellar HCC often also has a central scar. FNH is typically hypervascular with a prominent central artery and radiating branches in a stellate or spoke-wheel configuration with centrifugal flow. This is a unique characteristic of this lesion (Fig. 8-49), but hard to see without US contrast.[62,63]

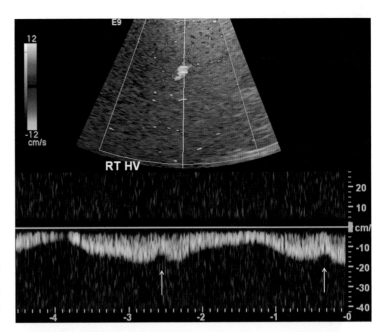

FIGURE 8-47 Spectral Doppler tracing of a hepatic vein in a patient with severe steatosis. The high degree of fatty infiltration compresses the intrahepatic vasculature. The hepatic vein flow profile has become damped. Nevertheless, a subtle A-wave effect can be perceived.

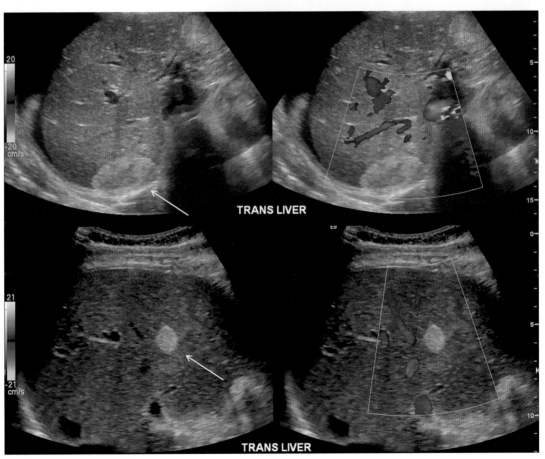

FIGURE 8-48 Transverse images of two haemangiomas (arrows) in a patient. The larger lesion shows irregularity in the echotexture. The smaller is more consistently hyperechoic. Neither lesion shows any flow with colour Doppler.

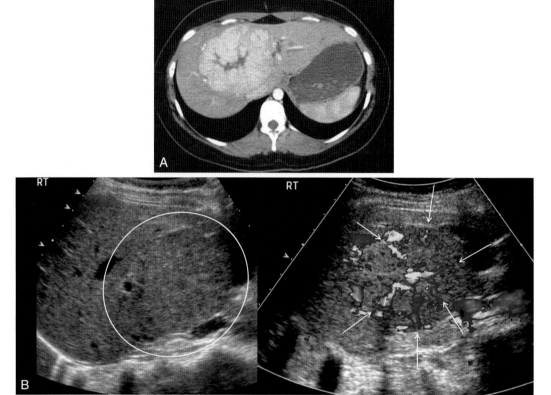

FIGURE 8-49 (A) Arterial phase of a contrast-enhanced CT scan through the upper liver. A briskly enhancing round mass with a central scar is clearly evident (encircled). (B) Ultrasound imaging and colour Doppler through the lesion reveals a mass with a faint central scar. With a little bit of imagination, one can see a spoke wheel distribution of the vasculature. Biopsy confirmed this lesion to be focal nodular hyperplasia. This diagnosis however, is made with much greater confidence when using ultrasound contrast or with contrast-enhanced MR or CT. (Figure courtesy of Paul Sidhu, MD.)

Adenoma

Hepatic adenoma, a rare benign liver tumour, is being seen with increasing frequency. In females it is related to oral contraceptive use, in males to anabolic steroids. Adenomas appear as solid masses with variable echogenicity due to differences in fat content or haemorrhage. Colour Doppler US sometimes demonstrates peripheral peritumoral and intratumoral vessels with spectral Doppler usually showing a flat or uncommonly, triphasic flow profile.[64] In a small percentage of females with hepatic steatosis, the condition can progress to liver adenomatosis in which the tumours tend to increase size. Sonographic diagnosis however is difficult because of the variety of appearance.

Infantile Haemangioendothelioma

Infantile haemangioendothelioma is a rare liver tumour of infancy. It commonly presents as multiple lesions scattered throughout the liver with areas of infarction, haemorrhage and occasionally calcification. The tumour is composed of anastomosing vascular channels lined by one or more layers of endothelial cells. The incidence of congestive heart failure is high because of arterial venous (AV) shunting within the masses. It is considered a benign tumour and most gradually regress after presentation. Some children, however, succumb to the congestive heart failure associated with the high degree of AV shunting. The ultrasound appearance of these lesions usually

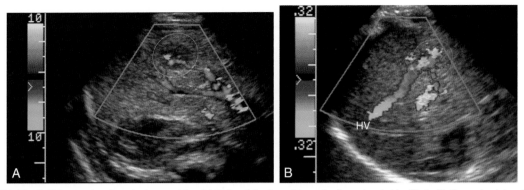

FIGURE 8-50 (A) Oblique colour Doppler image of the right lobe of the liver. A large feeding artery is identified with flow going into a tangled vascular malformation. (B) Longitudinal colour Doppler image. From the vascular malformation flow is seen draining into a large hepatic vein. Infantile haemangioendothelioma was confirmed at autopsy.

shows mixed or variable echogenicity. Large feeding arteries and draining veins (Fig. 8-50) can be perceived by colour Doppler with turbulent flow on spectral Doppler.

Monitoring Treatment of Portal Hypertension

SURGICAL PORTOSYSTEMIC SHUNTS

Numerous variants of surgical portosystemic shunting have been devised over the years including mesocaval, distal splenorenal (Warren), proximal splenorenal, portocaval, and mesoatrial shunts. As with any surgical anastomosis, stenosis or thrombosis may develop. Imaging of shunt integrity by Doppler ultrasound can be difficult because the shunt is usually retroperitoneal and hard to visualise. The sonographer must be informed of the exact type and location of the shunt in order to focus the examination in the correct region. If a prior CT or MR is available it should be reviewed prior to scanning. Brisk hepatofugal flow in the main portal vein is a secondary finding that predicts shunt patency, but the definitive diagnosis is made by direct visualisation of the shunt itself (Fig. 8-51). Spectral velocity measurement across the anastomosis, if possible, should show a velocity gradient of less than 4-fold. Invasive measurement of the pressure gradient across the anastomosis is definitive. Velocity gradients less than 4-fold tend to have insufficient pressure gradients to warrant the risk associated with balloon dilatation.

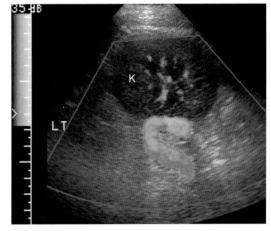

FIGURE 8-51 Oblique longitudinal view of the left flank focused at the upper pole of the left kidney; in a patient with a surgically created splenorenal shunt. A large candy-cane-shaped vessel is identified. The patient is status-post splenectomy with anastomosis of the distal splenic vein to the renal vein. Doppler confirms the anastomosis is widely patent. Fortuitously, the kidney provided a sonographic window in this patient. It is rare to be able to visualise surgical shunts this well.

TRANSJUGULAR INTRAHEPATIC PORTOSYSTEMIC SHUNTS

Treatment of portal hypertension and variceal bleeding by interventional diversion of portal flow as an alternative to surgery or sclerotherapy was first proposed in 1969.[65] Transjugular intrahepatic portosystemic shunt (TIPS) is a percutaneously created communication between the high-pressure portal system of a cirrhotic patient and the low-pressure hepatic veins. Its most important role is to divert blood flow away from potential life-threatening haemorrhage of oesophageal varices. Endoscopic sclerotherapy or banding of oesophageal varices has the ability to treat a focal bleed but does not resolve the underlying cause. A recent advance in TIPS design (covering the frame with a fabric sheath) has led to a re-evaluation of treatment priorities.[66]

In placing a TIPS a transparenchymal track is created between the hepatic vein and the portal vein. It is then dilated and a stent inserted to maintain patency. Although the TIPS is most often placed between the right hepatic vein and the right branch of the portal vein, a left hepatic vein to left portal vein route may be created for technical or anatomic reasons.

Pre-Procedural Assessment

Imaging evaluation is performed before TIPS placement to estimate liver size, evaluate for the presence of tumour, confirm patency of the portal vein and hepatic veins, rule out thrombosis, measure vessel size and search for the presence of portosystemic varices. This is best accomplished with CT angiography. Pre-procedural Doppler flow documentation provides a baseline for comparative appreciation of the results of the procedure; specifically changes in portal haemodynamics, spleen size and the amount of ascites. Any varices (especially left gastric and recanalised paraumbilical) should be identified prior to the procedure so that they may be occluded with coils.[67]

Post-Procedural Assessment

Unfortunately, TIPS complications are common; the most significant being progressive narrowing with compromised function and eventual thrombosis and occlusion. Clinical monitoring of TIPS function is insensitive. By the time clinical indicators such as ascites become evident, the TIPS is usually occluded. The best way to monitor a TIPS is with Doppler sonography at regular intervals. Prompt identification of a stenosis with timely intervention may prevent progression to thrombosis. A recently thrombosed TIPS may be recanalised successfully, but if the clot has time to mature then treatment usually requires placement of a second TIPS.[68]

An evaluation of a non-sheathed TIPS should be performed within 24 hours after its creation to confirm patency and establish baseline flow directions and velocities. Subsequent evaluation is conducted periodically thereafter. The frequency varies among centres, but most re-examine the shunt at 3 months post placement and then at 6-month intervals.

Optimum scanning parameters and normal US findings following TIPS have been described by a number of investigators.[69–72] Low-frequency transducers are necessary because of the increased echogenicity and sound-attenuating features of the cirrhotic liver, along with the fact that the shunt is deep within the body. Doppler gain should be set as high as possible, without encountering noise. The transducer is focused at the level of the shunt or vessel of interest. The sample volume is placed in the centre of flow with an angle of insonation less than 60° when feasible. This is not possible in the mid shunt, where the direction of flow runs perpendicular to the insonating beam. The pulse repetition frequency is set as low as possible, but avoiding aliasing. Scan parameters must be optimised to avoid a false-positive diagnosis of shunt thrombosis.[72]

Recent introduction of TIPS stents sheathed with thermo-mechanically expanded polytetrafluoroethylene (Gore-Tex) creates a unique problem for immediate post implantation imaging. The nature of the fabric causes trapping of air bubbles within its matrix. This air completely reflects sound and presents the appearance of an acutely thrombosed shunt. By 3–5 days after implantation this air becomes absorbed and visualisation of flow becomes possible. Doppler cannot be used to confirm patency in the immediate post-implant timeframe of a sheathed stent. The advantage of these stents is that the fabric prevents ingrowth of the neo-intimal hyperplasia often seen with traditional stents. Long-term patency rates are better.[73–75]

Normal Findings

The TIPS follow-up study begins with a survey of the liver to rule out development of tumour, fluid collections or biliary obstruction; and a quick look around the abdomen for ascites. The shunt is then localised, typically between the right portal and right hepatic veins. The stent should extend from within the portal vein, across the parenchyma, and into the hepatic vein.

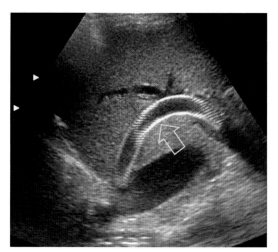

FIGURE 8-52 Greyscale longitudinal image of the right lobe of the liver. The TIPS catheter is seen coursing from the portal vein to the junction of the right hepatic vein with the inferior vena cava (arrow). This long shunt is composed of two stent elements. Note the subtle narrowing at the mid-shunt where the two stent elements overlap. The mesh-like appearance of the shunt is due to the echo reflection off the individual wire elements of the stents.

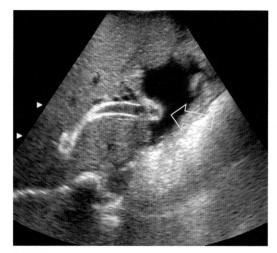

FIGURE 8-53 Transverse view of the TIPS at its junction with the inferior vena cava. The opening of the stent is seen projecting into the right atrium (arrow).

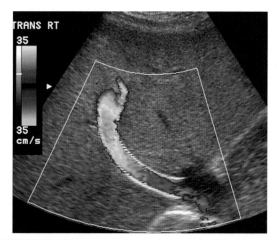

FIGURE 8-54 Oblique colour Doppler image of the TIPS. The entire lumen is saturated with colour indicating patency. Note the non-uniformity of colour encoding – a function of increased velocity at the area of stent overlap. Now turbulence is present, however.

The stent is highly echogenic and appears as two parallel, curvilinear lines, relatively uniform in diameter in its intraparenchymal course but slightly flared at the portal and hepatic vein ends (Fig. 8-52). Imaging sometimes reveals malposition of the stent as a result of inappropriate deployment, or subsequent migration down into the portal vein, or up into the right atrium (Fig. 8-53). Transplant surgeons should be made aware of caval or atrial deployment of the proximal TIPS end since this puts them at risk of contracting hepatitis from the stent wires sticking out of the liver during native hepatectomy prior to transplantation.

Flow within the stent is then evaluated by Doppler ultrasound. The presence of blood flow is easily confirmed, as the entire shunt lumen fills with colour due to the high-velocity flow (Fig. 8-54). Assuming a right portal to right hepatic vein TIPS, the velocity, flow direction and waveform are checked at the portal vein end, mid-shunt and hepatic vein end. The main portal vein and the left portal vein are assessed and the right hepatic vein is checked both proximal to and just beyond its junction with the stent (Fig. 8-55). Spectral Doppler evaluation should verify that the direction of flow in the shunt is from the portal vein to the hepatic

vein. Flow in the widely patent shunt should show standard hepatic vein periodicity throughout the shunt due to right atrial pressure changes being transmitted back through the shunt, against the direction of flow (Fig. 8-56). Periodicity is most pronounced at the hepatic vein end. In one study, half of the patients with patent TIPS demonstrated some periodicity at the hepatic vein end of the shunt, while the other half had high-velocity turbulent flow.[71] The presence of

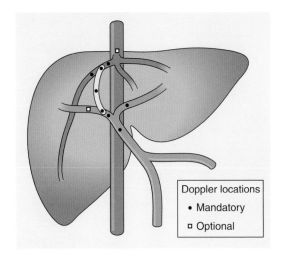

FIGURE 8-55 Illustration of the TIPS and its related vasculature in the standard right hepatic vein to right portal vein configuration. Circles indicate those points at which a Doppler tracing should be obtained in a complete TIPS ultrasound evaluation. (Figure courtesy of Gerald Mulligan, MD.)

the triphasic (hepatic venous) waveform at the portal vein end of the TIPS gives the examiner great confidence that the TIPS is widely patent.

Flow velocities in the shunt vary widely, but should not drop below 50 cm/s.[69,71,72] Flow across the shunt is usually quite turbulent, especially when multiple stent components are used, since overriding stents cause a relative narrowing of the shunt lumen. Velocities in the main portal vein are just as variable. Following TIPS insertion, the mean portal vein velocity has been reported to increase by two-to three-fold.[72] Hepatic arterial flow has also been shown to increase after TIPS, presumably because by decompressing the portal system, the TIPS removes resistance to arteriovenous shunting.[70]

In a properly functioning TIPS, flow direction in the portal system is towards the portal vein end of the stent. Therefore, flow in the main portal vein is hepatopetal and its velocity is typically brisk (between 20 and 60 cm/s). The faster the better, as long as one is not dealing with focal post-stenotic jet.[70] Flow in the left and right portal veins usually becomes hepatofugal, flowing out of the diseased liver and towards the inflow of the shunt (Fig. 8-57). Depending on the diameter of the narrowest shunt component and the severity of the liver disease, however, flow may continue to be hepatopetal into the parenchyma. This is most often seen when the TIPS ends short of the inferior vena cava and most proximal hepatic vein remains narrowed by the surrounding diseased liver. If the patient has a patent but not occluded paraumbilical vein, it will continue to shunt blood away from the liver. Flow in the left portal vein, therefore, continues in a hepatopetal direction despite normal TIPS function.

The Doppler data are recorded and maintained in a table format for follow-up (Fig. 8-58). Serial documentation provides the best means of identifying any

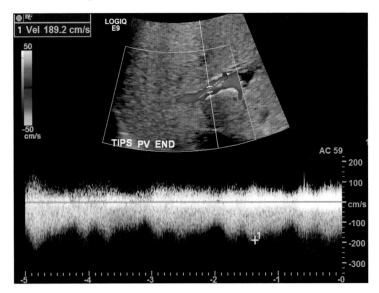

FIGURE 8-56 Doppler tracing obtained at the portal vein end of the TIPS. Note the presence of flow periodicity within the TIPS. The waveform is similar to that seen in hepatic veins. Identification of brisk flow and this degree of periodicity at the portal vein end of the stent is a confident indicator of a widely patent shunt.

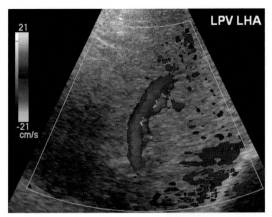

FIGURE 8-57 Colour Doppler image of the left portal vein and hepatic artery in a patient with an appropriately functioning TIPS. The flow in the hepatic artery is towards the transducer, therefore into the left lobe of the liver. The left portal vein flow, however, is away from the transducer, therefore hepatofugal and towards the inflow of the shunt. This is appropriate in a properly functioning TIPS.

variations in velocity and/or flow direction over time and these changes are the best early indicator of shunt compromise. If a branch of the portal vein changes flow direction over time from hepatofugal to hepatopetal, a significant flow-limiting lesion is assumed to have developed in the TIPS.

Shunt Stenosis

The two most common causes of TIPS compromise are neointimal hyperplasia within the shunt, or a focal stenosis at the hepatic vein end. Almost all non-sheathed TIPS have some degree of neointimal hyperplasia,

which is overgrowth of liver tissue combined with fibrosis through the stent mesh and into the lumen. As it progresses it limits flow through the TIPS and eventually occludes it. Beyond the point of maximum stenosis, a high-velocity jet may be perceived by Doppler (Fig. 8-59). Through the rest of the TIPS and the portal system, however, velocities decrease. With sufficient compromise, flow direction in the branch portal veins revert - to hepatopetal and eventually flow in the main portal vein may become hepatofugal.

Focal hepatic vein stenosis can occur where the proximal end of the TIPS abuts the hepatic vein. Focal irritation of the vein wall by the stent wires may cause a bar of granulation tissue to build up. This can obstruct outflow and decrease velocities throughout the shunt.[70] If the stent ends short of the inferior vena cava the non-stented segment of the vein remains narrow, continuing to obstruct outflow and resulting in a high-velocity jet. A key Doppler finding of this focal stenosis is flattening of the hepatic vein flow profile within the TIPS, combined with the presence of post-stenotic high-velocity jet above the point of narrowing (Fig. 8-60). The sonologist must therefore evaluate flow beyond the end of the stent, sometimes even as far as the right atrium.

Flow in all three hepatic veins is normally towards the heart but a stenosis at the junction of the TIPS and its host hepatic vein can compromise outflow. If severe, it causes reversal of flow within that hepatic vein. The path of least resistance for TIPS outflow becomes that hepatic vein with blood coursing back into the liver, percolating across the sinusoids and then returning to the heart via the other hepatic veins (Fig. 8-61).

Name:					ID:		
	VELOCITIES				**DIRECTIONS**		
Date	PV End	Mid	HV End	Main PV	Lt PV	HV↑TIPS	Comments

FIGURE 8-58 TIPS data sheet. Each patient receiving a TIPS should have a data sheet maintained with velocities and flow directions documented at each visit. Progressive compromise of the TIPS can then be more easily recognised as changes in velocities or a change in direction flow become manifest. Velocity measurement in the mid-TIPS tends to be the most erratic. A continuing decrease in main portal vein inflow velocity over the sequence of studies is the most definitive indicator of progressive shunt compromise.

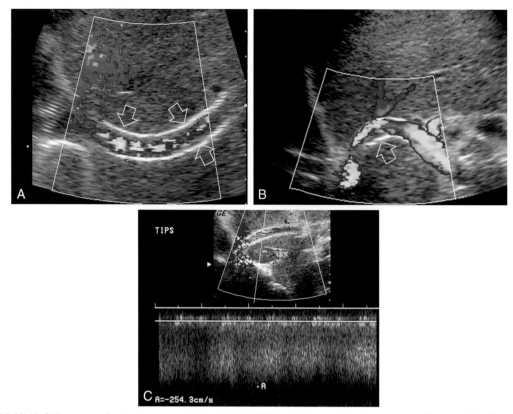

FIGURE 8-59 (A) Oblique colour Doppler image along the length of a TIPS shunt. Turbulent flow is seen across this shunt. Note the absence of flow along the shunt wall (arrows) indicating neointimal hyperplasia along almost the entire length of the TIPS. (B) Oblique colour Doppler image along the length of a TIPS shunt. Flow is seen throughout the TIPS. At the portal vein end it is relatively uniform. At the mid-TIPS, however, there is narrowing and turbulence with a discrete focus of neointimal hyperplasia compromising the lumen. (C) Oblique colour Doppler image along the length of a TIPS shunt. Spectral Doppler tracing at the mid-TIPS shows turbulent flow at the high velocity of greater than 2.5 m/s, well above the accepted normal upper limit of 1.2 m/s for the mid-TIPS. This is caused by a high velocity jet just beyond a focal stenosis.

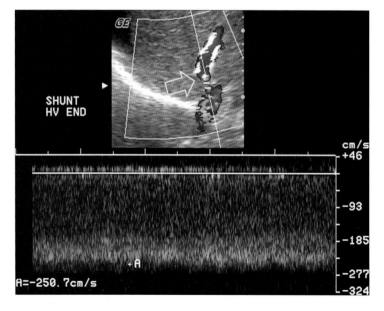

FIGURE 8-60 Spectral and colour Doppler image at the hepatic vein end of a TIPS catheter. Note on the colour image that the catheter ends short of the inferior vena cava. The diameter of the hepatic vein above the TIPS is relatively narrow (arrow). The spectral Doppler tracing shows a velocity of 2.5 m/s. This high-velocity jet is due to the persistent narrowing of the non-stented segment of the hepatic vein.

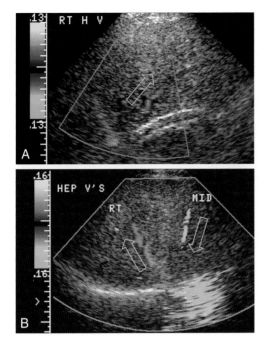

FIGURE 8-61 (A) Longitudinal colour Doppler image including the right hepatic vein and TIPS shunt. Note the poor colour saturation of the TIPS indicating poor flow. Colour signal from the right hepatic vein shows flow coursing towards the transducer, which is away from the inferior vena cava. This is a result of focal stenosis at the hepatic vein junction with the TIPS shunt. (B) Transverse colour Doppler image of the same patient. Flow in the right hepatic vein is indeed coursing away from the heart. Flow collateralises to the middle hepatic vein which has appropriate flow direction back towards the heart.

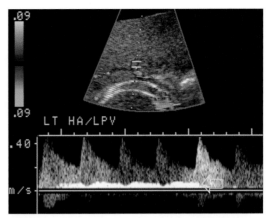

FIGURE 8-62 Spectral Doppler tracing of the left hepatic artery and portal vein including a portion of the TIPS stent. Absence of colour signal with the shunt indicates TIPS thrombosis. This is further reinforced by conversion back to a hepatopetal direction of flow in the left portal vein (arrow). Compare this to the hepatofugal left portal vein hepatic artery flow direction normally seen with a properly functioning TIPS as illustrated in Figure 8.57.

BOX 8-3 CRITERIA FOR COMPROMISED TIPS FUNCTION

- Shunt velocity of <50 cm/s

- Increase or decrease in shunt velocity of >50 cm/s compared with initial post-procedure value

- Focal region of increased velocity in the shunt or hepatic vein

- Conversion from hepatofugal to hepatopetal flow in left and right portal vein branches

- Hepatofugal flow in the main portal vein

- Conversion from periodicity within the TIPS to a flattened flow profile

Several investigators have attempted to determine flow velocities which define critical TIPS stenosis,[69,70,76] but reported findings have varied considerably. In one study, a velocity <50 cm/s at the portal venous end was 100% sensitive and 93% specific.[77] In another study, a velocity <50 cm/s in the middle segment of the TIPS was 78% sensitive and 99% specific.[78] The wide variability of reported TIPS velocity criteria underscores the merits of establishing individual patient baseline velocities soon after TIPS placement and using those as the foundation upon which to make a diagnosis. A change in velocity of ±50 cm/s from baseline is a reasonably sensitive and specific threshold value for predicting haemodynamically significant shunt compromise.[79] If there is significant flow compromise through the TIPS, main portal vein velocity decreases. Flow in the left portal vein may revert back to a hepatopetal direction (Fig. 8-62), representing a reversion to pre-TIPS haemodynamics (Box 8-3).[70,72,80,81]

Shunt Occlusion

If flow cannot be detected in the shunt and portal vein flow reverts to pre-TIPS velocity and direction, shunt occlusion is likely. The absence of flow by colour or power Doppler within the TIPS is a highly specific indicator of shunt thrombosis (Fig. 8-63). However, before concluding that the stent is occluded, meticulous scanning for slow flow should be performed.

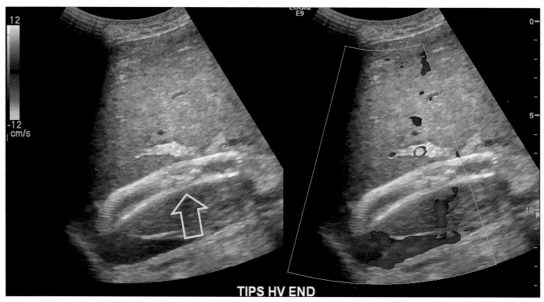

FIGURE 8-63 Ultrasound imaging and colour Doppler of a TIPS stent. Echogenic debris is seen within the TIPS (arrow). Absence of colour signal within the stent indicates complete TIPS thrombosis.

Colour Doppler settings (including pulse repetition frequency, gain and filtration) need to be optimised to differentiate true occlusion from very slow flow. A functioning TIPS, however, is not a low-flow system, so misinterpretation of thrombosis for technical reasons is rarely a problem. Identifying low flow or recent occlusion mandates TIPS revision. Indeed, repeat interventions are the key to long-term success of a TIPS.

REFERENCES

1. Sutherland T, Temple F, Lee WK, et al. Evaluation of focal hepatic lesions with ultrasound contrast agents. *J Clin Ultrasound* 2011;**39**(7):399–407.
2. Grenier N, Basseau F, Rey MC, et al. Interpretation of Doppler signals. *Eur Radiol* 2001;**11**(8):1295–307.
3. Altinkaya N, Koc Z, Ulusan S, et al. Effects of respiratory manoeuvres on hepatic vein Doppler waveform and flow velocities in a healthy population. *Eur J Radiol* 2011;**79**(1):60–3.
4. Kruskal JB, Newman PA, Sammons LG, et al. Optimizing Doppler and color flow US: application to hepatic sonography. *Radiographics* 2004;**24**(3):657–75.
5. Baik SK. Haemodynamic evaluation by Doppler ultrasonography in patients with portal hypertension: a review. *Liver Int* 2010;**30**(10):1403–13.
6. Sacerdoti D, Merkel C, Bolognesi M, et al. Hepatic arterial resistance in cirrhosis with and without portal vein thrombosis: relationships with portal hemodynamics. *Gastroenterology* 1995;**108**(4):1152–8.
7. Ohta M, Hashizume M, Kawanaka H, et al. Prognostic significance of hepatic vein waveform by Doppler ultrasonography in cirrhotic patients with portal hypertension. *Am J Gastroenterol* 1995;**90**(10):1853–7.
8. Iwao T, Toyonaga A, Shigemori H, et al. Hepatic artery hemodynamic responsiveness to altered portal blood flow in normal and cirrhotic livers. *Radiology* 1996;**200**(3):793–8.
9. Goyal N, Jain N, Rachapalli V, et al. Non-invasive evaluation of liver cirrhosis using ultrasound. *Clinical Radiol* 2009;**64**(11):1056–66.
10. Lafortune M, Madore F, Patriquin H, et al. Segmental anatomy of the liver: a sonographic approach to the Couinaud nomenclature. *Radiology* 1991;**181**(2):443–8.
11. Gallix BP, Taourel P, Dauzat M, et al. Flow pulsatility in the portal venous system: a study of Doppler sonography in healthy adults. *AJR Am J Roentgenol* 1997;**169**(1):141–4.
12. Wood MM, Romine LE, Lee YK, et al. Spectral Doppler signature waveforms in ultrasonography: a review of normal and abnormal waveforms. *Ultrasound Q* 2010;**26**(2):83–99.
13. Gielecki J, Zurada A, Sonpal N, et al. The clinical relevance of coeliac trunk variations. *Folia Morphol* 2005;**64**(3):123–9.
14. Oppo K, Leen E, Angerson WJ, et al. Doppler perfusion index: an interobserver and intraobserver reproducibility study. *Radiology* 1998;**208**(2):453–7.
15. Abu-Yousef MM. Normal and respiratory variations of the hepatic and portal venous duplex Doppler waveforms with simultaneous electrocardiographic correlation. *J Ultrasound Med* 1992;**11**(6):263–8.
16. Shapiro RS, Winsberg F, Maldjian C, et al. Variability of hepatic vein Doppler tracings in normal subjects. *J Ultrasound Med* 1993;**12**(12):701–3.
17. McNaughton DA, Abu-Yousef MM. Doppler US of the liver made simple. *Radiographics* 2011;**31**(1):161–88.
18. Iwao T, Toyonaga A, Oho K, et al. Value of Doppler ultrasound parameters of portal vein and hepatic artery in the diagnosis of

cirrhosis and portal hypertension. *Am J Gastroenterol* 1997;**92**(6):1012–17.

19. Westra SJ, Zaninovic AC, Vargas J, et al. The value of portal vein pulsatility on duplex sonograms as a sign of portal hypertension in children with liver disease. *AJR Am J Roentgenol* 1995;**165**(1):167–72.

20. Kuo CH, Changchien CS, Tai DI, et al. Portal vein velocity by duplex Doppler ultrasound as an indication of the clinical severity of portal hypertension. *Changgeng Yi Xue Za Zhi* 1995;**18**(3):217–23.

21. Berzigotti A, Piscaglia F. Ultrasound in portal hypertension – part 1. *Ultraschall Med* 2011;**32**(6):548–68.

22. Berzigotti A, Piscaglia F, Education E. Professional Standards C. Ultrasound in portal hypertension–part 2–and EFSUMB recommendations for the performance and reporting of ultrasound examinations in portal hypertension. *Ultraschall Med* 2012;**33**(1):8–32.

23. Barakat M. Portal vein pulsatility and spectral width changes in patients with portal hypertension: relation to the severity of liver disease. *Br J Radiol* 2002;**75**(893):417–21.

24. Rector Jr WG, Hoefs JC, Hossack KF, et al. Hepatofugal portal flow in cirrhosis: observations on hepatic hemodynamics and the nature of the arterioportal communications. *Hepatology* 1988;**8**(1):16–20.

25. Abu-Yousef MM, Milam SG, Farner RM. Pulsatile portal vein flow: a sign of tricuspid regurgitation on duplex Doppler sonography. *AJR Am J Roentgenol* 1990;**155**(4):785–8.

26. Loperfido F, Lombardo A, Amico CM, et al. Doppler analysis of portal vein flow in tricuspid regurgitation. *J Heart Valve Dis* 1993;**2**(2):174–82.

27. Berzigotti A, Ashkenazi E, Reverter E, et al. Non-invasive diagnostic and prognostic evaluation of liver cirrhosis and portal hypertension. *Dis Markers* 2011;**31**(3):129–38.

28. Gorg C, Riera-Knorrenschild J, Dietrich J. Pictorial review: Colour Doppler ultrasound flow patterns in the portal venous system. *Br J Radiol* 2002;**75**(899):919–29.

29. Robinson KA, Middleton WD, Al-Sukaiti R, et al. Doppler sonography of portal hypertension. *Ultrasound Q* 2009;**25**(1):3–13.

30. Gupta D, Chawla YK, Dhiman RK, et al. Clinical significance of patent paraumbilical vein in patients with liver cirrhosis. *Dig Dis Sci* 2000;**45**(9):1861–4.

31. Amitrano L, Guardascione MA, Brancaccio V, et al. Risk factors and clinical presentation of portal vein thrombosis in patients with liver cirrhosis. *J Hepatol* 2004;**40**(5):736–41.

32. Ponziani FR, Zocco MA, Campanale C, et al. Portal vein thrombosis: insight into physiopathology, diagnosis, and treatment. *World J Gastroenterol* 2010;**16**(2):143–55.

33. Sorrentino P, D'Angelo S, Tarantino L, et al. Contrast-enhanced sonography versus biopsy for the differential diagnosis of thrombosis in hepatocellular carcinoma patients. *World J Gastroenterol* 2009;**15**(18):2245–51.

34. Raby N, Meire HB. Duplex Doppler ultrasound in the diagnosis of cavernous transformation of the portal vein. *Br J Radiol* 1988;**61**(727):586–8.

35. Pozniak MA, Baus KM. Hepatofugal arterial signal in the main portal vein: an indicator of intravascular tumor spread. *Radiology* 1991;**180**(3):663–6.

36. Hidajat N, Stobbe H, Griesshaber V, et al. Imaging and radiological interventions of portal vein thrombosis. *Acta Radiol* 2005;**46**(4):336–43.

37. Mhanna T, Bernard P, Pilleul F, et al. Portal vein aneurysm: report of two cases. *Hepatogastroenterology* 2004;**51**(58):1162–4.

38. Maher MM, Tonra BM, Malone DE, et al. Portal venous gas: detection by gray-scale and Doppler sonography in the absence of correlative findings on computed tomography. *Abdom Imaging* 2001;**26**(4):390–4.

39. Balci A, Karazincir S, Sumbas H, et al. Effects of diffuse fatty infiltration of the liver on portal vein flow hemodynamics. *J Clin Ultrasound* 2008;**36**(3):134–40.

40. Joynt LK, Platt JF, Rubin JM, et al. Hepatic artery resistance before and after standard meal in subjects with diseased and healthy livers. *Radiology* 1995;**196**(2):489–92.

41. Han SH, Rice S, Cohen SM, et al. Duplex Doppler ultrasound of the hepatic artery in patients with acute alcoholic hepatitis. *J Clin Gastroenterol* 2002;**34**(5):573–7.

42. Tanaka K, Numata K, Morimoto M, et al. Elevated resistive index in the hepatic artery as a predictor of fulminant hepatic failure in patients with acute viral hepatitis: a prospective study using Doppler ultrasound. *Dig Dis Sci* 2004;**49**(5):833–42.

43. Falkoff GE, Taylor KJ, Morse S. Hepatic artery pseudoaneurysm: diagnosis with real-time and pulsed Doppler US. *Radiology* 1986;**158**(1):55–6.

44. Finley DS, Hinojosa MW, Paya M, et al. Hepatic artery pseudoaneurysm: a report of seven cases and a review of the literature. *Surg Today* 2005;**35**(7):543–7.

45. Ocran K, Rickes S, Heukamp I, et al. Sonographic findings in hepatic involvement of hereditary haemorrhagic telangiectasia. *Ultraschall Med* 2004;**25**(3):191–4.

46. Memeo M, Scardapane A, De Blasi R, et al. Diagnostic imaging in the study of visceral involvement of hereditary haemorrhagic telangiectasia. *La Radiol Med* 2008;**113**(4):547–66.

47. Erden A. Budd-Chiari syndrome: a review of imaging findings. *Eur J Radiol* 2007;**61**(1):44–56.

48. Kew MC, Hodkinson HJ. Membranous obstruction of the inferior vena cava and its causal relation to hepatocellular carcinoma. *Liver Int* 2006;**26**(1):1–7.

49. Barakat M. Non-pulsatile hepatic and portal vein waveforms in patients with liver cirrhosis: concordant and discordant relationships. *Br J Radiol* 2004;**77**(919):547–50.

50. Janssen HL, Tan AC, Tilanus HW, et al. Pseudo-Budd-Chiari syndrome: decompensated alcoholic liver disease mimicking hepatic venous outflow obstruction. *Hepatogastroenterology* 2002;**49**(45):810–12.

51. Zhang Y, Yin J, Duan Y, et al. Assessment of intrahepatic blood flow by Doppler ultrasonography: relationship between the hepatic vein, portal vein, hepatic artery and portal pressure measured intraoperatively in patients with portal hypertension. *BMC Gastroenterol* 2011;**11**:84.

52. Mahgerefteh SY, Sosna J, Bogot N, et al. Radiologic imaging and intervention for gastrointestinal and hepatic complications of hematopoietic stem cell transplantation. *Radiology* 2011;**258**(3):660–71.

53. Coy DL, Ormazabal A, Godwin JD, et al. Imaging evaluation of pulmonary and abdominal complications following hematopoietic stem cell transplantation. *Radiographics* 2005;**25**(2):305–17.

54. Abu-Yousef MM. Duplex Doppler sonography of the hepatic vein in tricuspid regurgitation. *AJR Am J Roentgenol* 1991;**156**(1):79–83.

55. Jeong WK, Kim KW, Kim MY, et al. Increase of modified retrograde to antegrade flow ratio on Doppler ultrasounds of the hepatic vein indicating tricuspid regurgitation during follow-up of liver transplantation: correlation with echocardiographic results. *Transplant Proc* 2009;**41**(10):4238–42.

56. Tchelepi H, Ralls PW. Ultrasound of focal liver masses. *Ultrasound Q* 2004;**20**(4):155–69.

57. Kudo M. Diagnostic imaging of hepatocellular carcinoma: recent progress. *Oncology* 2011;**81**(Suppl. 1):73–85.

58. Murakami T, Imai Y, Okada M, et al. Ultrasonography, computed tomography and magnetic resonance imaging of hepatocellular carcinoma: toward improved treatment decisions. *Oncology* 2011;**81**(Suppl. 1):86–99.

59. Tochio H, Kudo M. Afferent and efferent vessels of premalignant and overt hepatocellular carcinoma: observation by color Doppler imaging. *Intervirology* 2004;**47**(3–5):144–53.

60. Gaiani S, Casali A, Serra C, et al. Assessment of vascular patterns of small liver mass lesions: value and limitation of the different Doppler ultrasound modalities. *Am J Gastroenterol* 2000;**95**(12):3537–46.

61. Bhatnagar G, Sidhu HS, Vardhanabhuti V, et al. The varied sonographic appearances of focal fatty liver disease: review and diagnostic algorithm. *Clin Radiol* 2012;**67**(4):372–9.

62. Hussain SM, Terkivatan T, Zondervan PE, et al. Focal nodular hyperplasia: findings at state-of-the-art MR imaging, US, CT, and pathologic analysis. *Radiographics* 2004;**24**(1):3–17.

63. Soresi M, Carroccio A, Campagna P, et al. Diagnosis of focal nodular hyperplasia. Role of imaging techniques. *Ann Ital Med Int* 2002;**17**(2):95–101.

64. Choi BY, Nguyen MH. The diagnosis and management of benign hepatic tumors. *J Clin Gastroenterol* 2005;**39**(5):401–12.

65. Rosch J, Hanafee WN, Snow H. Transjugular portal venography and radiologic portacaval shunt: an experimental study. *Radiology* 1969;**92**(5):1112–14.

66. Bhogal HK, Sanyal AJ. Using transjugular intrahepatic portosystemic shunts for complications of cirrhosis. *Clin Gastroenterol Hepatol* 2011;**9**(11):936–46.

67. Saad N, Darcy M, Saad W. Portal anatomic variants relevant to transjugular intrahepatic portosystemic shunt. *Tech Vasc Interv Radiol* 2008;**11**(4):203–7.

68. Darcy M. Evaluation and management of transjugular intrahepatic portosystemic shunts. *AJR Am J Roentgenol* 2012;**199**(4):730–6.

69. Feldstein VA, Patel MD, LaBerge JM. Transjugular intrahepatic portosystemic shunts: accuracy of Doppler US in determination of patency and detection of stenoses. *Radiology* 1996;**201**(1):141–7.

70. Foshager MC, Ferral H, Finlay DE, et al. Color Doppler sonography of transjugular intrahepatic portosystemic shunts (TIPS). *AJR Am J Roentgenol* 1994;**163**(1):105–11.

71. Longo JM, Bilbao JI, Rousseau HP, et al. Transjugular intrahepatic portosystemic shunt: evaluation with Doppler sonography. *Radiology* 1993;**186**(2):529–34.

72. Surratt RS, Middleton WD, Darcy MD, et al. Morphologic and hemodynamic findings at sonography before and after creation of a transjugular intrahepatic portosystemic shunt. *AJR Am J Roentgenol* 1993;**160**(3):627–30.

73. Charon JP, Alaeddin FH, Pimpalwar SA, et al. Results of a retrospective multicenter trial of the Viatorr expanded polytetrafluoroethylene-covered stent-graft for transjugular intrahepatic portosystemic shunt creation. *J Vasc Interv Radiol* 2004;**15**(11):1219–30.

74. Hausegger KA, Karnel F, Georgieva B, et al. Transjugular intrahepatic portosystemic shunt creation with the Viatorr expanded polytetrafluoroethylene-covered stent-graft. *J Vasc Interv Radiol* 2004;**15**(3):239–48.

75. Maleux G, Nevens F, Wilmer A, et al. Early and long-term clinical and radiological follow-up results of expanded-polytetrafluoroethylene-covered stent-grafts for transjugular intrahepatic portosystemic shunt procedures. *Eur Radiol* 2004;**14**(10):1842–50.

76. Dodd 3rd GD, Zajko AB, Orons PD, et al. Detection of transjugular intrahepatic portosystemic shunt dysfunction: value of duplex Doppler sonography. *AJR Am J Roentgenol* 1995;**164**(5):1119–24.

77. Chong WK, Malisch TA, Mazer MJ, et al. Transjugular intrahepatic portosystemic shunt: US assessment with maximum flow velocity. *Radiology* 1993;**189**(3):789–93.

78. Mituzani P, Saxon R, Alexander P. Duplex US screening after transjugular intrahepatic portosystemic shunt placement. *Radiology* 1993;**189**(P)(Suppl.):254.

79. Wachsberg RH. Doppler ultrasound evaluation of transjugular intrahepatic portosystemic shunt function: pitfalls and artifacts. *Ultrasound Q* 2003;**19**(3):139–48.

80. Zemel G, Katzen B, Grubbs G. Sonographic indicators of unsuccessful transjugular intrahepatic portosystemic shunt placement. *Radiology* 1994;**193**(P)(Suppl.):254.

81. Middleton WD, Teefey SA, Darcy MD. Doppler evaluation of transjugular intrahepatic portosystemic shunts. *Ultrasound Q* 2003;**19**(2):56–70.

Chapter 9

The Kidneys

Therese M. Weber, Michelle L. Robbin and Mark E. Lockhart

Renal Vascular Doppler Ultrasound

Ultrasound is the imaging modality of choice for evaluation of the kidneys, especially in patients with borderline renal function, the incidence of which is increasing. In comparison with other modalities, ultrasound has the distinct advantage of providing clinically diagnostic information without the need for ionising radiation or contrast agents. The combination of spectral, colour, and/or power Doppler is extremely helpful in renal vasculature evaluation.

CLINICAL CONSIDERATIONS

Common clinical indications for renal ultrasound include renal insufficiency and renal failure. Specifically, the request to exclude renal obstruction as the aetiology of acute renal failure leads the list. Doppler ultrasound is not routinely performed to evaluate acute renal failure but may be prompted by certain clinical indicators (Box 9-1) or greyscale findings. Colour and spectral Doppler is more commonly used in the native kidneys for evaluation of unexplained or uncontrolled hypertension caused by renal artery stenosis (RAS) or for determination of vessel patency. In hypertensive patients, some authors suggest Doppler should be reserved for those patients with a strong clinical suspicion for RAS who are likely to benefit from intervention.[1] As will be shown, there are many other vascular abnormalities than can be demonstrated by Doppler, and these can present with a wide variety of symptoms or signs.

TECHNICAL CONSIDERATIONS

Renal Doppler ultrasound can be one of the most challenging vascular ultrasound examinations. Extensive training and experience in performance and interpretation of the study will reduce examination time, improve study quality, and optimise diagnostic accuracy. A dedicated quality control programme is an important mechanism to assess accuracy and to review cases in which an incorrect diagnosis was made. The goal of this review process should be to improve the quality of future studies.

One common challenge in renal vascular ultrasound is direct visualisation of the proximal renal arteries. Overlying bowel gas may completely obscure the renal vascular origins and result in a nondiagnostic study. To improve the likelihood of a diagnostic study, we request that patients be fasting for at least 6 to 8 hours, when possible, to decrease bowel gas. Another limitation is the deep location of the native renal vessels, especially in obese patients, and utilisation of appropriate sonographic windows may be helpful. Graded transducer pressure can bring the transducer closer to the arteries and simultaneously displace overlying gas. However, the renal arteries occasionally may not be directly visualised despite optimal technique; in some of these technically difficult cases, the identification of segmental arterial waveform abnormalities may still allow successful diagnosis of RAS.

Main Renal Artery Evaluation

Doppler evaluation of the renal arteries should not occur without a thorough greyscale examination of the kidneys. Greyscale imaging can provide useful information about renal size and cortical thickness and should be part of the initial series of images. For Doppler image acquisition, a preliminary scan of the abdominal aorta is performed with colour Doppler in the transverse plane beginning at the level of the superior mesenteric artery (SMA) to locate the main renal arteries, which typically originate within 2 cm

CLINICAL CRITERIA USED TO SELECT WHO SHOULD BE EVALUATED FOR RENAL ARTERY STENOSIS (RAS)

- Hypertension with clinical concern for renal artery stenosis
- Hypertension uncontrolled by medical therapy
- Hypertension with abrupt onset
- Hypertension after ACE inhibitor
- Hypertension with discrepant renal size on greyscale US
- Audible abdominal bruit
- Patient with aortic aneurysm
- Patient with aortic dissection
- Patient with renal insufficiency at clinical risk for RAS
- Follow-up of known RAS after vascular therapy

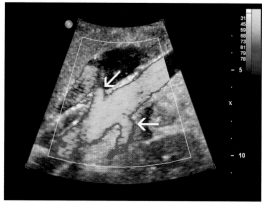

FIGURE 9-2 Normal renal arteries. Longitudinal power Doppler shows the aorta and both renal artery origins in normal location (arrows) with appearance termed as a 'banana peel'.

of the SMA (Fig. 9-1). Transverse images may be obtained from a midline approach with the patient supine or rolled into the left lateral decubitus position. The imager can localise the right renal artery passing posterior to the IVC then rotate the transducer while maintaining the artery in view. Also, the transducer can be placed longitudinally lateral to the rectus muscle resulting in a 'banana peel' image (Fig. 9-2), in which the aorta is the banana and the renal artery is the banana skin on each side, being peeled off the banana. If the main renal arteries cannot be demonstrated from the midline approach, a right or left lateral approach is used to follow each artery centrally from the renal hilum. Regardless of the technique used to

identify the renal artery origin, the entire main renal artery should be visualised sonographically. Lack of visibility of even a 10 mm segment of main renal artery will limit the sensitivity of the direct method for RAS. This is especially relevant in younger patients in whom fibromuscular dysplasia is a concern; stenosis in these patients may not be near the renal artery origins (described later). As part of the direct Doppler evaluation, the peak systolic velocity with angle correction should be measured at the renal artery origin, mid and distal artery, and at any region of turbulent disorganised flow with aliasing on colour Doppler.

Accessory renal arteries occur commonly (approximately 30% of kidneys), but are not always demonstrated sonographically. In fact, studies suggest that only 21–41% of accessory renal arteries are visualised by Doppler evaluation.[2,3] This low success rate has prompted some individuals to argue that sonographic evaluation for RAS is not sensitive enough as a screening study. However, Bude et al. found that less than 1% of accessory renal arteries were the only stenotic artery,[4] which essentially negates the significance of not visualising an accessory renal artery.

As mentioned earlier, the deep location of main renal arteries often limits their direct evaluation, and it will drive the choice of transducer. Lower-frequency transducers will have better sonographic depth penetration, with a trade-off of decreased spatial resolution. As a general rule, the highest-frequency transducer that allows good demonstration of the artery and arterial waveform is preferable.

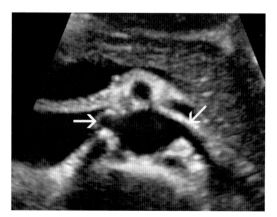

FIGURE 9-1 Normal renal arteries. Greyscale transverse image of the aorta demonstrates normal origins of the renal arteries (arrows).

Greyscale visualisation of the renal arteries should be optimised prior to colour and spectral Doppler evaluation. Doppler gain should be adjusted for flow detection by increasing the gain to a level just below the appearance of colour artifact in adjacent structures. Pulse repetition frequency, or velocity scale, is the frequency of sampling, and under-sampling may underestimate peak velocities. In newer systems, built-in software can automatically optimise these parameters, with manual adjustment occasionally required by the sonographer. For spectral Doppler, the Doppler gate should be set to include the entire arterial lumen and angled to the direction of flow. The angle of insonation should be maintained at 60 degrees or less. As angulation increases to 80–90 degrees, the confidence in the measured velocity decreases, as the cosine of the angle of insonation approaches zero. This yields large differences in measured velocity for a small variation in the relative angle of flow.

Segmental Intrarenal Artery Evaluation

When the main renal artery is not well seen in its entirety, evaluation of the segmental intrarenal arteries may allow a non-diagnostic direct examination to become diagnostic for RAS.[5,6] We always examine the segmental arteries even when the main renal arteries are well seen, because the segmental artery waveform morphology may be useful in detecting concomitant renal parenchymal disease.

A posterior flank approach reduces the distance from the transducer to the segmental arteries. Of note, the liver and spleen should not be used as a window to improve visualisation of the kidney, as the vessels are closer to a zero degree angle with the transducer positioned using a more posterior approach. The upper, interpolar, and lower pole segmental arteries are individually studied. A heel–toe technique is commonly applied in which one edge of the transducer is angled into the skin to align the targeted segmental artery flow as close to the transducer angle of insonation (theta less than 20 degrees) as possible to enhance the signal quality. This can enhance the definition of the early systolic peaks. Electronic beam steering can also be used to better align angulation of the insonating beam to enhance waveform morphology.

Characteristics of the spectral Doppler tracing in normal segmental intrarenal arteries should include rapid upstroke to an early systolic peak with gentle decrease in flow velocity during late systole and diastole (Fig. 9-3). Persistent antegrade flow throughout the cardiac cycle should be present without return to baseline. The resistive index (RI), calculated as:

$$\frac{\text{Peak systolic velocity (PSV)} - \text{End diastolic velocity (EDV)}}{\text{Peak systolic velocity (PSV)}}$$

is a common parameter for characterisation of arterial flow. The RI is inversely proportionate to the relative amount of diastolic flow. For instance, an end diastolic

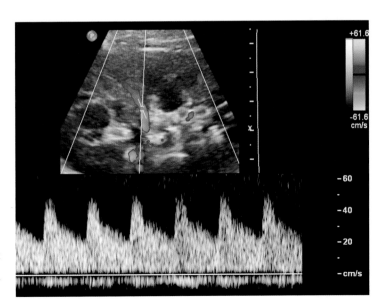

FIGURE 9-3 Normal segmental artery waveform. Colour Doppler shows normal colour flow without aliasing. Spectral Doppler shows rapid upstroke and smooth velocity decline with persistent flow throughout the cardiac cycle.

velocity that is 20% of the peak flow will result in RI of 0.80. The upper limit of RI in normal adults has been reported as less than 0.70,[7] but concern for pathology is not often raised until the RI is 0.75–0.80, or higher. Furthermore, the RI may be affected by other factors such as heart rate, Valsalva, and arterial compliance. In fact, RIs greater than 0.70 are common in elderly patients.[8] The impact of systemic vascular disease in chronic renal dysfunction is significant. It has been recently suggested that the renal RI measurement does not distinguish local from systemic vascular damage. A new potential ultrasound measurement, the difference of RIs between the spleen and kidney, may allow more specific evaluation of renal parenchymal damage.[9] However, this study has not yet been further validated or widely applied in practice.

Anatomy of the Native Kidneys

ARTERIAL ANATOMY

The renal arteries typically arise from the abdominal aorta caudal to the level of the SMA. The right renal artery usually originates from the anterolateral aspect of the aorta, while the left renal artery usually originates from the posterolateral aspect. As noted earlier, approximately 30% of patients will have more than one renal artery.[10] Accessory renal arteries usually arise from the aorta caudal to the main renal artery to supply the renal lower pole, but occasionally will course cranially to supply the upper pole. Rarely, accessory arteries may arise from an iliac artery or even the SMA. Renal anomalies such as horseshoe or pelvic kidney almost always have multiple renal arteries, which may arise from the aorta or iliac arteries.

The main renal artery divides into dorsal and ventral rami that course posterior and anterior to the renal pelvis. The anterior and superior aspects of the kidney are typically supplied by the larger ventral division. The posterior and inferior portions of the kidney are supplied by the smaller dorsal division. The junction of these ventral and dorsal divisions creates a relatively avascular plane (Brodel's line), which is the preferred track of percutaneous nephrostomy placement, and should be considered when performing a renal biopsy.

The branching pattern of the renal arteries progresses symmetrically to the renal cortex (Fig. 9-4).

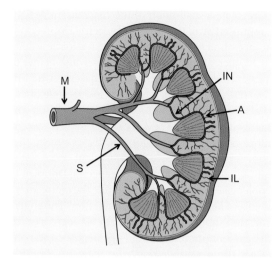

FIGURE 9-4 Renal arterial branching. Line drawing demonstrates the normal arterial branching from the main artery (M) to the segmental (S), interlobar (IN), arcuate (A), and interlobular (IL) arteries.

Segmental branches arise from the dorsal and ventral rami and run along the infundibulae before dividing into interlobar arteries. These interlobar arteries course between the pyramids, and then branch into arcuate arteries, which run along the bases of medullary pyramids. Within the cortex, small interlobular arteries course outward toward the surface of the kidney.

VENOUS ANATOMY

The renal venous anatomy parallels the arterial anatomy. Normal venous flow on spectral Doppler has a relatively low velocity. Its waveform is driven by right atrial activity. Accessory left renal veins are less frequent than accessory renal arteries; however, accessory right renal veins are quite common. Left venous anomalies may be seen in approximately 11% of patients.[11] Variants most commonly include the retroaortic and circumaortic renal veins (Fig. 9-5), and these may be clinically relevant even beyond filter placement. In a recent study by Karazincir et al., the incidence of retroaortic left renal vein was found to be significantly higher in patients with varicocele, compared with controls[12] (see Fig. 9-24 in the varicocele section).

The left renal vein receives drainage from the inferior phrenic, capsular, ureteric, adrenal and gonadal

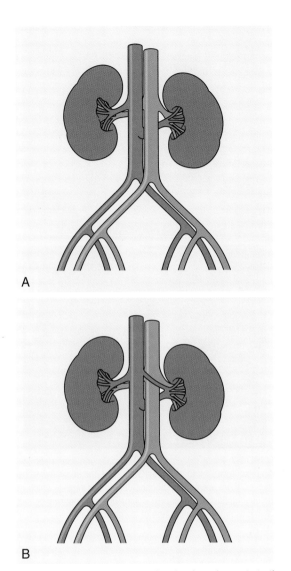

A

B

FIGURE 9-5 Renal vein variants. Line drawings demonstrate the anatomic appearance of a retroaortic (A), and circumaortic (B) left renal vein.

veins and flows across midline into the normal IVC. In patients with a left-sided IVC, the left common iliac vein continues cranially as the left IVC and drains into the inferior aspect of the left renal vein. The right renal vein is shorter than the left and courses obliquely into the IVC. The right renal vein receives capsular and ureteric veins; however, the right inferior phrenic and gonadal veins enter directly into the IVC. Valves may be present within the renal veins, but their reported incidence varies greatly. Renal vein varices may be secondary to renal vein thrombosis or portal hypertension, or they may be idiopathic. Like varicoceles, renal varices are more common on the left than the right. In cases of left renal vein thrombosis, the varices may extend through the inferior phrenic, adrenal, gonadal, and ureteric veins. On the right, the only common branch is the ureteric vein.

Renal Failure and Obstruction

Doppler can play a supportive role in the diagnosis or exclusion of renal obstruction in patients with acute renal failure. Identification of a dilated renal collecting system is fairly easy with ultrasound. The difficulty, however (in the absence of prior examinations) is the differentiation of an acutely obstructed high-pressure system versus that of a low-pressure, chronically dilated system. It has been suggested that elevated resistive index may help differentiate between severe acute urinary obstruction and chronic dilatation.[13–15] The RI of the obstructed kidney may be elevated relative to the normal contralateral kidney. An RI difference of greater than 0.10 between the non-obstructed and obstructed kidney is the suggested threshold for diagnosis of acute obstructed uropathy. However, intrarenal autoregulatory hormonal systems counteract the mechanical effect of the high-pressure collecting system pressing upon the parenchyma. This rapidly modifies the resistance to flow, reducing sensitivity of the test. In the setting of partial obstruction or less severe obstruction, this finding also lacks sensitivity.[16,17] As an aside, in cases of chronic renal disease without obstruction, elevated RI > 0.80 has been shown to be associated with worsening renal function and mortality.[18]

Another Doppler tool to assist in the evaluation of urinary obstruction can be performed within the bladder. In cases with suspected renal obstruction, sonographic evaluation for a ureteral jet should be a component of the renal ultrasound examination (Fig. 9-6). Although entry of urine into the urinary bladder is not synchronous, demonstration of three or more ureteral jets by Doppler on one side without a single pulse of flow from the contralateral side implies obstruction of the non-pulsing ureter.

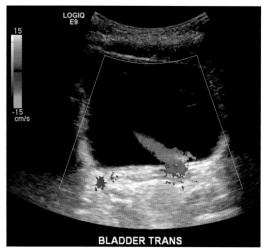

FIGURE 9-6 Normal ureteral jet. Transverse colour Doppler image shows a linear 'jet' of colour projecting into the bladder lumen. This represents the rapid flow of urine into the bladder secondary to ureteral peristalsis.

Renal Infection

Renal ultrasound examination is not routinely requested in cases of renal infection and ultrasound findings are quite variable in these cases. Renal parenchymal infection may be global or focal and the route of spread may be ascending or blood-borne. More common ultrasound findings, not consistently seen, are enlargement or altered echogenicity of the affected kidney. The presence of perinephric fluid would add confidence. Demonstration of altered blood flow, with reduction of Doppler indices and perfusion in an affected renal segment adds confidence to the diagnosis of focal pyelonephritis.

Nephrolithiasis

Colour Doppler evaluation should be a routine component of the renal ultrasound examination when nephrolithiasis is suspected. Greyscale alone has poor sensitivity for small renal stones. Using colour Doppler, twinkle artifact[19] can increase confidence in the presence of renal, ureteral or bladder stones (Fig. 9-7). The irregular surface of the calculus causes a Doppler shift which manifests as a noisy colour and spectral signal. This helps confirm that a bright echogenic focus within the renal hilum is indeed a calculus,

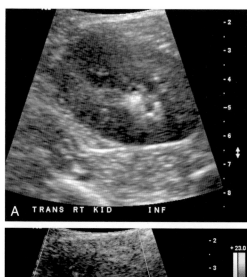

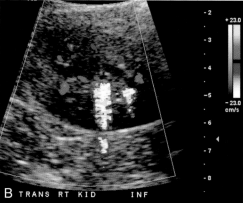

FIGURE 9-7 Renal calculus. (A). Greyscale ultrasound shows an echogenic focus in the calyceal region of the renal lower pole. However, there are other echogenic foci in this region, which may represent additional stones. (B) Colour Doppler confirms presence of two calculi with visualisation of 'twinkle' artifact.

rather than bright echogenic renal hilar adipose tissue. This technique should be used to demonstrate the presence of the stone, not to measure size of the stone. This is an especially useful adjunct to evaluate for distal ureteral stone with endovaginal technique when a dilated upper renal collecting system is identified in pregnancy (Fig. 9-8).

Renal Tumours

Greyscale ultrasound is the primary sonographic technique for detection of a renal tumour, but colour Doppler can provide additional information for

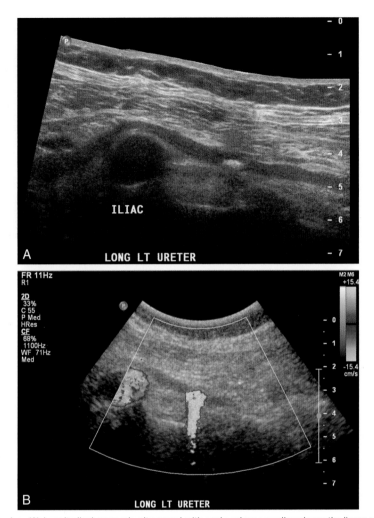

FIGURE 9-8 Ureteral calculus. (A) Longitudinal greyscale ultrasound with sepia colour encoding shows the linear anechoic distal ureter with a shadowing echogenic focus. (B) Colour Doppler confirms the presence of a ureteral stone with 'twinkle' artifact.

surgical planning. Colour Doppler may be useful in intraoperative ultrasound examinations when trying to precisely identify the depth of tumour invasion (Fig. 9-9). Colour Doppler may also be helpful to confirm the extent of renal cell tumour invasion into the inferior vena cava (Fig. 9-10). This may be helpful for surgical planning by clearly delineating the cranial extent of tumour. Colour Doppler can help confirm whether tumour involves the intrahepatic portion of the IVC, which would significantly increase the complexity of surgical removal. The presence of arterial signal within the thrombus confirms it as tumour thrombus (versus bland thrombus).

Renal Vascular Abnormalities

RAS/HYPERTENSION

Renal vascular disease is an uncommon cause of hypertension; however, it is potentially curable, and is most commonly considered in young adult patients with abrupt onset of hypertension and uncontrolled or rapidly accelerating hypertension. Stenotic renovascular disease has two primary aetiologies, atherosclerosis and fibromuscular dysplasia. In older patients the underlying aetiology is most frequently renal ostial atherosclerotic disease. The second most common aetiology is fibromuscular dysplasia, which is an

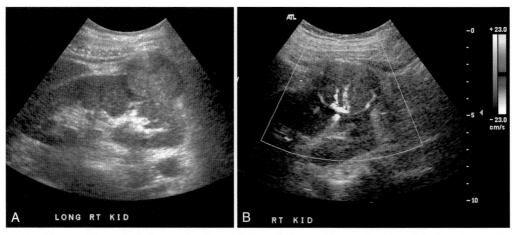

FIGURE 9-9 Renal tumour. (A) Longitudinal greyscale ultrasound demonstrates a solid exophytic mass arising from the renal lower pole. (B) Colour Doppler clearly depicts the margins of the tumour and the presence of vessels along its periphery. This allows better definition of the depth of invasion to aid in surgical planning.

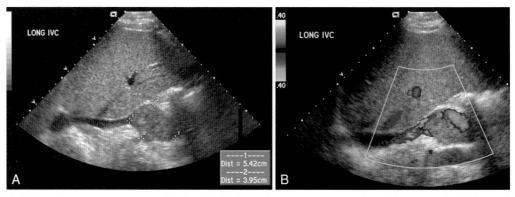

FIGURE 9-10 Renal tumour venous extension into the IVC. (A) Greyscale image shows expansion of the infrahepatic IVC by a solid lesion (calipers). (B) The addition of colour Doppler helps delineate the cranial extent of the tumour thrombus.

uncommon disorder seen most frequently in younger women, and unlike atherosclerotic lesions, generally responds well to angioplasty.[20,21] The role of imaging is influenced by the potential benefit of intervention.[1] Although renal artery stenosis can be identified with imaging, recent studies suggest that simply the identification of stenosis does not justify invasive treatment by stenting. Two recent randomised trials, including the ASTRAL study, have shown no benefit to revascularisation of atherosclerotic lesions, with regards to either blood pressure or renal function.[22,23] The ASTRAL study found that there was

no significant difference in two randomised cohorts of patients between medical management versus stent therapy for the treatment of RAS. The long-standing ischaemic insult to the renal parenchyma with associated cholesterol crystal embolisation causes significant damage that does not benefit from reestablishment of more normal flow through the main renal artery. Evaluation of renal perfusion in the presence of stenosis may be more useful to select patients who will benefit from intervention. Some authors have suggested Doppler measurement of resistive index, with high resistance behind a stenosis indicating significant parenchymal damage. A patient with a low-resistance tardus-parvus waveform may, however, still benefit. Recent advances in MR perfusion technology allow measurement of perfusion/diffusion and tissue oxygenation, making it more accurate in this prediction.

The results of the ASTRAL trial have stirred much controversy in the literature. Recent reviews suggest there still may be a role for imaging and stenting in patients with acute-onset hypertension or rapidly accelerating hypertension. This is suggested for those patients in whom parenchymal renal damage has not yet advanced to the point of irreversible hypertension.

Although CT and MR angiography are probably used more frequently for evaluation of RAS in most institutions, ultrasound is an ideal initial screening study because of the lack of ionising radiation or contrast administration. In ultrasound programmes experienced with renal vascular ultrasound, recent studies have shown the sensitivity and specificity of Doppler ultrasound for RAS is up to 95% and 90%, respectively.[24]

There are two main methods for sonographic detection of RAS: direct demonstration of RAS and indirect assessment of the downstream effect of the stenosis on the segmental renal arteries[25] (Box 9-2). Greyscale findings are first considered and a renal length disparity greater than 2 cm with cortical thinning should raise concern for the diagnosis. Visualisation of turbulent flow within the renal artery on colour Doppler suggests an area of stenosis.[26] Increased velocities in the focal area of stenosis may appear as colour aliasing if the

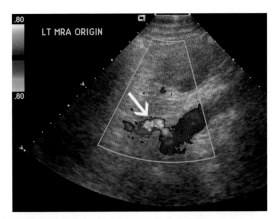

FIGURE 9-11 Renal artery stenosis. Turbulent flow may appear as 'aliasing' on colour Doppler (arrow) as elevated velocities wrap around into the lower colour scale.

velocity is beyond the scale limits and wraps into the other end of the colour scale (Fig. 9-11), and should lead to close evaluation with spectral Doppler in this area. Spectral Doppler confirmation of RAS relies primarily on demonstration of elevated PSV and demonstration of disturbed flow distal to the lesion.

Varying criteria have been suggested for the direct spectral Doppler diagnosis of RAS, which has resulted in controversy. A PSV of greater than 200 cm/s (Fig. 9-12) has been suggested for Doppler diagnosis of 60% diameter reduction of the renal artery.[27,28] In a recent meta-analysis, PSV was the best critical factor in diagnosing RAS, with sensitivity and specificity of 85% and 92%, respectively.[29] The ratio of the renal artery PSV to the aortic PSV (RA/Ao) is another criterion suggested for diagnosis of RAS. An RA/Ao PSV ratio of greater than 3.5:1 (Fig. 9-13) suggests significant RAS, yielding 91% sensitivity and 91% specificity.[30] An elevated ratio of peak renal artery systolic velocity to distal renal artery systolic velocity has also been suggested as a criterion for diagnosis of RAS.[31,32] One study of 187 renal arteries with angiographic correlation also showed an absolute renal interlobar PSV of less than 15 cm/s resulted in 87% and 91% sensitivity and specificity, respectively, for Doppler diagnosis of 50% stenosis.[32] Jian-Chu et al. have recently studied the impact of atherosclerosis and age on Doppler sonographic parameters for the diagnosis of RAS and suggest that use of the renal-aortic ratio and renal-interlobar ratio diagnostic

BOX 9-2 SUMMARY OF DOPPLER PARAMETERS FOR DIAGNOSIS OF RAS

- Elevated peak systolic velocity (PSV)
- Elevated PSV ratio of renal artery relative to aorta
- Focal aliasing in renal artery on colour Doppler due to turbulent flow
- Asymmetry of segmental artery resistive indices relative to contralateral kidney
- Segmental artery loss of early systolic peaks
- Segmental artery delayed systolic acceleration (tardus)
- Segmental artery low peak velocity (parvus)

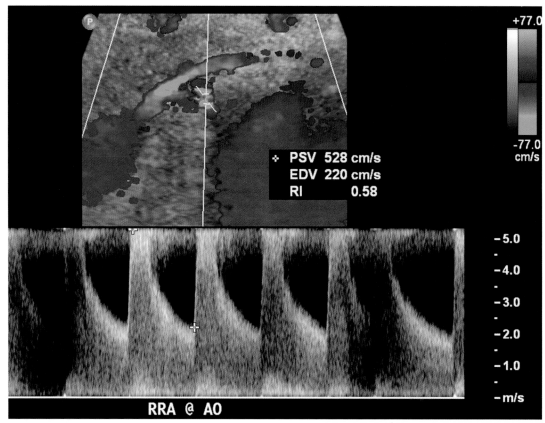

+77.0

PSV 528 cm/s
EDV 220 cm/s
RI   0.58

-77.0
cm/s

-5.0
-
-4.0
-
-3.0
-
-2.0
-
-1.0
-
-m/s

RRA @ AO

FIGURE 9-12 Renal artery stenosis. Duplex Doppler shows a region of colour Doppler aliasing (Doppler gate), and the peak systolic velocity measures 528 cm/s, which is above the 200 cm/s threshold.

thresholds differ in patients older versus younger than 46 years. Other sonographic criteria were not substantially affected by patient age in their study.[33]

The indirect method of RAS assessment of segmental renal artery waveforms becomes important when the entire length of the main renal artery cannot be directly seen with ultrasound. Stavros et al.[5,34] have suggested that normal intrarenal waveform morphology with early systolic peak in the upper, interpolar, and lower pole segmental renal arteries may be used to adequately exclude significant RAS. This normal compliance peak (Fig. 9-14) is not present when there is flow-limiting stenosis in the proximal artery, although others have found this sign less sensitive.[35]

Another criterion of RAS is prolonged acceleration time of greater than 0.07 second. Acceleration time is the time interval from onset of systole to the early

systolic peak. In blunted waveforms, this early peak may be absent, and the measurement should extend from onset of systole to the first point of deflection.[36] The presence of the tardus–parvus waveform morphology is helpful in the diagnosis of severe RAS; however, its absence does not exclude RAS.[37] The tardus–parvus spectral waveform is defined by the slow upstroke (the tardus) and spectral broadening with blunting of the systolic peak (the parvus) (Fig. 9-15). It is important to note that in patients with atherosclerotic disease, vessel compliance may be diminished, making the tardus–parvus waveform morphology less obvious.[38]

A less common criterion suggested for diagnosis of RAS is excessive difference in RI of the two kidneys (≥ 0.07).[5,39] For lesser degrees of stenosis, the abnormal kidney will show lower RIs beyond the point of stenosis due to post-stenotic dilatation. However, as

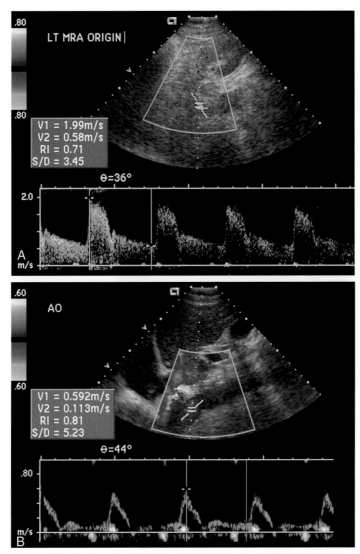

FIGURE 9-13 Renal artery stenosis. (A) Duplex Doppler of renal artery demonstrates borderline peak systolic velocity, 199 cm/s. (B) Spectral Doppler waveform of the aorta shows peak velocity is 59 cm/s. The calculated renal artery-aortic peak systolic velocity ratio of 3.72 is above the 3.5 threshold, suggesting significant stenosis.

the stenosis becomes more flow limiting, there may not be persistence of flow throughout the cardiac cycle, resulting in a high RI.

Another potential application of Doppler is for follow-up to assess for restenosis in patients after stent placement for RAS (Fig. 9-16). This may be ordered due to worsening renal function or even when clinical signs of restenosis are absent. In a study of 64 stented patients without clinical suspicion of restenosis, 22 patients had elevated PSV of greater than 200 cm/s and had significantly worsened rate of renal function decline than those patients with PSV of less than 200 cm/s.[40] In 6 of 11 of these patients with this criterion who underwent angiography despite the lack of clinical suspicion, all had restenosis of greater than 70% at angiography.

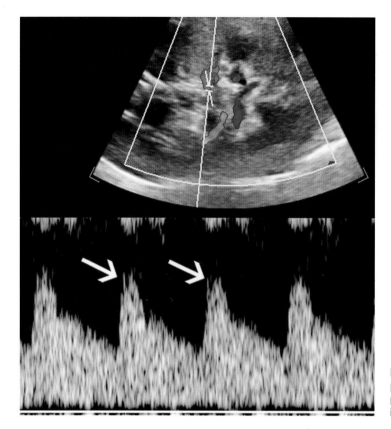

FIGURE 9-14 Normal segmental artery compliance peak. Duplex Doppler shows an early systolic small peak (arrows) at the point of peak systolic velocity in the absence of upstream stenosis.

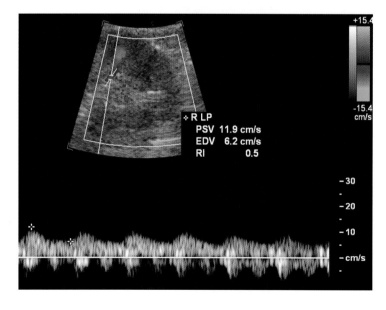

FIGURE 9-15 Renal artery stenosis. On duplex Doppler of a lower pole segmental artery, the delayed systolic acceleration (tardus) and small waveform (parvus) are consistent with upstream stenosis and further main renal artery evaluation is warranted if a stenosis has not yet been directly visualised.

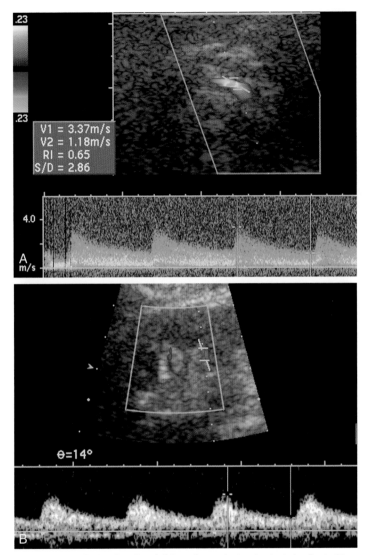

FIGURE 9-16 Restenosis after stenting. (A) Duplex Doppler of right main renal artery in stented patient with recurrent hypertension shows elevated PSV in region of colour aliasing. (B) Spectral Doppler of a segmental renal artery demonstrates tardus-parvus waveform.

INTRARENAL VASCULAR DISEASE

Intrarenal vascular disease such as polyarteritis nodosa (PAN), Wegener's granulomatosis, and scleroderma cannot routinely be diagnosed with renovascular Doppler ultrasound. Renal artery thrombosis, embolisation, ischaemia and infarction should be detectable by Doppler ultrasound. Visible structural renal vascular lesions may include renal artery aneurysm (RAA) or arteriovenous malformation.

RENAL ARTERY THROMBOSIS

Complete thrombosis of the native renal artery is uncommon except in the setting of stents or bypass grafts for abdominal aortic aneurysm repair, or in the setting of trauma. In the setting of trauma, there may be avulsion of the renal artery with or without extravasation. Traumatic dissection of the artery can also result in arterial occlusion, and can have similar Doppler findings as renal artery avulsion. Asymmetric

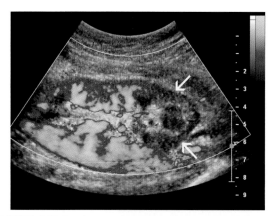

FIGURE 9-17 Renal artery thrombosis. No parenchymal flow is visible in the lower pole (arrows) on power Doppler. When there is absence of normal flow on routine colour Doppler, then power Doppler should be performed due to its higher sensitivity for slow flow.

lack of flow may involve the entire kidney or a segment, dependent on the level of the abnormality. Colour Doppler can show a perfusion defect, but power Doppler is often used to characterise any slow flow in this region. If no flow is identified, optimisation of the Doppler settings should be performed using the contralateral kidney prior to an additional insonation of the affected kidney.

A regional lack of power Doppler flow in the renal parenchyma with wedge-shaped appearance suggests segmental infarction (Fig. 9-17). Search for other similar abnormalities in the contralateral kidney or other organs should be performed since this may be due to showering of emboli from a remote source.

RENAL ARTERY ANEURYSM

The diagnosis of renal artery aneurysm or pseudoaneurysm is most commonly made by CT or MRI. However, there are findings on Doppler that may be seen in this abnormality. It may appear as a vascular structure that is fusiform, eccentric, and saccular. RAA commonly arise from a branch point within the artery. On colour Doppler, there may be circular flow with a 'yin-yang' appearance (Fig. 9-18). A portion of the aneurysm may be thrombosed. It is common for RAA to have peripheral calcifications, and these may limit sonographic evaluation of central flow.

ARTERIOVENOUS FISTULA AND MALFORMATIONS (AVF AND AVM)

Arteriovenous fistula in the native kidney is rare except in cases of prior renal biopsy and will not be suspected sonographically if colour or power Doppler is not evaluated. Colour or power Doppler characteristically will show a large tortuous cluster of vessels. Spectral Doppler waveforms of the renal arteries feeding the fistula will show high velocity and low resistance (Fig. 9-19). The main renal vein may be dilated and arterialised waveforms may be found in veins near the fistula (Fig. 9-20).

VENOUS DISEASE
Renal Vein Thrombosis

Renal vein thrombosis (RVT) of the native kidneys is seen more commonly in the paediatric population than in adults. In adults, the underlying aetiology may include dehydration and nephrotic syndrome,[41] hypercoagulable state, or trauma to the renal vein. Visualisation of renal vein flow with Doppler is critical in patients with clinical suspicion for acute RVT. It is important to demonstrate the entire renal vein before excluding renal vein thrombosis because the native kidney may develop collaterals quickly.

The diagnosis of RVT is based upon demonstration of thrombus filling the renal vein (Fig. 9-21) or non-occlusive thrombus surrounded by venous flow. In some cases, the vein may be expanded by the thrombus. The absence of flow in the renal vein without demonstration of thrombus may suggest RVT; however, demonstration of low-level colour signal within the vein on Doppler does not exclude the possibility of non-occlusive or occlusive renal vein thrombus. Monophasic venous waveforms are abnormal but not specific for RVT.[42] Because of the potential for thrombus to extend cranially within the IVC (Fig. 9-22) and the effect on clinical management, the IVC should be imaged as part of the sonographic examination when evaluating for RVT.

Renal vein thrombus may also be seen in patients with renal cell carcinoma if there is tumour extension into the renal vein. In these cases arterial flow may be seen within the thrombus on spectral Doppler.

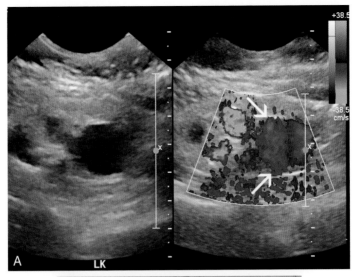

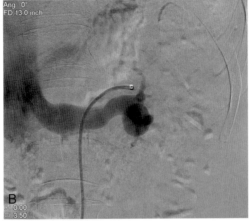

FIGURE 9-18 Renal artery aneurysm. (A) Split image shows anechoic round structure on greyscale with flow on colour Doppler. The circular flow on colour Doppler (arrows), termed the 'yin-yang' sign, can be seen with aneurysm or pseudoaneurysm. (B) On angiography, the typical round vascular structure of an aneurysm is confirmed.

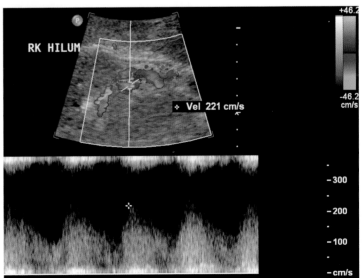

FIGURE 9-19 Arteriovenous fistula. Spectral Doppler shows high-velocity pulsatile arterial flow with low resistance near the renal hilum.

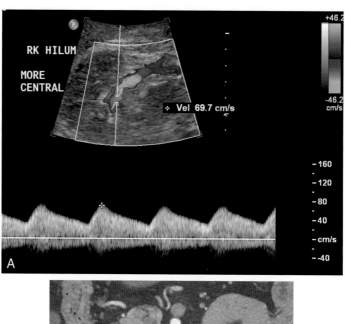

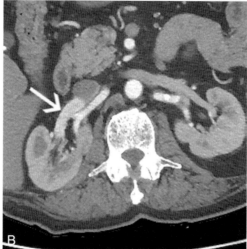

FIGURE 9-20 Arteriovenous fistula. (A) Spectral Doppler demonstrates arterialised venous flow with high velocities and low resistance. (B) CT angiography shows early enhancement of right renal vein (arrow), compared with the left renal vein.

Nutcracker Syndrome

The 'nutcracker' phenomenon results from compression of the left renal vein between the superior mesenteric artery and the aorta and may lead to left renal vein hypertension, haematuria, and varix formation. It is important to remember that a distended left renal vein may be seen in some of the normal population by CT, MR, or ultrasound. Therefore, other criteria should be applied, including a high Doppler velocity ratio

(Fig. 9-23) and high venous diameter ratio as described in recent literature.[43] Due to the complexity of the potential surgical repair, measurement of a pressure gradient between the IVC and the left renal vein may be needed as confirmation before clinically significant renal vein compression is diagnosed. Visualisation of blood from the ureteral orifice on retrograde ureteroscopy may also be supportive. Colour flow Doppler may provide noninvasive evidence of renal vein

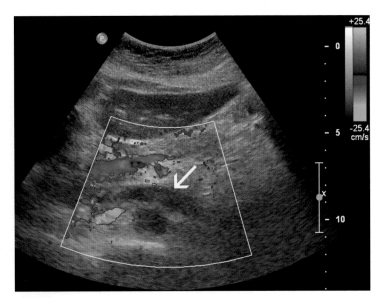

FIGURE 9-21 Renal vein thrombus. On colour Doppler, low-level echoes fill the left renal vein with absence of complete Doppler flow filling of the lumen (arrow).

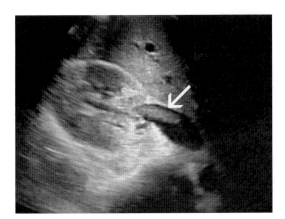

FIGURE 9-22 Renal vein thrombus. Greyscale image of the right renal vein shows linear thrombus (arrow) extending into the IVC. In this patient, the thrombus was mobile during cardiac pulsations, worrisome for potential subsequent embolisation.

compression with peak velocity ratio greater than 5:1 when collateral veins are demonstrated. On CT, there may be a sharp change in venous calibre as the vein crosses the SMA, usually with a 'beaked' appearance.

Varicocele Formation

Varicocele is dilatation of the pampiniform venous plexus seen on testicular ultrasound examination,

and is more common on the left due to anatomical factors of angle of insertion of the gonadal vein into the left renal vein and potential for compression of the left renal vein by the SMA. The primary type of varicocele is associated with incompetent valves, and the secondary type is associated with increased venous pressure due to obstructed venous outflow. Isolated right varicocele is uncommon and should warrant further evaluation of the right retroperitoneal area and kidney to exclude a right renal hilar mass or adenopathy compressing venous outflow. Diagnosis of varicocele is made on testicular ultrasound examination when the veins in the spermatic cord area are dilated to greater than 2 to 3 mm in diameter (Fig. 9-24). Rarely, the varix may be intratesticular in location. In some cases, colour Doppler of the dilated veins may show intraluminal thrombus. Reversal of venous flow at rest with increased reversed flow during Valsalva is suggestive of the diagnosis, but in some patients there may only be reversal during Valsalva.[44] Techniques used to improve detection of varicocele include Valsalva or standing position. As noted earlier, a recent study by Karazincir et al. showed the incidence of retroaortic left renal vein was significantly higher in patients with varicocele compared with controls.[12]

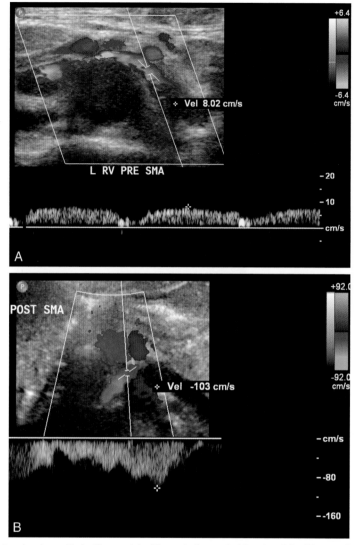

FIGURE 9-23 Renal vein nutcracker. In a patient with unexplained haematuria, spectral Doppler of the (A) preaortic left renal vein demonstrates normal low-velocity flow, 8 cm/s. (B) As the vein crosses between the aorta and SMA (Doppler gate), there is visible narrowing with elevated peak systolic velocity, 103 cm/s.

Summary

Ultrasound plays an important role in the diagnosis and management of renal disease. Ultrasound also plays an extremely important role in the initial evaluation for RAS. The quality and accuracy of

vascular ultrasound is dependent on the volume of cases, as well as the skill and experience of the sonographers and sonologists interpreting the examination. The high attention to detail required in performing and interpreting renal vascular ultrasound examinations will continue to limit its widespread

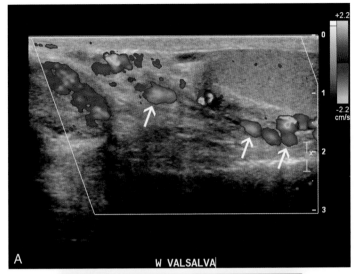

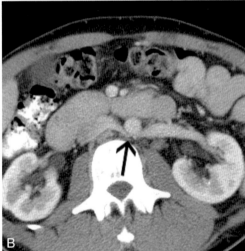

FIGURE 9-24 Varicocele. (A) Colour Doppler shows dilatation and increased flow within the vessels (arrows) of the spermatic cord and scrotum during Valsalva measuring greater than 3 mm diameter. In the setting of borderline findings, standing position of the patient may accentuate the finding. (B) CT in the same patient shows retroaortic left renal vein (black arrow).

application, as compared to CTA and MRA examinations. However, renal vascular ultrasound will continue to offer the strong advantage of not requiring potentially nephrotoxic intravenous contrast agents in patients with diminished renal function or acute renal failure. Future improvements in ultrasound technology and more widespread practice of optimal techniques should be able to keep up with the predicted increase in patients with renal insufficiency.

REFERENCES

1. O'Neill WC, Bardelli M, Yevzlin AS. Imaging for renovascular disease. *Semin Nephrol* 2011 May;**31**(3):272–82.
2. Aytac SK, Yigit H, Sancak T, Ozcan H. Correlation between the diameter of the main renal artery and the presence of an accessory renal artery: sonographic and angiographic evaluation. *J Ultrasound Med* 2003 May;**22**(5):433–9; quiz 440–2.
3. Halpern EJ, Nazarian LN, Wechsler RJ, et al. US, CT, and MR evaluation of accessory renal arteries and proximal renal arterial branches. *Acad Radiol* 1999 May;**6**(5):299–304.

4. Bude RO, Forauer AR, Caoili EM, Nghiem HV. Is it necessary to study accessory arteries when screening the renal arteries for renovascular hypertension? *Radiology* 2003 Feb;**226**(2):411–16.

5. Stavros T, Harshfield D. Renal Doppler, renal artery stenosis, and renovascular hypertension: direct and indirect duplex sonographic abnormalities in patients with renal artery stenosis. *Ultrasound Q* 1994;**12**(4):217–64.

6. Radermacher J, Chavan A, Schaffer J, et al. Detection of significant renal artery stenosis with colour Doppler sonography: combining extrarenal and intrarenal approaches to minimize technical failure. *Clin Nephrol* 2000 May;**53**(5):333–43.

7. Platt JF. Duplex Doppler evaluation of native kidney dysfunction: obstructive and nonobstructive disease. *AJR Am J Roentgenol* 1992 May;**158**(5):1035–42.

8. Tublin ME, Bude RO, Platt JF. Review. The resistive index in renal Doppler sonography: where do we stand? *AJR Am J Roentgenol* 2003;Apr;**180**(4):885–92.

9. Grun OS, Herath E, Weihrauch A, et al. Does the measurement of the difference of resistive indexes in spleen and kidney allow a selective assessment of chronic kidney injury? *Radiology* 2012 Sep;**264**(3):894–902.

10. Cochran ST, Krasny RM, Danovitch GM, et al. Helical CT angiography for examination of living renal donors. *AJR Am J Roentgenol* 1997 Jun;**168**(6):1569–73.

11. Kawamoto S, Montgomery RA, Lawler LP, Horton KM, Fishman EK. Multidetector CT angiography for preoperative evaluation of living laparoscopic kidney donors. *AJR Am J Roentgenol* 2003 Jun;**180**(6):1633–8.

12. Karazincir S, Balci A, Gorur S, Sumbas H, Kiper AN. Incidence of the retroaortic left renal vein in patients with varicocele. *J Ultrasound Med* 2007 May;**26**(5):601–4.

13. Gottlieb RH, Luhmann Kt, Oates RP. Duplex ultrasound evaluation of normal native kidneys and native kidneys with urinary tract obstruction. *J Ultrasound Med* 1989 Nov;**8**(11):609–11.

14. Platt JF, Rubin JM, Ellis JH. Acute renal obstruction: evaluation with intrarenal duplex Doppler and conventional US. *Radiology* 1993 Mar;**186**(3):685–8.

15. Shokeir AA, Abdulmaaboud M. Resistive index in renal colic: a prospective study. *BJU Internat* 1999 Mar;**83**(4):378–82.

16. Chen JH, Pu YS, Liu SP, Chiu TY. Renal hemodynamics in patients with obstructive uropathy evaluated by duplex Doppler sonography. *J Urol* 1993 Jul;**150**(1):18–21.

17. Gurel S, Akata D, Gurel K, Ozmen MN, Akhan O. Correlation between the renal resistive index (RI) and nonenhanced computed tomography in acute renal colic: how reliable is the RI in distinguishing obstruction? *Am J Roentgenol: official journal of the American Institute of Ultrasound in Medicine* 2006 Sep;**25**(9):1113–20; quiz 1121–3.

18. Radermacher J, Ellis S, Haller H. Renal resistance index and progression of renal disease. *Hypertension* 2002 Feb;**39**(2 Pt 2):699–703.

19. Lee JY, Kim SH, Cho JY, Han D. Colour and power Doppler twinkling artifacts from urinary stones: clinical observations and phantom studies. *AJR Am J Roentgenol* 2001 Jun;**176**(6):1441–5.

20. Dworkin LD, Cooper CJ. Clinical practice. Renal-artery stenosis. *New Engl J Med* 2009 Nov 12;**361**(20):1972–8.

21. Safian RD, Textor SC. Renal-artery stenosis. *New Engl J Med* 2001 Feb 8;**344**(6):431–42.

22. Bax L, Woittiez AJ, Kouwenberg HJ, et al. Stent placement in patients with atherosclerotic renal artery stenosis and impaired renal function: a randomized trial. *Ann Intern Med.* 2009 Jun 16;**150**(12):840–8.

23. Wheatley K, Ives N, Gray R, et al. Revascularisation versus medical therapy for renal-artery stenosis. *New Engl J Med* 2009 Nov 12;**361**(20):1953–62.

24. Bokhari SW, Faxon DP. Current advances in the diagnosis and treatment of renal artery stenosis. *Rev Cardiovasc Med* 2004 Fall;**5**(4):204–15.

25. Lockhart ME, Robbin ML. Renal Vascular Imaging: Ultrasound and Other Modalities. *Ultrasound Q* 2007;**23**(4):279–92. http://dx.doi.org/10.1097/ruq.0b013e31815adf4c.

26. Helenon O, el Rody F, Correas JM, et al. Colour Doppler US of renovascular disease in native kidneys. *Radiographics* 1995 Jul;**15**(4):833–54.

27. Olin JW, Piedmonte MR, Young JR, DeAnna S, Grubb M, Childs MB. The utility of duplex ultrasound scanning of the renal arteries for diagnosing significant renal artery stenosis. *Ann Intern Med* 1995 Jun 1;**122**(11):833–8.

28. Pellerito JSZW. Ultrasound assessment of native and renal vessels and renal allografts. In: WJ Z, editor. *Introduction to Vascular Ultrasonography.* Philadelphia, Pennsylvania, United States of America: Saunders Elsevier; 2005.

29. Williams GJ, Macaskill P, Chan SF, et al. Comparative accuracy of renal duplex sonographic parameters in the diagnosis of renal artery stenosis: paired and unpaired analysis. *AJR Am J Roentgenol* 2007 Mar;**188**(3):798–811.

30. Soares GM, Murphy TP, Singha MS, Parada A, Jaff M. Renal artery duplex ultrasonography as a screening and surveillance tool to detect renal artery stenosis: a comparison with current reference standard imaging. *J Ultrasound Med* 2006 Mar;**25**(3):293–8.

31. Chain S, Luciardi H, Feldman G, et al. Diagnostic role of new Doppler index in assessment of renal artery stenosis. *Cardiovasc Ultrasound* 2006;**4**:4.

32. Li JC, Wang L, Jiang YX, et al. Evaluation of renal artery stenosis with velocity parameters of Doppler sonography. *J Ultrasound Med* 2006 Jun;**25**(6):735–42; quiz 743–4.

33. Li JC, Xu ZH, Yuan Y, et al. Impact of atherosclerosis and age on Doppler sonographic parameters in the diagnosis of renal artery stenosis. *J Ultrasound Med* 2012 May;**31**(5):747–55.

34. Stavros AT, Parker SH, Yakes WF, et al. Segmental stenosis of the renal artery: pattern recognition of tardus and parvus abnormalities with duplex sonography. *Radiology* 1992 Aug;**184**(2):487–92.

35. Postma CT, Bijlstra PJ, Rosenbusch G, Thien T. Pattern recognition of loss of early systolic peak by Doppler ultrasound has a low sensitivity for the detection of renal artery stenosis. *J Human Hypertens* 1996 Mar;**10**(3):181–4.

36. Halpern EJ, Needleman L, Nack TL, East SA. Renal artery stenosis: should we study the main renal artery or segmental vessels? *Radiology* 1995 Jun;**195**(3):799–804.

37. Kliewer MA, Tupler RH, Carroll BA, et al. Renal artery stenosis: analysis of Doppler waveform parameters and tardus-parvus pattern. *Radiology* 1993 Dec;**189**(3):779–87.

38. Demirpolat G, Ozbek SS, Parildar M, Oran I, Memis A. Reliability of intrarenal Doppler sonographic parameters of renal artery stenosis. *J Clin Ultrasound* 2003 Sep;**31**(7):346–51.

39. Bude RO, Rubin JM, Platt JF, Fechner KP, Adler RS. Pulsus tardus: its cause and potential limitations in detection of arterial stenosis. *Radiology* 1994 Mar;**190**(3):779–84.

40. Girndt M, Kaul H, Maute C, Kramann B, Kohler H, Uder M. Enhanced flow velocity after stenting of renal arteries is associated with decreased renal function. *Nephron Clin Pract* 2007;**105**(2): c84–c9.

41. Llach F, Papper S, Massry SG. The clinical spectrum of renal vein thrombosis: acute and chronic. *Am J Med* 1980 Dec;**69**(6):819–27.

42. Mulligan SA, Koslin DB, Berland LL. Duplex evaluation of native renal vessels and renal allografts. *Semin Ultrasound CT MR* 1992 Feb;**13**(1):40–52.

43. Kurklinsky AK, Rooke TW. Nutcracker phenomenon and nutcracker syndrome. *Mayo Clin Proc* 2010 Jun;**85**(6):552–9.

44. Tasci AI, Resim S, Caskurlu T, Dincel C, Bayraktar Z, Gurbuz G. Colour Doppler ultrasonography and spectral analysis of venous flow in diagnosis of varicocele. *Eur Urol* 2001 Mar;**39** (3):316–21.

Chapter 10

Solid Organ Transplantation

Myron A. Pozniak

Introduction

The number of transplant candidates on waiting lists for organs continues to increase each year. The shortage of organs remains a major problem for patients with end-stage liver, renal failure and diabetes mellitus. Graft and patient survival rates following solid organ transplantation continue to improve due to refinements in surgical technique, advances in human leukocyte antigen typing for recipient/donor matching[1] new and improved immunosuppressive agents[2,3] refinements in national coordinated organ-sharing systems, improvements in recipient immune system desensitisation and advances in non-invasive transplant monitoring. As the number of transplant recipients grows, it is important for anyone responsible for providing imaging services to at least have a basic understanding of transplantation and its complications since there is an increasing incidence of transplant recipients presenting for emergency care to non-transplant centres. Chances for graft survival are significantly improved with timely identification of the aetiology of transplant dysfunction, allowing prompt medical and/or surgical intervention when necessary.

Renal Transplantation

Quality of life after successful renal transplantation significantly improves for patients in dialysis-dependent end-stage renal disease. Renal allograft and patient survival rates continue to improve. In the United States 1-year graft survival currently approximates 91.2% for deceased donor and 96.3% for living-donor kidney transplants.[4] When screening laboratory test results indicate renal transplant dysfunction, imaging studies are often required to evaluate renal morphology and perfusion. Doppler ultrasound is an ideal tool for this purpose because it is non-invasive, readily available, and can detect and distinguish many of the vascular

complications that can be the cause of transplant dysfunction. The application of Doppler ultrasound to functional problems, such as rejection or acute tubular necrosis, however, is limited.

Examination of the transplant kidney requires careful attention to scan technique and awareness of potential pitfalls. A complete sonographic examination of the renal transplant should cover the points listed in Box 10-1. The most common abnormal findings, which may be demonstrated, are listed in Box 10-2.

ULTRASOUND ANATOMY OF THE RENAL TRANSPLANT

In most cases, the isolated transplant kidney is positioned retroperitoneally in the right iliac fossa with an end-to-side anastomosis of the renal vasculature to the common or external iliac artery and vein (Fig. 10-1). If the patient has undergone a simultaneous renal–pancreas transplant, then the kidney is usually intraperitoneal within the left flank. The transplanted ureter is implanted directly into the superior surface of the bladder or to the native ureter (see Fig. 10-34A). In approximately 20% of transplants, because of variation in donor anatomy, multiple arterial or venous anastomoses may be required. Because numerous technical variations exist in the way kidneys are transplanted, it is very important that the sonologist is familiar with the surgical technique common to their institution and the specific anatomical details of the patient being scanned. If the patient's surgical anatomy varies from standard, proper documentation and communication of the surgical record is very important in ensuring correct understanding and interpretation of imaging findings and Doppler flow profiles. Ideally, if the transplant has variant

BOX 10-1 RENAL TRANSPLANT SONOGRAPHIC EXAMINATION CHECKLIST

- Review any available prior imaging studies. Review the surgical record, especially with regard to the vasculature

- Evaluate the renal collecting system. If dilated, make certain that the bladder is empty

- Measure the renal length. Report any change

- Look for perinephric fluid collections. Record any change in size if previously seen

- Check for a lymphocele

- Verify uniform parenchymal perfusion by power Doppler. Look at the intrarenal waveform with spectral Doppler. Check for tardus-parvus or alterations in resistance

- Examine the main renal artery, particularly near its anastomosis (especially if a tardus parvus waveform is observed within the transplanted kidney)

- Verify renal vein patency

BOX 10-2 RENAL TRANSPLANT SONOGRAPHIC FINDINGS AND POSSIBLE CAUSES

INCREASE IN SIZE OF TRANSPLANTED KIDNEY
- Hypertrophy of the kidney
- Allograft rejection
- Postoperative infection
- Renal vein thrombosis

REDUCTION IN SIZE OF TRANSPLANTED KIDNEY
- Ischaemia
- Chronic rejection

INCREASED RENAL ARTERIAL FLOW RESISTANCE
- Compressive effect by transducer, adjacent mass or fluid collection
- Infection
- Advanced stages of rejection
- High-grade obstruction
- Acute tubular necrosis
- Renal vein thrombosis

DECREASED RENAL ARTERIAL FLOW RESISTANCE
- Renal artery stenosis
- Severe aortoiliac atherosclerosis
- Arteriovenous fistula

RENAL COLLECTING SYSTEM DILATATION
- Obstructive hydronephrosis
- Ureteral anastomosis stenosis
- Chronic distention of flaccid denervated system
- Sequela of prior obstructive episode
- Bladder outlet obstruction (neurogenic bladder)

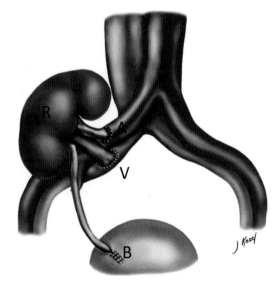

FIGURE 10-1 Artist rendering of a renal transplant (R) located in the right iliac fossa. The transplant renal artery is typically anastomosed to the common iliac artery (A). The transplant renal vein anastomosis is to the common iliac vein (V). The ureter is connected to the urinary bladder (B).

vascular anatomy, a drawing is recorded by the surgical team which shows the orientation of the kidney and its vasculature, the number and location of anastomoses, and any other atypical anatomical information.

DOPPLER ULTRASOUND TECHNIQUE

Successful Doppler evaluation of the transplanted kidney can only be accomplished when scan quality is optimal. This requires equipment that provides high

Doppler sensitivity. The examiner must optimise Doppler settings, since improper adjustment can result in misdiagnosis of thrombosis. Angle of insonation should approximate the orientation of the vascular pedicle. Scanning should be done with minimal transducer pressure since compression of the kidney can elevate perceived inflow resistance.

Ultrasound examination of the kidney should first confirm its appropriate location and the absence of any significant fluid collections. Colour Doppler is then used to identify the renal vascular pedicle. Spectral Doppler is applied to the main renal artery, main renal vein and intrarenal segmental or intralobar branches at the mid, upper, and lower poles. If any inflow compromise is suspect to all or part of the kidney, then power Doppler can be applied to confirm uniform vascular perfusion to the organ[5] (Fig. 10.2A–D).

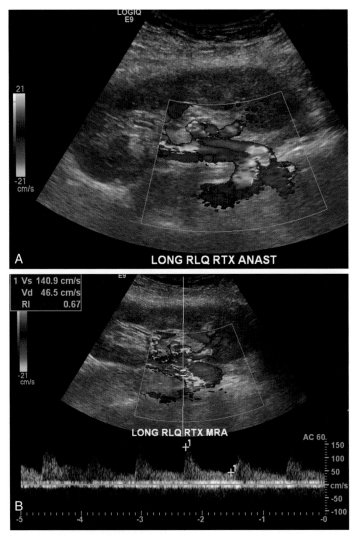

FIGURE 10-2 Longitudinal colour, spectral and power Doppler images of a normal renal transplant. (A) Colour Doppler image of the vascular pedicle reveals the anastomosis. The vessels often become curved in their course as the organ is nestled into the iliac fossa. (B) spectral Doppler tracing of the renal artery shows a brisk upstroke in systole. The resistive index is appropriate at between 60 to 70%.

Continued

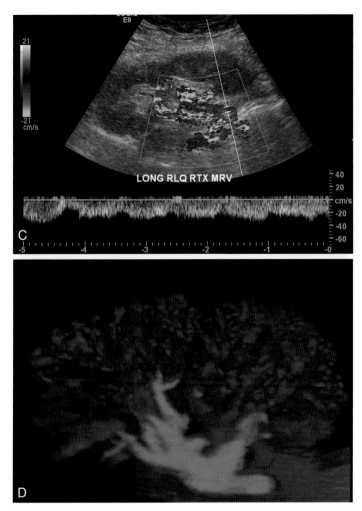

FIGURE 10-2—CONT'D (C) Normally, the renal vein flow profile shows an element of cardiac periodicity. This presence of periodicity in the renal vein helps reinforce anastomotic patency. (D) 3-D rendering of a power Doppler evaluation shows uniform distribution of flow out to the capsular surface of this normal renal transplant.

Scale Setting (Pulse Repetition Frequency [PRF])

For the initial scan, the colour and spectral Doppler scales should be set relatively low to localise the renal vasculature with colour Doppler and then demonstrate appropriate excursion on the spectral Doppler tracing. If aliasing occurs, the examiner can always increase the PRF until the optimal level for that particular vessel is displayed.

Doppler Gain

The gain should be set at the highest level possible without creating noise in the image or tracing.

Filtration Level

The Doppler filter reduces noise in both colour and spectral modes. If the filtration level is set too high, it can eradicate the display of slow flow. Initially, filtration should be at a low setting and only increased incrementally when the low setting does not allow for an effective examination.

Optimising Angle of Insonation Relative to Vessel Orientation

To ensure proper perception of flow by colour Doppler, or accurate measurement of the spectral velocity, the angle of insonation should be less than 60°. Finding an appropriate angle can be especially problematic when examining transplanted kidneys because their vessels may be extremely tortuous and a committed search for a suitable Doppler window is required.[6]

Minimising Transducer Pressure

Often the imaging study is limited because intervening adipose tissue increases the distance from the patient's skin to the transplanted kidney or there is gas in overlying bowel. By applying sufficient pressure, fat or bowel loops can be displaced. Doing so, however, will compromise the Doppler examination as the renal parenchyma also becomes compressed and inflow can be impeded (Fig. 10-3). This results in elevation of the resistive index. Thus, care must be taken not to apply excess pressure to the kidney or its associated vasculature, so that any diagnosis made on the basis of the resistive index or velocity measurement is accurate.[7]

COMPLICATIONS OF RENAL TRANSPLANTATION

Functional Complications

Functional complications include hyperacute rejection, perioperative ischaemia, acute tubular necrosis, acute rejection, chronic rejection and drug toxicity (most commonly immunosuppressive agents). Imaging techniques, including ultrasound with Doppler, are limited in their ability to identify and distinguish these complications.[8]

With hyperacute rejection (humeral-mediated rejection), graft failure occurs rapidly (within minutes of implantation) secondary to the presence of preformed circulating antibodies. This condition is typically observed in patients who have been sensitised by a previous transplant organ or a blood transfusion. This diagnosis is usually made in the operating suite, within minutes of unclamping the vascular pedicle to the newly implanted organ. Extremely high resistance to inflow can be expected on spectral Doppler.

Acute rejection is a cellular-mediated process, whereby the immune system attacks the foreign renal allograft. Acute rejection is controlled by the use of steroids, cyclosporine, tacrolimus, sirolimus and other immunosuppressive agents. Occasional elevation in a transplant recipient's immune status (triggered by viral illness or non-compliance with the immunosuppressive drug regimen) can result in an acceleration of acute rejection to a critical level. The kidney becomes oedematous and swollen, intracapsular pressure rises, and eventually resistance to vascular perfusion increases (Fig. 10-4). Although early investigators proposed that resistive index elevation was useful in identifying acute rejection as the cause of kidney transplant dysfunction, subsequent laboratory and clinical studies have shown it to be unreliable, and acute rejection remains a pathological diagnosis. Indeed, in a canine study it has been found that resistive index actually decreases in the mild to moderate stages of acute rejection.[9] During the early to mid-stages of rejection, the physical effects of increased intrarenal pressure are counteracted by intrarenal hormonal autoregulatory mechanisms. Elevation of resistive index, therefore, does not manifest until the process of acute rejection is quite severe.[9] If a scan being performed in anticipation of transplant biopsy identifies the kidney to be oedematous and swollen with loss of central sinus fat echo and very high resistive indices, thought should be given to deferring the biopsy. Puncturing the capsule of a tense rejecting kidney may cause it to rupture.

Resistive index is rarely affected in the mild to moderate stages of acute rejection and when it is, its specificity is low. It is not until acute rejection progresses to severe levels that the resistive index becomes consistently elevated. Elevation of resistive index, however, can also occur from many other causes such as hydronephrosis, acute tubular necrosis, infection and compression of the kidney by an adjacent mass or fluid collection. Thus, specificity for the diagnosis of acute rejection by Doppler ultrasound is unacceptably low and renal biopsy is still needed to establish the diagnosis.[9,10]

Chronic rejection is a multifactorial process, mostly antibody-mediated, but the pathophysiology is not entirely understood. Doppler indices rarely show any significant alteration in flow profiles with chronic rejection.[11]

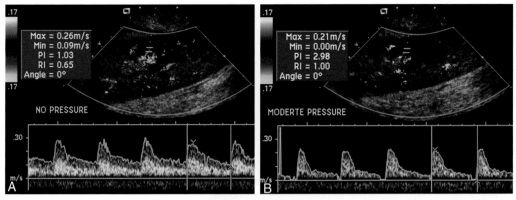

FIGURE 10-3 (A) Renal transplant interlobar artery spectral Doppler tracing acquired with gentle transducer contact. Note the normal waveform and 65% resistive index. (B) When moderate pressure is applied with the transducer, the tracing of the same artery now exhibits an elevated resistive index of 100%. Transducer pressure alone is responsible for this increase in vascular impedance and resultant elevation of resistance.

Perioperative ischaemia can result in transient compromise of renal function, particularly at the level of the distal tubules which are most sensitive to hypoxia. This condition is self-limiting and typically resolves within 1–2 weeks of transplantation. The medullary pyramids are oedematous and therefore appear enlarged and hypoechoic, and spectral Doppler shows an increase in the resistive index. Although the imaging and Doppler findings may suggest acute tubular necrosis, specificity is low[9] (Fig. 10-5).

Anatomic Complications

These include haematomas, seromas, urinomas, abscesses, lymphoceles, obstructive hydronephrosis, focal masses, arterial and venous stenosis or thrombosis, and intrarenal arteriovenous fistula and pseudoaneurysm.[12,13] Unlike functional complications, most anatomic complications are readily identified by ultrasound.

Perinephric fluid is a common sequela of renal transplantation and is not considered significant if it is crescentic in shape, and decreases in size over time. Most fluid collections are haematomas or seromas, which weep from tissue around the transplant. Urinomas are relatively uncommon and usually are the result of breakdown at the ureteral anastomosis to the bladder. Doppler examination is of limited value in these cases. High-pressure collections, such as haematoma

after biopsy or organ rupture may exert mass effect upon the kidney and locally affect haemodynamics. In this case, Doppler may reveal a high-resistance spectral tracing adjacent to the fluid pocket (Fig. 10-6).

A rounded, expansile collection with internal debris and associated signs of infection usually represent an abscess. Sonographic specificity is low, however, and computed tomography (CT) is considered a better imaging study for this purpose, especially to determine its extent and percutaneous drainage potential. Occasionally colour Doppler may reveal hyperaemia of the tissues surrounding the abscess.

Lymphoceles usually manifest at about 6–8 weeks postoperatively and are seen as rounded, lobulated collections near the vascular anastomoses. They are the result of surgical disruption of iliac lymphatic channels when the vascular anastomosis to the transplanted kidney is created. An expanding lymphocele may cause ureteric compression and hydronephrosis. If a lymphocele becomes large enough, it may compress or kink the renal vascular pedicle. In this situation, Doppler examination may show findings similar to arterial or venous stenosis[14] (Fig. 10-7).

Intraperitoneal renal transplantation typically when combined with pancreas transplantation results in a mobile kidney. Occasionally ptosis or rotation and torsion of the kidney may occur along its vascular pedicle. This may result in arterial inflow and venous outflow narrowing or obstruction[15] (Fig. 10-8).

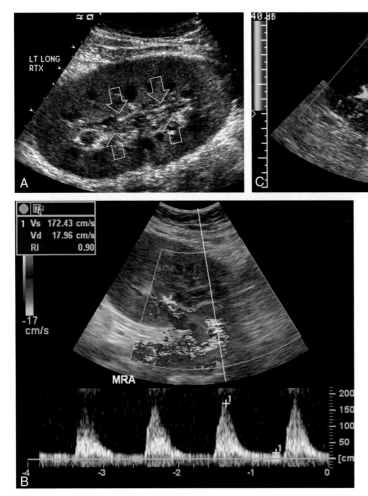

FIGURE 10-4 (A) Longitudinal grey scale image of a transplanted kidney. Note the rounded globular configuration of the kidney. The central hilar space (arrows) is compressed due to oedema and swelling; and the central hilar fat has been displaced. (B) Spectral Doppler tracing at the main renal artery level shows a resistive index of 90%. Biopsy confirmed severe acute rejection. (C) Power Doppler image of a severely rejecting renal transplant shows the main central vasculature and a few interlobar vessels but no flow can be seen out to the periphery. The high resistance generated by the rejection process results in this colour Doppler 'pruned tree' appearance. Contrast this to the appearance of normal renal power Doppler flow in Figure 10-2D.

Transient dilatation of the collecting system as a result of ureteral anastomotic oedema frequently occurs immediately after renal transplantation or removal of the ureteral stent. The presence of a dilated transplant collecting system does not automatically signify an obstructed system under pressure, as the denervated, flaccid collecting system can become markedly dilated, particularly when the urinary bladder is distended. Platt et al.[16] proposed that the identification of an elevated resistive index was useful in distinguishing obstructive hydronephrosis from chronic, low-pressure dilatation of the transplant collecting system. Although this observation may be sensitive, its specificity is very poor because of the many other factors that similarly affect renal haemodynamics.

Nuclear scintigraphy or the Whitaker test are more specific for differentiating high-pressure obstructive hydronephrosis from low-pressure distention of a flaccid renal transplant collecting system.

The transplanted ureter is normally anastomosed to the superior surface of the bladder. Occasionally, colour Doppler can identify the ureteral jet from the transplanted ureter. The posteriorly directed flow of urine may initially confuse the unexperienced examiner (Fig. 10-9).

Although uncommon, urinary tract calcifications can develop within a transplant kidney. When evaluating a renal transplant with hydronephrosis, the dilated ureter should be followed toward the anastomosis. If intraluminal debris is identified. The application of

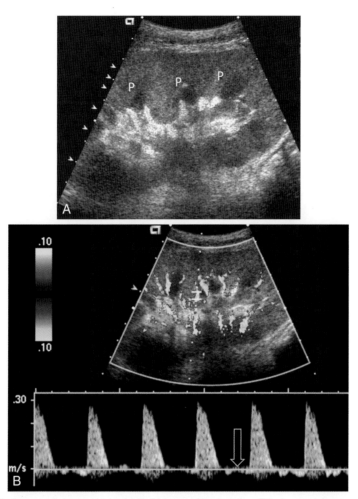

FIGURE 10-5 (A) Longitudinal grey scale image obtained with 24 hours of implantation. This deceased donor organ experienced prolonged ischaemic time. Note that the kidney has an appropriate contour and the sinus fat is preserved. The medullary pyramids (P), however, are prominent, hypoechoic and oedematous. (B) Spectral and colour Doppler image of the same kidney. The resistive index approximates 100%. This combination of findings in the appropriate clinical situation is consistent with acute tubular necrosis. This is common immediately after transplantation but can also be seen with drug toxicity.

colour Doppler may reveal twinkle artifact. This helps identify the abnormality as a calculus (Fig. 10-10).

Vascular Complications

Following renal transplantation, vascular complications are observed in less than 10% of recipients; however, when present, they are associated with a high morbidity and mortality. Complications include renal artery or vein stenosis, compression, kink, thrombosis, intrarenal arteriovenous fistula and pseudoaneurysm. If identified promptly, they can often be successfully repaired prior to transplant failure. Doppler

sonography is a very effective, non-invasive tool for identifying significant vascular complications.[17–19]

Renal Transplant Artery Stenosis. This is most often observed within 1–2 cm of the anastomosis, usually as a result of vessel wall ischaemia due to disruption of the vasa vasorum within the artery wall. Stenosis should be suspected if a tardus parvus waveform and relatively low-resistance flow are noted in the intrarenal branches. A tardus parvus waveform is characterised by a delayed upstroke in systole (prolonged acceleration time >0.07 s), rounding of the systolic

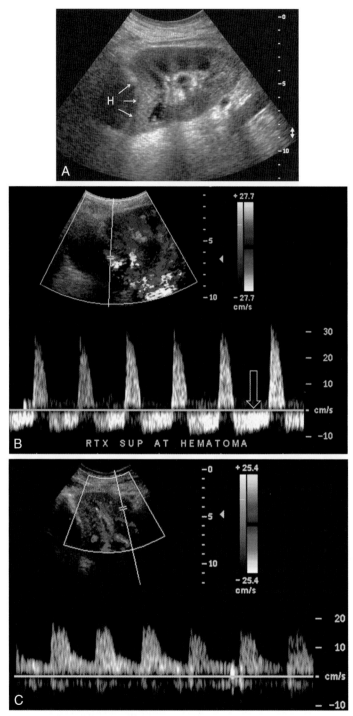

FIGURE 10-6 (A) Longitudinal grey scale image of a renal transplant within 24 hours of an upper pole biopsy. The biopsy was complicated by haemorrhage (H). Blood accumulated in the subcapsular space and severely compressed the upper pole of this kidney (arrows). (B) Spectral Doppler tracing obtained of an interlobar artery just adjacent to the high-pressure haematoma reveals extremely high resistive index with reverse flow in diastole. (C) Spectral Doppler tracing at the opposite (lower pole) of this same kidney shows a normal low resistance flow profile. The compressive haematoma exerts local mass effect and elevates resistance to flow.

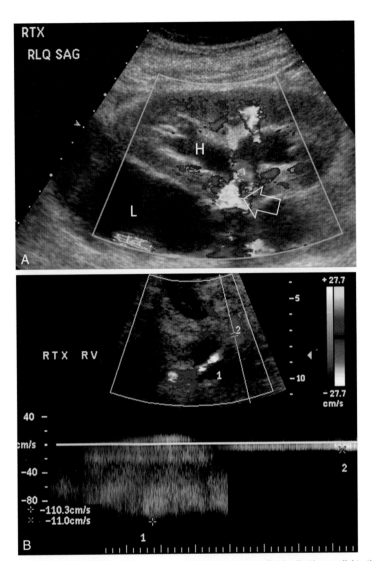

FIGURE 10-7 (A) Longitudinal colour Doppler image of this renal transplant shows a large fluid collection medial to the kidney, surrounding the renal vascular pedicle. This is a lymphocele (L) and it has caused distortion of the pedicle. Colour aliasing can be seen in the renal artery (arrow). There is also obvious hydronephrosis (H) caused by compression of the ureter. (B) Spectral Doppler tracing of the renal vein shows marked compression where it courses past the lymphocele (#1), the measured velocity at this area is 1.1 m/s; whereas within the kidney (proximal to the lymphocele (#2)) the velocity is only 0.1 m/s. This 10-fold velocity gradient identifies this as a significant renal venous outflow obstruction.

peak and obliteration of the early systolic notch. A flow velocity approximating 2 m/s with associated distal turbulence near the renal artery anastomosis is diagnostic of renal artery stenosis (Fig. 10-11). If an intrarenal tardus parvus waveform is observed, but a stenosis cannot be identified at the level of the renal artery anastomosis, the examiner should conduct a thorough examination from the renal hilum through the iliac artery in search of inflow compromise (Fig. 10-12). With severe renal artery stenosis the intra-arterial waveforms become flattened to the point that systolic diastolic velocity variation becomes difficult to perceive. Subtle pulsatile flow is enough to document the patency of the artery and avoid misdiagnosis of thrombosis. This is further reinforced by identifying outflow in the renal vein (Fig. 10-13).

A long-standing undiagnosed stenosis can develop post-stenotic dilatation. Imaging and colour Doppler reveal a characteristic focal area of expansion of the artery. This usually incorporates the high-velocity post-stenotic jet (Fig. 10-14).

Approximately 20% of transplanted kidneys require more than one arterial anastomosis due to the presence of accessory arteries. If one of these

vessels becomes compromised, then perfusion to the subtended segment of the kidney is decreased. Again, a tardus parvus waveform is seen, this time limited to the segment perfused by the affected artery. If thrombosis of this artery occurs, then the subtended area shows no flow on colour or power Doppler and an arterial tracing will not be identified by spectral Doppler. The area affected will vary

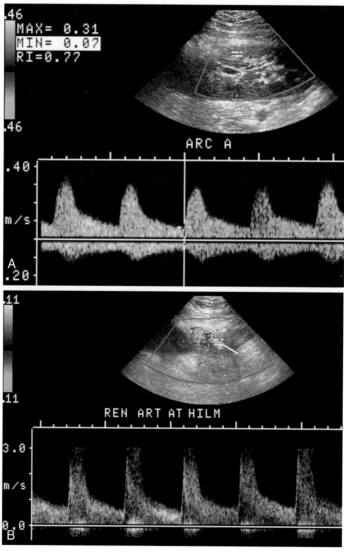

FIGURE 10-8 (A) Colour Doppler image along the long axis of an intraperitoneal renal transplant with a spectral Doppler tracing of an arcuate artery. The waveform shows a tardus parvus configuration indicating arterial inflow compromise. (B) Doppler of the main renal artery at the hilum reveals a high-velocity jet approximating 3 m/s.

Continued

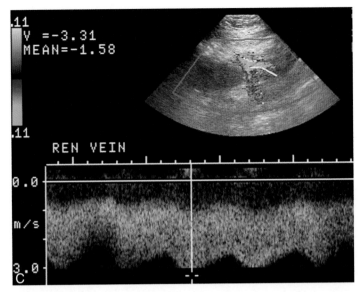

FIGURE 10-8—CONT'D (C) Immediately adjacent to the main renal artery, the main renal vein tracing also shows turbulent high-velocity flow. This finding of high-velocity, turbulent Doppler tracings in both artery and vein identifies partial torsion of the renal vascular pedicle with a twisting compromise of the main artery and vein. Fortuitously this was only partial torsion of the kidney and was corrected with surgical detorsion and nephropexy. Torsion of an intraperitoneal transplant kidney has been reported to result in infarction.

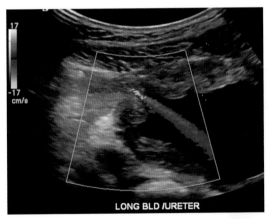

FIGURE 10-9 Colour Doppler image of the urinary bladder. The transplanted ureter is normally anastomosed to the anterior superior bladder wall. Flow of urine is seen through the anastomosis manifesting as a jet, but pointing posteriorly; not in the direction we are accustomed to seeing ureteral jets.

depending on the anatomic vascular distribution (Fig. 10-15).

Renal parenchymal scarring secondary to chronic rejection may result in focal stenosis within branch arteries. This should be suspected if there is irregular distribution of flow on colour Doppler through the kidney. Segmental or interlobar renal artery stenosis can be confirmed by the presence of intrarenal high-velocity flow. Because these lesions are typically multiple and distal, treatment options are limited.[20]

A similar appearance can be seen with scarring after transplant biopsy. If the biopsy needle is guided centrally toward the renal hilum, there is a greater chance of vessel injury. Direct puncture of a major artery usually becomes immediately manifest as an area of turbulence on colour Doppler, a rapidly expanding haematoma, or brisk haematuria due to an arteriourteral fistula. Biopsy in close proximity to a major artery may present with a delayed segmental perfusion defect as scarring results in progressive compromise of flow to that portion of kidney.

Renal Transplant Artery Thrombosis. Thrombosis of the main renal transplant artery is a rare event. It is typically due to a technical problem with the surgical anastomosis or an occlusive kink. Doppler fails to demonstrate any arterial inflow.

Severe acute rejection may cause microvascular thrombosis. Colour and power Doppler will show no flow within the kidney. Flow may still be present

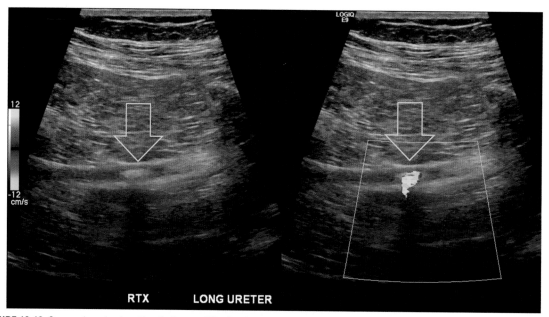

FIGURE 10-10 Grey scale and colour Doppler image of the distal transplanted ureter. An echogenic focus within the ureter causes shadowing. The application of colour Doppler manifests twinkle artifact and helps confirm the diagnosis of a ureteral calculus.

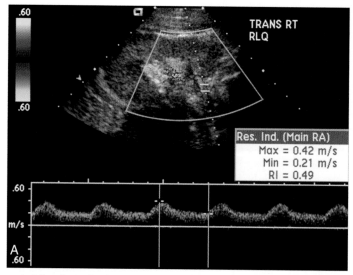

FIGURE 10-11 (A) Renal transplant Doppler tracing in a hypertensive recipient with elevated serum creatinine. The renal arterial waveform manifests tardus parvus configuration with a slow systolic upstroke, and a rounded systolic peak with low resistance. These findings suggest a more proximal stenosis.

Continued

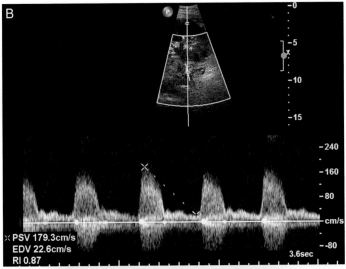

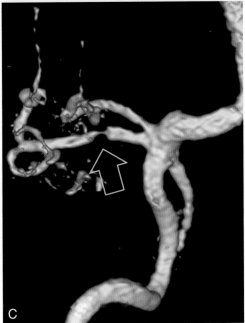

FIGURE 10-11—CONT'D (B) Spectral Doppler tracing closer to the anastomosis of the main renal artery to the iliac artery. Note the high-velocity (1.79 m/s), turbulent flow characteristic of renal artery stenosis. (C) MR angiogram of this transplanted kidney actually revealed a double arterial anastomosis. The lower pole artery has a high-grade stenosis (arrow) within 1 cm of its anastomosis.

in the segmental or interlobar branches, but spectral Doppler shows very high resistance because the flow has nowhere to go (Fig. 10-16). It may be difficult to differentiate the two aetiologies, but the non-rejecting kidney with arterial thrombosis is typically not as swollen and oedematous as the acutely rejecting thrombosed kidney that is congested with inflammation.[21]

The spectral Doppler tracing of renal vein flow in microvascular thrombosis may be very confusing.

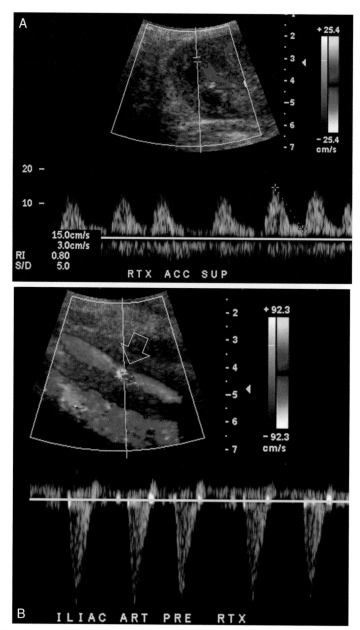

FIGURE 10-12 (A) Spectral Doppler tracing of a transplant main renal artery. Tardus parvus changes were identified but an anastomotic stenosis could not be identified. (B) The exam was extended to include a spectral Doppler tracing of the external iliac artery. A high-velocity jet is identified with velocities of >3 m/s. An atheromatous lesion in the right iliac artery in this diabetic recipient was responsible for the inflow compromise to the renal transplant.

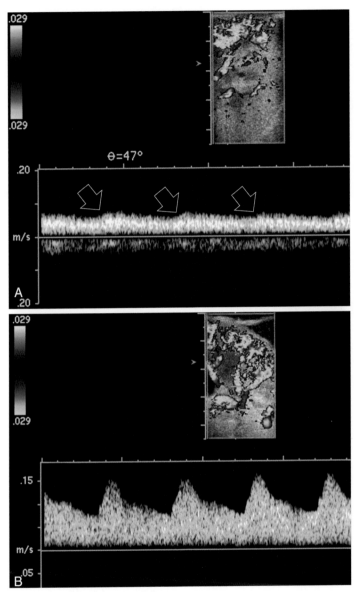

FIGURE 10-13 Intraoperative spectral and colour Doppler ultrasound of a recent renal transplant recipient being reoperated because of poor renal function. Preoperative Doppler examination suggested arterial stenosis. (A) Direct contact scanning on the kidney showed an abnormal spectral Doppler tracing of a segmental artery with only a very subtle undulation in the arterial waveform (towards the transducer). A high-grade proximal inflow compromise wiped out the expected systolic/diastolic arterial velocity variation. (The tracing below the baseline is an adjacent vein.) (B) A kink of the vascular pedicle was identified and as the artery was surgically manipulated the spectral Doppler tracing suddenly normalised.

The blood within the main renal vein is typically sloshing back and forth with cardiac periodicity transmitted down the inferior vena cava (IVC) with little, if any, total antegrade progress.

Renal Transplant Vein Stenosis. Renal vein stenosis is an uncommon complication following kidney transplantation, but when present, it is a significant cause of graft dysfunction (Figs 10-17 and 10-7B). Venous

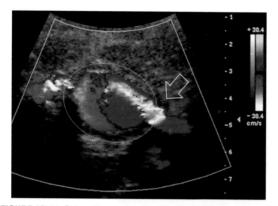

FIGURE 10-14 Colour Doppler image along the long axis of the main renal artery. A focal area of stenosis with a high-velocity jet presents as focal turbulence and aliasing. Sacular dilatation of the transplant artery represents a post-stenotic aneurysm and reveals a swirling flow pattern. Flow continues on towards the kidney in the more distal normal-calibre artery.

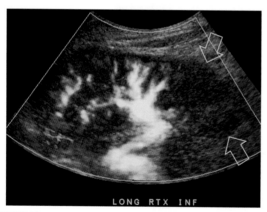

FIGURE 10-15 Longitudinal power Doppler image of the lower pole of a renal transplant recipient with hypertension. There is complete absence of flow at the lower pole. This renal transplant required two arterial anastomoses. Thrombosis of the lower pole artery was suggested and confirmed at angiography.

stenosis may be seen as a focal narrowing with associated dilatation of the proximal vein. However, to confirm the diagnosis of a significant stenosis, there should be at least a four-fold velocity gradient across the lesion. If the gradient is less than four-fold, it is usually not clinically significant, even though it may have a dramatic appearance on the Doppler images.[22]

Renal Transplant Vein Thrombosis. Renal transplant vein thrombosis is also a relatively rare post-transplantation complication. It typically presents within the first week following surgery. It is more likely to occur when there is technical difficulty with the venous anastomosis. It may occur with preservation injury, or it may evolve during an episode of severe acute allograft rejection. Extremely high resistance (resistive index typically greater than 100%) will be seen on the renal arterial waveforms with spectral Doppler. In most cases, thrombosis results in partial rather than complete occlusion of the vein and some renal venous outflow can be detected with spectral Doppler. To prevent a false-negative diagnosis, it is important that the examiner conduct a careful imaging and colour Doppler evaluation of the vein when arterial resistance greater than 100% is observed[23,24] (Fig. 10-18).

Intrarenal Arteriovenous Fistulae and Pseudo-aneurysms. These are typically the result of renal transplant biopsy. The true incidence of these complications varies from centre to centre depending on biopsy technique (operator experience). Arteriovenous fistulae manifest as a flash of colour, or 'visible thrill', in the adjacent parenchyma when the kidney is examined at normal colour Doppler settings. This phenomenon is caused by vibration of the surrounding tissues due to the rapidly flowing blood through the fistula. It is often possible to distinguish the feeding artery and the enlarged draining vein by adjusting the colour Doppler to higher velocity settings. Spectral Doppler tracings will demonstrate a high-velocity, low-resistance flow within the feeding artery. Turbulent, pulsatile (arterialised) flow will be present in the draining segmental vein. If the arteriovenous fistula is large enough, it may be possible to observe pulsatile flow within the main renal vein (Fig. 10-19).

Pseudoaneurysms are typically the result of a biopsy that captured partial thickness of an arterial wall. Therefore, they are extremely rare. On imaging they usually appear as a pulsating cyst, or a rounded collection of paravascular fluid. Colour Doppler, however, immediately reveals that the 'cyst' is not simple (Fig. 10-20). Spectral Doppler tracings show to-and-fro blood flow at the neck of the pseudoaneurysm and a distorted, turbulent, pulsatile waveform can be observed within the pseudoaneurysm. The majority of intrarenal arteriovenous fistulae and pseudoaneurysms resolve spontaneously, but if they

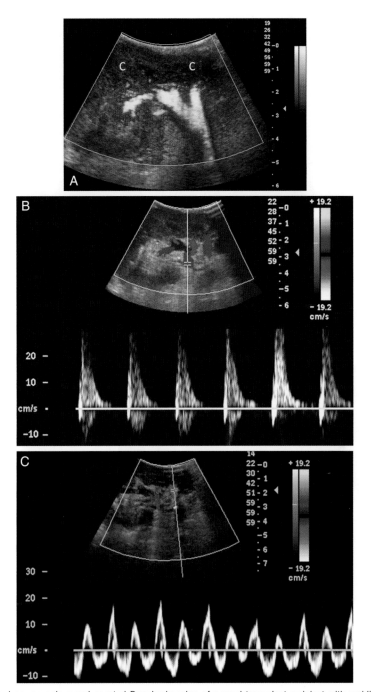

FIGURE 10-16 Longitudinal power, colour and spectral Doppler imaging of a renal transplant recipient with rapidly rising creatinine levels. (A) Power Doppler image shows central flow within the hilum of the kidney, but no flow within the renal parenchyma. (B) Spectral Doppler tracing of the artery shows a brisk spike in systole but no flow during diastole. (C) The renal vein spectral Doppler waveform has a to-and-fro pattern. When comparing relative flow above and below the baseline, it becomes evident that they are relatively equivalent and there is little antegrade flow. Due to renal microvascular thrombosis, the flow within the vein is stagnant, only moving to-and-fro in response to venous pressure changes transmitted from the right atrium. Contrast this to a tracing of a normal renal vein.

Continued

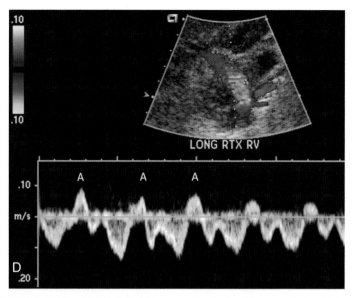

FIGURE 10-16—CONT'D (D) The retrograde component of flow known as the A-wave (A) occurs during atrial systole. But this component is relatively small in comparison to the flow below the baseline that is returning toward the heart.

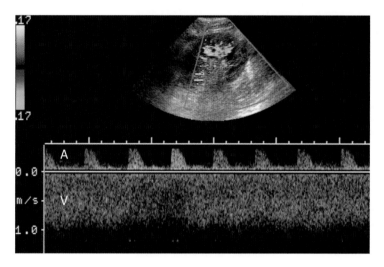

FIGURE 10-17 Spectral Doppler tracing of the renal vascular pedicle incorporating both the main renal artery (above the baseline) and main renal vein (below). Note the high velocity in the vein approximating 1 m/s. Note the corresponding high-resistance arterial waveform. Renal vein stenosis due to scarring was identified at surgery.

increase in size over a period of time, angiographic embolisation may be necessary. They may steal so much flow as to lead to renal transplant ischaemia.[22]

Liver Transplantation

Liver transplant outcomes analysis shows continued improvement in survival rates. As of 2011, in the US, 62,500 liver transplant recipients were living with a functioning graft.[4] Graft function and survival is enhanced by prompt identification of structural or functional abnormalities by timely imaging and rapid intervention when appropriate.[25]

PREOPERATIVE ASSESSMENT

Preoperative assessment of a potential transplant candidate consists of confirmation of vascular patency,

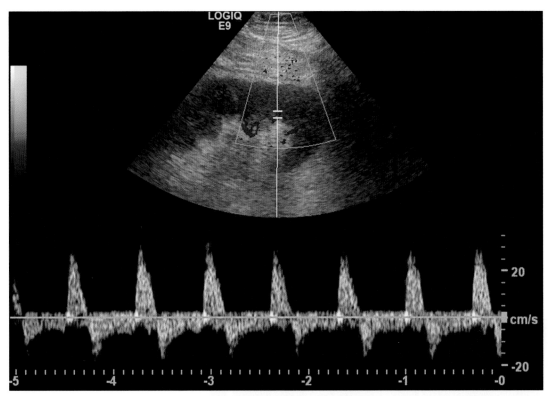

FIGURE 10-18 Spectral Doppler tracing of the main renal transplant artery in a recent recipient with a rapidly rising creatinine. The arterial waveform reveals to-and-fro flow with a large retrograde component. The resistive index measures approximately 140%. No flow could be identified by spectral or colour Doppler in the renal veins. Complete venous thrombosis was confirmed at angiography.

mapping native vascular anatomy, quantification of diseased liver volume, identification of vascular collaterals secondary to portal hypertension and a search for intra- or extrahepatic malignancy. There are many ways to accomplish this including angiography and ultrasound, but currently CT angiography is the favoured method for the adult. Some centres rely on Doppler and magnetic resonance imaging (MRI), especially for the paediatric candidate.[26] A complete sonographic examination of the liver transplant candidate should cover the points listed in Box 10-3.

POSTOPERATIVE ASSESSMENT

The major complications of liver transplantation are rejection, vascular stenosis or kink, thrombosis, biliary leak or obstruction, and recurrence of unexpected neoplasm. Acute rejection is clinically monitored

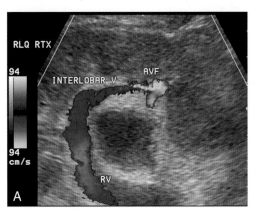

FIGURE 10-19 (A) Colour Doppler image of a renal transplant approximately 2 weeks after biopsy. A focus of increased flow is present in the mid-kidney which is drained by a large vein with robust flow.

Continued

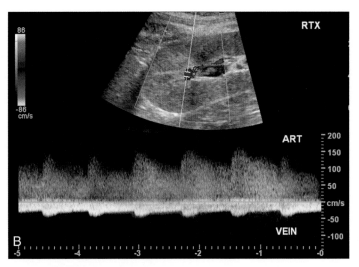

FIGURE 10-19—CONT'D (B) Spectral Doppler tracing obtained at the biopsy site reveals turbulent, high-velocity low-resistance arterial waveform; and arterialisation of the venous outflow. This is characteristic of an arteriovenous fistula.

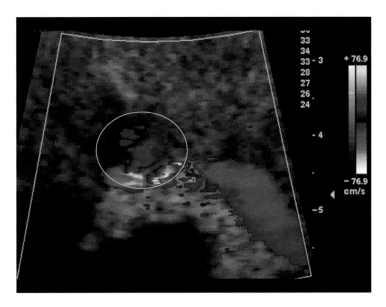

FIGURE 10-20 Colour Doppler image of a renal transplant six weeks after biopsy. A rounded focus of increased flow in a swirling pattern is present. This appearance is characteristic for a post-biopsy pseudoaneurysm.

by serum liver enzymes, bilirubin, and ammonia levels. Diagnosis is established by biopsy. Ultrasound and Doppler have little to offer in the diagnosis of acute hepatic rejection. Doppler ultrasound, however, plays a key role in monitoring for potential vascular complications.

A complete sonographic examination of the liver transplant recipient should cover the points listed in Box 10-4. Evaluation of the newly transplanted liver requires a precise understanding of the surgical anatomy. Many variations are possible including segmental or reduced-size transplantation, especially in the paediatric population.[27,28] Variations of the arterial anastomoses are necessary when the donor hepatic arterial anatomy is anomalous. Variations of venous anastomoses are necessary when the recipient portal vein is thrombosed. The sonologist must be aware of any variations in surgical anatomy so that a thrombosed accessory hepatic artery or a stenotic jump graft is not overlooked (Fig. 10-21). This is especially important in living related transplants.[29]

The liver transplant ultrasound examination should include a general survey of the abdomen and pelvis in order to identify and quantify any haematomas or fluid collections. The liver parenchyma is then examined to rule out any focal abnormality, specifically any fluid collection, area of infarction or possible neoplasm. The biliary system should be evaluated to rule out obstruction or sludge accumulation, especially in a patient with hepatic artery thrombosis. The intra- and extrahepatic arteries are checked to confirm patency and the waveforms are analysed to rule out stenosis. Patency of the portal vein is confirmed and the Doppler waveform analysed, particularly across the anastomosis (Fig. 10-22). Patency of the three hepatic veins is confirmed and their waveforms are evaluated. Finally, the IVC is checked with special attention to the upper anastomosis (Fig. 10-23).

ABNORMAL FINDINGS

The most common abnormal findings encountered in liver transplantation are listed in Box 10-5.

The hepatic artery anastomosis is technically difficult and problems, such as stenosis, kink, thrombosis and fistula formation, have the most significant impact on liver transplant success as they predispose to biliary stricture, infarction, biloma, and subsequent intrahepatic abscess formation.

Doppler findings of hepatic artery inflow compromise include an intrahepatic tardus parvus waveform (slow upstroke and low-resistance flow) and a high-velocity jet with turbulence just beyond the point of stenosis or kink. A focal high-velocity jet in the hepatic artery in excess of 200 cm/s or greater than three times the velocity in the prestenotic hepatic artery indicates clinically significant stenosis. The identification of an intrahepatic tardus parvus waveform with low resistance flow (<60% RI), a prolonged upstroke in systole (>0.08 s) and rounding of the systolic peak, should force a careful survey along the anticipated course of the hepatic artery for a high-velocity jet (Fig. 10-24). It has been shown that searching for the tardus parvus waveform pattern is highly predictive for hepatic artery inflow compromise.[30] In the paediatric population, the finding of hepatic arterial resistive index <60% is highly predictive of impending hepatic artery thrombosis due to stenosis.[31] Although an intrahepatic arterial tracing may be demonstrated, it should be remembered that a severe stenosis may still lead

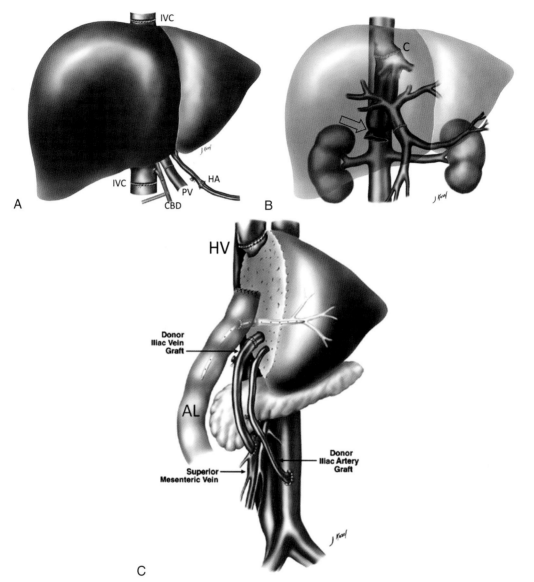

FIGURE 10-21 Three artist renderings of liver transplant variants. (A) An in-line liver transplant has a total of five anastomoses. In the porta hepatis, there are anastomoses of the hepatic artery (HA), portal vein (PV), and bile duct (CBD). The recipient inferior vena cava is resected with the explant liver. The donor inferior vena cava is implanted in-line with an upper and lower IVC anastomosis (IVC). (B) The piggyback technique requires the same three anastomoses in the porta hepatis. The recipient inferior vena cava remains in place. The explant native liver is stripped off of the inferior vena cava. The donor liver is then placed over and hooked up to the recipient inferior vena cava via a cloaca (C) formed from the recipient hepatic vein ostia. The lower end of the donor cava is ligated (arrow) effectively turning it into an accessory hepatic vein. (C) The reduced or donor liver transplant has the most complicated anatomy. The hepatic artery and portal vein frequently require a jump graft (JGs) (an interposed length of donor vasculature). The biliary system is often drained via an afferent loop (AL) of bowel. The hepatic vein draining the transplanted segment is anastomosed to the inferior vena cava usually via a donor hepatic vein (HV).

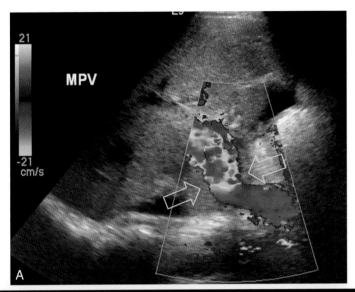

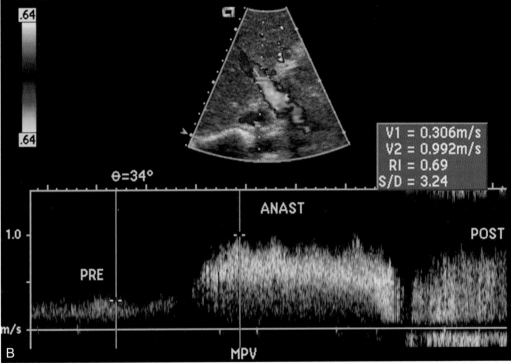

FIGURE 10-22 Colour Doppler image of the porta hepatis (A). The anastomosis between donor and recipient portal vein is evident by the angulation and subtle change in calibre which cause the focal aliasing at that level (arrows). Spectral Doppler tracing (B) across the anastomosis and on either side reveals the velocity changes are relatively insignificant (less than fourfold).

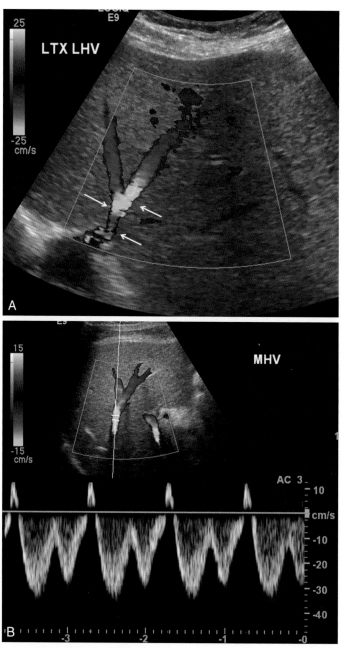

FIGURE 10-23 Longitudinal colour Doppler image of the left hepatic vein as it approaches the IVC anastomosis (A). This vein is patent with flow in the appropriate direction. Aliasing however is evident as the veins narrow near the anastomosis (arrows). Spectral Doppler tracing of the same patient's middle hepatic vein (B) reveals normal cardiac periodicity transmitting into the liver. Since this waveform must propagate against the direction of flow, its presence within the liver effectively rules out significant hepatic venous outflow obstruction, specifically the caval anastomosis is appropriately patent.

BOX 10-5 DIFFERENTIAL DIAGNOSIS OF ULTRASOUND FINDINGS IN THE TRANSPLANTED LIVER

DIFFUSELY IRREGULAR PARENCHYMAL ECHOTEXTURE

- Ischaemia or necrosis secondary to hepatic artery stenosis or thrombosis
- Infection or abscess
- Recurrent hepatitis
- Post-transplantation lymphoproliferative disorder or lymphoma
- Geographic or diffuse fatty infiltration
- Hepatocellular carcinoma
- Diffusely metastatic neoplasm

FOCAL PARENCHYMAL ABNORMALITY

- Abscess
- Infarction
- Recurrent neoplasm
- Intraductal air secondary to choledochojejunostomy or sphincterotomy
- Intraductal sludge or calculi

HIGH-RESISTANCE FLOW IN HEPATIC ARTERY

- Preservation injury – common during the first few days after transplantation
- Organ compression by adjacent mass or fluid collection
- Hepatic venous outflow obstruction
- Severe hepatocellular disease

LOW-RESISTANCE FLOW IN HEPATIC ARTERY

- Hepatic artery stenosis
- Severe aortoceliac atherosclerotic disease
- Diaphragmatic crus sling effect
- Intrahepatic arteriovenous fistula
- Arteriobiliary fistula

FLATTENING OF HEPATIC VEIN WAVEFORM

- Hepatic parenchymal disease, including rejection
- Stenosis or kink of the upper inferior vena cava anastomosis

to biliary ischaemia, or may progress to complete thrombosis.

Absence of an arterial signal in the porta hepatis on spectral and colour Doppler ultrasound should lead one to suspect hepatic artery thrombosis. Since this is a diagnosis based on the absence of the arterial Doppler tracing, great care must be taken to ensure proper Doppler settings. Scanning by a second experienced sonologist is encouraged, since this ultrasound diagnosis usually requires arteriography. Use of ultrasound echo-enhancing agents if available is encouraged to better define a weak arterial signal and hopefully decrease the rate of false-positive diagnosis of hepatic artery thrombosis, thereby reducing the frequency of arteriography.[32,33]

Early hepatic artery thrombosis (eHAT), defined as occurring within a week of transplantation, has an incidence of 4.4%. It is a major cause of graft loss (53.1%) and mortality (33.3%) in the early postoperative period. The incidence of eHAT is significantly higher in children (8.3%) than in adults (2.9%).[34,35]

Studies of patients with hepatic artery stenosis and thrombosis have identified certain factors that place patients at a higher risk and warrant more frequent Doppler screening. These factors include bench reconstruction of anatomical variants, the use of an interposition graft, and retransplantation.[36]

Collateralisation commonly develops in cases of hepatic artery thrombosis which are treated conservatively. A reestablished intrahepatic arterial signal can be detected by Doppler ultrasound as early as 2 weeks after the thrombosis. This typically manifests as a thready tracing with a tardus parvus appearance and can be seen in as many as 40% of patients with documented hepatic artery thrombosis, especially in children.

Within the first few days of transplantation, the hepatic artery tracing often shows a relatively high-resistance waveform. This is a common manifestation of ischaemic reperfusion injury (the anoxia and traumatic insult sustained by the liver during recovery, handling, preservation and surgery). It has been shown to be more common with older donor age and more prolonged ischaemic time[37] (Fig. 10-25). The high resistance is due to vasospasm and can be reversed with provocative testing with vasodilatory agents such as nifedipine. One must be cautious, however, to ensure that the transplant recipient is stable

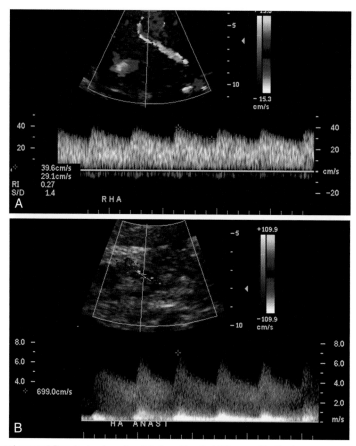

FIGURE 10-24 (A) Colour and spectral Doppler tracing of an intrahepatic arterial flow profile. Tardus parvus pattern with a delayed upstroke in systole, rounded systolic curve and relatively low-resistance flow (0.27) is indicative of insufficient hepatic arterial inflow and suggests stenosis. The examiner should carefully walk the sample volume down the hepatic artery and out of the liver looking for the anticipated point of stenosis. (B) In this case a high-velocity jet measuring almost 7 m/s is identified at the point of stenosis in the subhepatic space.

enough to tolerate this drug as a diagnostic challenge since it causes a systemic drop in blood pressure. Augmenting the Doppler exam with this challenge, however, may obviate the need for an arteriogram if hepatic arterial inflow is compromised to the point where it appears to be occluded (Fig. 10-26). The spasm typically resolves within a few days of transplantation and resistance returns to a normal range.[38] A delayed finding of high resistance, beyond 3–5 days, is a poor prognostic indicator and some of these patients will develop arterial thrombosis.[39] The exact cause of thrombosis is not always apparent and in numerous cases is presumed to be secondary to immunological causes and rejection.

At the time of implantation, there must be sufficient length of all of the vasculature to create the anastomoses. A longer pedicle is easier to work with, however, if the vessels are too long a kink may occur as the liver is placed into the subdiaphragmatic fossa and the abdominal wall is closed. Clinically the patient presents with liver dysfunction. A stenosis may be suspect on spectral Doppler. Colour or power Doppler may reveal the tortuosity. Three-dimensional CT angiography provides 'the big picture' and suggests if a stent or reoperation is the best treatment (Fig. 10-27).

Arteriovenous fistulas are a rare complication of transplantation and are most often the result of a biopsy. US imaging alone rarely reveals an abnormality,

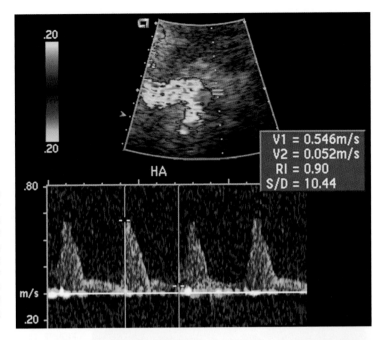

FIGURE 10-25 Spectral Doppler tracing of the hepatic artery on day one after liver transplantation shows a very high-resistance waveform with sharp spikes in systole and very little flow during diastole. Finding high resistance in the hepatic artery soon after surgery is common. It is secondary to ischaemic injury related to the surgical procedure. Rarely does this progress to thrombosis, but more often evolves into a normal-resistance waveform as the oedema and vasospasm subsides.

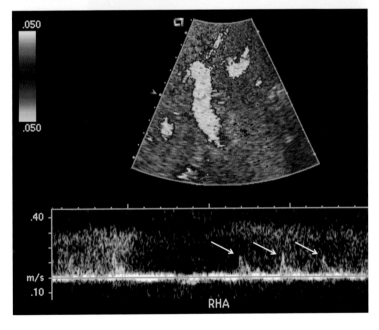

FIGURE 10-26 Spectral Doppler tracing of the porta hepatis on the first postoperative day. The hepatic artery was extremely difficult to identify (arrows). Because of the thready, high-resistance flow due to severe vasospasm this patient should be monitored closely. Ultrasound contrast or a provocative test with vasodilating agents could be considered to more confidently confirm arterial patency.

but colour Doppler shows the localised flash artefact. When Doppler settings are adjusted for high velocities, the feeding artery and draining vein are seen. Spectral Doppler reveals a low-resistance arterial waveform with high diastolic velocity.

The donor portal vein is usually anastomosed end-to-end with the recipient portal vein. Variations may be required if the recipient portal vein is thrombosed, hypoplastic, or of insufficient length. Because the vessel is relatively large, flow alterations on colour Doppler are

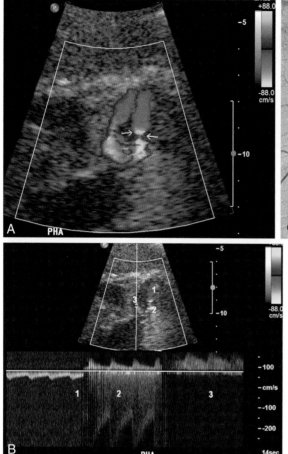

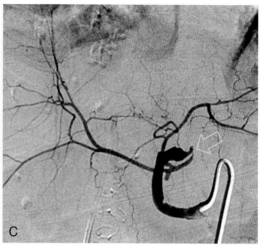

FIGURE 10-27 Intrahepatic Doppler of this liver transplant recipient showed a severe tardus-parvus waveform. (A) Colour Doppler image of the subhepatic space shows an unusual loop of the hepatic artery (B) Spectral Doppler tracing of the hepatic artery across this loop shows slow inflow, followed by an extremely high-velocity jet, followed by the tardus-parvus configuration. (C) A selective catheter angiogram of the hepatic artery reveals a kink (arrow) due to excessive vessel length in the subhepatic space. Reoperation was necessary to straighten the kink and promptly resolved the arterial inflow compromise.

rather striking (Fig. 10-28). Not all flow disturbances perceived by colour Doppler are haemodynamically significant and clinically significant compromise of portal vein flow is relatively rare. When it occurs, it is usually due to mismatch between the diameter of the recipient and donor portal veins, to excessive vessel length causing kink, or to a stenosis. If portal vein stenosis is suspected, the velocity gradient across the anastomosis should be measured by spectral Doppler. A velocity gradient of less than fourfold is unlikely to be significant. Nevertheless, anastomotic compromise can lead to portal vein thrombosis. This can be treated by surgical thrombectomy, angioplasty or thrombolytic infusion. Prompt identification is mandatory to avoid retransplantation.[40,41]

Post-transplantation portal vein thrombosis is quite rare and most often attributed to technical factors. It is more likely to occur in the paediatric recipient, especially after split liver transplantation.[42,43] Prompt detection with frequent Doppler evaluation and aggressive surgical treatment in selected cases are required to avoid graft loss or mortality.

If slow velocity is identified in the portal vein (<1 m/s), it may be due to increased intrahepatic resistance from rejection, or to redirected flow from collateral steal phenomenon. This occurs when large varices remain unligated, shunting blood from the portal system to the systemic circulation, bypassing the liver.[44]

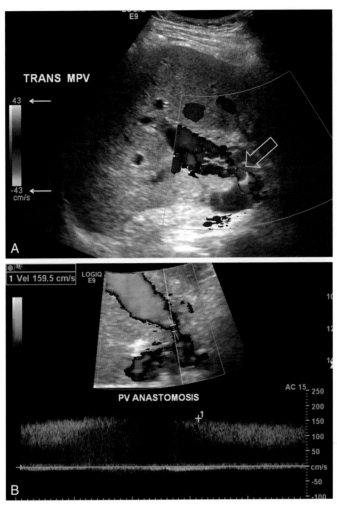

FIGURE 10-28 (A) Colour Doppler image of the portal vein in the region of the anastomosis. Note the area of narrowing at the point of anastomosis where the vein significantly narrows and colour aliasing is present throughout the vessel, despite the relatively high PRF setting (arrows). A post-stenotic jet with turbulence, eddy currents and post-stenotic dilatation is present. (B) Power Doppler does a better job of showing the focal stenosis. Spectral Doppler measured the velocity at 1.6 m/s. This was well over the threshold of the fourfold velocity gradient between pre- and post-stenotic velocities.

A pulsatile waveform in the portal vein may be observed within the first few weeks after transplantation, especially in patients who received small grafts. This pulsatile flow is due to capillary leak and often disappears without any treatment. It may, however, represent vascular complication such as arterioportal fistula.[45]

The donor IVC has a long intrahepatic course and is therefore transplanted along with the liver. The IVC may be inserted in-line with both supra- and infrahepatic

anastomoses; the native intrahepatic IVC being excised with the diseased liver. Currently the surgical technique of choice retains the native IVC of the recipient in place and the upper end of the donor IVC is anastomosed end-to-side to the native IVC at the confluence of the hepatic veins of the explanted liver. The lower end of the donor IVC is oversewn, which functionally converts it into an accessory hepatic vein. Relative flow volumes through this vessel are much less than when it served as the IVC, therefore clot may be seen partially filling the lumen

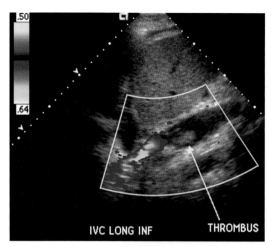

FIGURE 10-29 Longitudinal colour Doppler image of donor inferior vena cava. This liver is anastomosed with a piggy back technique, therefore the flow within the donor inferior vena cava is only a fraction of what it was previously. As a result clot has formed partially filling the lumen (arrow).

(Fig. 10-29). This should not cause concern as long as some flow can be perceived. This type of anastomosis is referred to as a 'piggyback'.[46]

The incidence of hepatic vein complications in partial liver transplantation is more frequent than that in whole liver transplantation. Any compromise of the upper caval anastomosis, from either stenosis or kinking, may cause hepatic venous outflow obstruction. This has been reported to occur in about 2% of recipients. In rare cases, poor graft function can cause swelling of the liver with subsequent obstruction and thrombosis of the vena cava. Ultrasound findings include marked damping, or complete flattening of the hepatic vein velocity profile with complete loss of periodicity, distension of the hepatic veins and a high-velocity jet with turbulence just above the caval anastomosis[47] (Fig. 10-30).

Hepatic vein or caval anastomotic stricture may be treated with balloon dilatation or endovascular stent placement. If these fail, then surgical intervention with a patch venoplasty of the anastomosis can be performed.[48] Ideally, after a successful procedure hepatic vein calibre should decrease and cardiac periodicity should return to the hepatic vein flow profile.[49] Loss of periodicity may also be due to compression of the hepatic veins by the surrounding liver tissue by oedema in the early postoperative period (typically due to preservation injury) or by oedema in the later postoperative period related to rejection.[50]

Due to the potential for a size mismatch between the donor and recipient cava, it is difficult to confidently diagnose a haemodynamically significant stenosis. A persistent monophasic hepatic vein flow profile is highly suggestive for hepatic outflow obstruction, but it is not specific. On the other hand, the presence of periodicity within the hepatic vein tracing on Doppler ultrasound can confidently exclude the significant outflow obstruction.[51] With hepatic vein outflow obstruction, the portal vein flow becomes altered. Increased periodicity may be present in the moderate stage; reversal of flow may occur with severe outflow obstruction.

In those patients with an in-line IVC, compromise of the lower anastomosis may present as lower extremity oedema and renal failure. Ultrasound and colour Doppler imaging of the anastomosis may reveal a kink or focal stenosis with a relatively high-velocity jet. As with a piggyback procedure, a size mismatch between the donor and recipient vessels may produce a relatively high-velocity jet and a less than three-fold velocity increase at the anastomosis is seldom clinically significant.

Several authors have studied the possibility of predicting acute liver transplant rejection by identifying changes in the hepatic vein waveform.[52] During rejection, hepatocellular oedema and inflammatory infiltration cause swelling and increase the pressure within Glisson's capsule. This reduces the compliance of the liver and results in a damped hepatic vein waveform. Unfortunately there are other causes of hepatocellular oedema, such as cholangitis, hepatitis and upper IVC anastomotic stenosis which produce similar damping, thereby limiting the specificity of this finding. The diagnosis of rejection is best made by needle biopsy. Ultrasound and colour Doppler guidance should be used to guide the biopsy needle into the liver, but away from the large central vessels. Nevertheless, a biopsy-related arteriovenous fistula may develop. The majority resolve on their own, but if they persist, it can lead to hepatocellular dysfunction as arterial inflow is shunted away from the liver parenchyma. Doppler evaluation will reveal high-velocity low-resistance

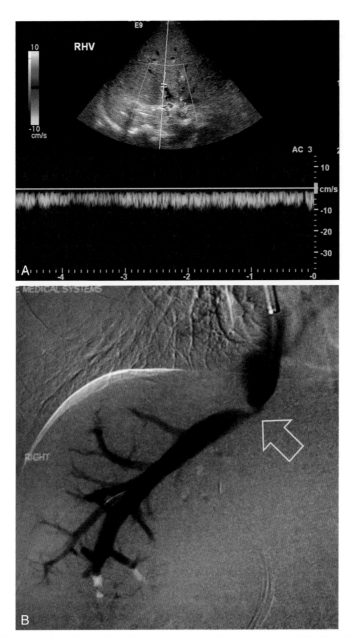

FIGURE 10-30 (A) Spectral Doppler tracing of the right hepatic vein shows complete absence of periodicity. Since this tracing is acquired within a few centimetres of the heart, one should expect to see velocity variation influenced by right atrial contraction. Its absence, along with moderate prominence of the veins, indicates hepatic venous outflow obstruction either due to organ shift and kink or stenosis. (B) A hepatic venogram identified the focal stenosis. Balloon angioplasty was subsequently performed.

arterial inflow to the fistula and arterialisation of the venous outflow (Fig. 10-31).

Hepatocyte transplantation is now performed at some centres as a temporising bridge until a donor liver can be acquired for the candidate. Patients undergo intraportal infusion of cryopreserved, matched human allogenic hepatocytes. Portal vein thrombosis with liver failure and death has been reported as a complication of this

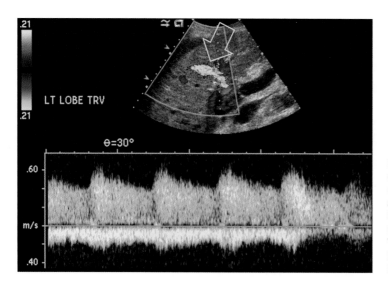

FIGURE 10-31 Colour and spectral Doppler image of the liver transplant recipient that previously had undergone liver transplant biopsy. A prominent artery with markedly increased velocity and aliasing is seen in the mid-liver. Doppler tracing shows markedly increased velocity with turbulence. Venous outflow on the same tracing shows arterialisation of the waveform. This represents a post-biopsy arteriovenous fistula.

treatment. Portal vein Doppler ultrasound during and after cell infusion is mandatory for these patients.[53,54]

Pancreas Transplantation

The first documented human pancreas transplant was performed in 1966 at the University of Minnesota. The goal was to improve glycaemic control without the need for exogenous insulin, thereby minimising or preventing diabetes-mellitus-related complications. There was a steady growth of pancreas transplantation until the year 2004. Since then the frequency has decreased, primarily due to improvements in insulin delivery systems.

In the USA, the current 1-year pancreas graft survival rate (when combined with a renal transplant) is 84.8%. As of 2011, in the US 9500 pancreas transplant recipients were living with a functioning graft.[4] Despite the remarkable improvements made in graft survival rates for all types of pancreatic transplantation, the high prevalence of graft loss caused by immunological rejection and surgical complications continues to be a problem. The technical failure rate approximates 8%, with vascular thrombosis being the dominant cause. Infection, pancreatitis, bleeding, anastomotic leak and rejection are other causes of transplant failure.[55]

The transplanted pancreas is one of the more difficult organs to monitor by any imaging modality. Ultrasound evaluation of the pancreas transplant can be very difficult. Because the pancreas does not have a discrete investing capsule, it is difficult to define its margins with sonography. Taken out of its normal anatomical location, it becomes even more difficult to perceive, especially when camouflaged among bowel loops. Furthermore, in the absence of an adjacent liver, determining its relative echogenicity is impossible. With inflammation of the pancreas and associated oedema of adjacent tissues, the already hard to define pancreas becomes even more indistinct.

The one intrinsic anatomical landmark helpful in determining that one is indeed looking at the pancreas is the pancreatic duct; but it is not always conspicuous. Identification of the pancreas may be improved by use of colour or power Doppler. It identifies flow within the gland and the adjacent transplanted splenic artery and vein. This helps it stand out against the background of bowel loops (Fig. 10-32 A,B).

The pancreas transplant is typically implanted intraperitoneally in the right pelvis using a midline incision, simultaneously with the same donor's kidney in the left pelvis. Organ harvesting of a deceased donor typically sends the major vascular pedicle with the liver. This leaves the pancreas with two unlinked arterial trunks (gastroduodenal and splenic) each requiring an arterial jump-graft. This is accomplished with a Y-graft from the donor's common, external and internal iliac arteries (Fig. 10-33). One branch of the Y-graft is sutured to the donor superior mesenteric artery, whereas the donor splenic artery is anastomosed to

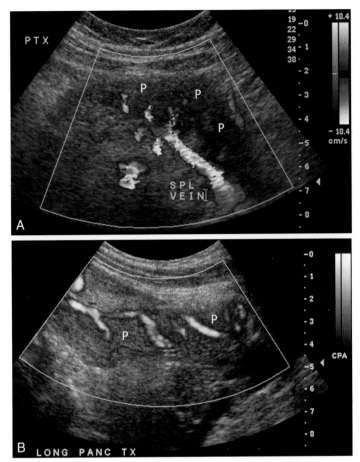

FIGURE 10-32 Colour Doppler image of the transplant pancreas (P). (A) The vascular pedicle to the transplant pancreas is a prominent feature that helps to distinguish it from the surrounding bowel loops. (B) Setting scan parameters for slower velocities can depict branch vasculature within the pancreas transplant. This of course may be difficult when there is robust peristalsis in adjacent bowel loops.

the other limb. Intraoperatively, the common iliac trunk of the donor Y-graft is then anastomosed to the recipient iliac artery. The donor portal vein is anastomosed to either a systemic vein or the portal venous system.[56]

Many sonographic patterns of pancreas transplant dysfunction have been described, including focal or diffuse inhomogeneity of echo texture; increased or decreased overall echogenicity and graft swelling. Unfortunately, none of these imaging findings is pathognomonic for any one complication of the pancreas transplant. In general, acute inflammatory changes tend to result in an oedematous swollen pancreas and a chronic insult tends to result in a small echogenic gland. These characteristics, however, do not help in solving the immediate clinical dilemma, specifically, differentiation between pancreatitis, rejection and vascular compromise.

A complete sonographic examination of the pancreas transplant recipient should cover the points listed in Box 10-6. When examining a pancreas transplant recipient, it is mandatory that the sonologist know the anatomic details of that patient's transplant (Fig. 10-34 A,B). Urological and metabolic complications occur frequently in the bladder-drained pancreas transplant recipient. Approximately 25% of bladder-drained pancreas allografts ultimately undergo enteric

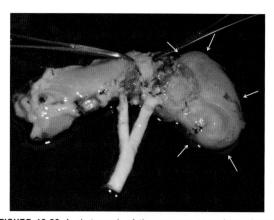

FIGURE 10-33 A photograph of the pancreas transplant prior to implantation, after creation of the donor vascular 'Y' graft. The head of the pancreas gets its blood supply from the gastroduodenal artery, and the body and tail from the splenic artery. This graft, harvested from the donor common iliac bifurcation, is created to establish arterial blood supply from a single recipient anastomosis. Note the duodenal stump along the head of the pancreas (arrows).

BOX 10-6 PANCREAS TRANSPLANT – SONOGRAPHIC EXAMINATION CHECKLIST

- Review the surgical record, especially with regard to the vasculature and drainage technique. Review any available prior imaging studies
- Evaluate organ echotexture. Make certain it is uniform throughout
- Rule out pancreatic duct dilatation
- Rule out peripancreatic fluid collections
- Examine the main artery to the transplant, particularly near its anastomosis
- Rule out pseudocyst
- Verify venous patency, particularly with high-resistance arterial inflow to the organ
- Verify uniform parenchymal perfusion by colour and power Doppler

conversion for these complications. Therefore, enteric drainage is now the preferred conduit for managing pancreatic exocrine secretions (amylase and lipase).

Unfortunately, the pancreas allograft is particularly prone to complications and early graft failure. Since the recipients are diabetics, they already have multiple medical and vascular issues. Additionally, the pancreas is a relatively low-flow organ relative to the vascular pedicle supplying it. Since the splenic artery and vein end blindly (the donor spleen is removed), there is an increased possibility of developing clot. If not properly anticoagulated, partial thrombosis may progress to complete organ thrombosis. Consequently, Doppler sonography is mandatory in searching for vascular complications including thrombosis, or anastomotic stricture.[57] Non-visualisation of flow within the organ is the ultimate disappointment. The Doppler tracing usually shows pan-diastolic reversal of arterial flow within the graft with an RI greater than 1.0 (Fig. 10-35). If identified promptly, however, thrombolytic therapy alone, or in combination with surgical thrombectomy, has been reported to succeed in restoring transplant perfusion. Early diagnosis of pancreas transplant vascular complications is of paramount importance for appropriate treatment and organ salvage.[58,59] Resistive indices (RIs) are otherwise quite variable when acquired within the transplant pancreas, thus limiting its clinical usefulness.

The digestive enzymes are typically drained into the gut via the duodenal stump, but if a leak occurs fluid may extend to the pancreas vasculature predisposing to pseudoaneurysm formation, especially in the region of the anastomosis. Pseudoaneurysms can also develop after biopsy, pancreatitis or graft infection. Arterial flow within a perianastomotic fluid collection, the presence of swirling blood on colour Doppler, and a to-and-fro spectral Doppler waveform indicate a transplant pedicle pseudoaneurysm (Fig. 10-36). Rupture of transplant-associated pseudoaneurysm has been described and is a life-threatening event.[60,61]

The pancreas, as with any other transplanted organ, requires occasional biopsy and this increases the risk of arteriovenous fistula (AVF). Doppler findings are similar to AVFs in other locations (Fig. 10-37A,B). AVFs are often clinically silent, although pancreatic endocrine insufficiency, pain, and a bruit over the graft can be presenting features. High-flow AVF may compromise graft perfusion, causing a 'steal phenomenon'. This may result in organ ischaemia.[62]

Although ultrasound is excellent in identifying parapancreatic fluid collections, the finding is basically non-specific. Abscess, haematoma or liquefied phlegmon

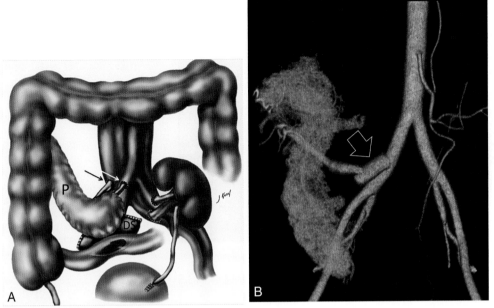

FIGURE 10-34 Artist rendering of a combined renal pancreas transplant. (A) Typically the pancreas (P) is transplanted on the right with an interposed duodenal stump (DS) between pancreas and ileum. The splenic artery and vein, which serve as the vascular pedicle for the pancreas transplant, are anastomosed to the common iliac artery and inferior vena cava. (B) With multiorgan donation harvesting of the vascular pedicle with the liver often leaves the pancreas requiring an interposition graft. This is typically accomplished with donor iliac artery. Branches are connected to the remnants of the splenic and gastroduodenal arteries, perfusing the body and the head of the pancreas respectively. Interposition jump grafts can be quite creative with the goal of establishing good perfusion to the end organ. Again, transmission of the surgical record is critical to the imager trying to understand complex surgical anatomy to the organ they are being asked to study. 3-D CTA of a pancreas transplant with an interposition graft added to establish appropriate length of the arterial conduit.

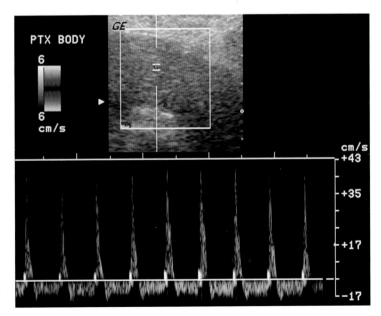

FIGURE 10-35 Power and spectral Doppler image of the pancreas. Despite optimised settings, no colour flow can be identified within the gland. A spectral Doppler tracing of the feeding artery shows extremely high resistance with spike of systolic inflow and reversed outflow throughout diastole. This is usually the result of venous outflow obstruction due to thrombosis or a kink. Microvascular thrombosis, secondary to severe acute rejection, can have a similar appearance.

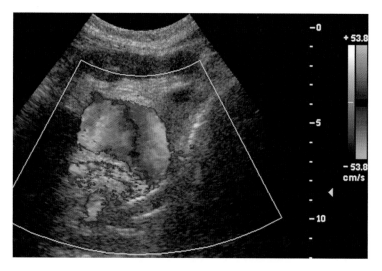

FIGURE 10-36 Colour Doppler image near the anastomosis of the pancreatic vascular pedicle. A rounded collection of colour flow with the classic swirl pattern identifies pseudoaneurysm of the anastomosed splenic artery.

may all have a similar ultrasound appearance of complicated, debris-filled, irregular collections (Fig. 10-38 A,B). The true extent of these collections is better evaluated by CT since bowel gas does not limit visualisation. Furthermore, follow-up CT examinations can be more reliably compared than ultrasound studies. The source of a fluid collection is best evaluated by a CT contrast study or by aspiration.

Rejection affects about 40% of pancreas transplants. Unfortunately, imaging findings lack specificity. Preliminary reports suggested that elevation of the resistive index could predict pancreas transplant rejection.

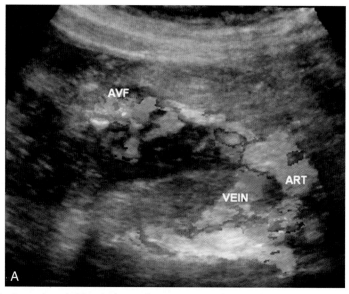

FIGURE 10-37 3-D rendered colour and spectral Doppler image of a pancreas several weeks after a biopsy. (A) The colour Doppler image shows a feeding artery and large draining vein from a focus of tortuous vascularity.

Continued

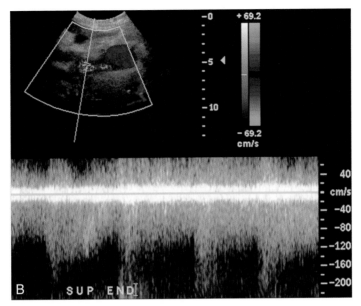

FIGURE 10-37—CONT'D (B) Spectral Doppler tracing shows high-velocity, turbulent, low-resistance arterial flow in the area of flash artifact. This was an arteriovenous fistula; a complication of the biopsy.

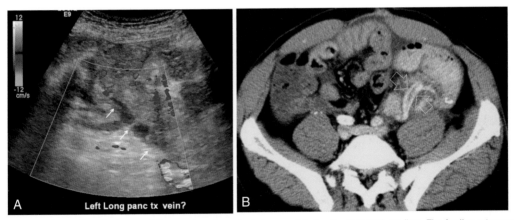

FIGURE 10-38 (A) Colour Doppler image of the pancreas transplant shows a tubular structure with no flow. The feeding artery was easily identified so the sonologist questioned whether this might represent clot within the vein. (B) Venous phase image from a CT angiogram reveals a tubular filling defect within the splenic vein (arrow) draining this pancreas transplant. The small amount of venous outflow from the pancreas is insufficient to flush this large-calibre vein which used to drain the spleen as well.

Unfortunately this is not the case, as many rejecting transplants have normal resistive indices. Since the pancreatic graft lacks a capsule, the rejection process will not generate enough intraparenchymal pressure to cause a consistently measurable elevation of vascular resistance. The key role of ultrasound in rejection is to guide the pancreas transplant biopsy. It must identify a safe path to the organ, free of overlying intestine or mesentery. Doppler needs to identify the pancreatic vascular pedicle which must be avoided. The biopsy is monitored in real time, and delayed imaging and Doppler are useful to identify complications.[63]

Post-Transplantation Lymphoproliferative Disorder

Post-transplantation lymphoproliferative disorder (PTLD) is a rare but serious complication following solid organ transplantation. The most commonly accepted theory for the pathophysiology of PTLD is that Epstein–Barr virus (EBV)-induced B-cell proliferation, unopposed by the pharmacologically suppressed immune system, causes plasma cell hyperplasia, leading to premalignant polymorphic B-cell proliferation and eventually malignant monoclonal lymphoma. If untreated, it can be fatal.[64] Reduction or cessation of immunosuppression is the best treatment and usually results in tumour regression. Early diagnosis prior to the development of frank lymphoma is very important and these patients have a much better prognosis. In a large study of PTLD in renal transplant recipients, the incidence was 2% of 1383 patients; but it contributed to death in over 50% of these cases.[65]

The liver is the organ most frequently involved by PTLD. It can appear as a focal mass, diffuse infiltration, or a periportal mass.[66] PTLD can affect the transplanted kidney and may manifest as a focal renal mass or diffuse infiltration.[67] The pancreas transplant may be involved, and can present as diffuse enlargement of the allograft or as a focal mass which may be confused with pancreatitis or acute rejection.[68]

Since ultrasound is often the first imaging study performed when laboratory tests suggest transplant dysfunction, it plays an important role in the early diagnosis of PTLD. It may detect urinary or biliary obstruction associated with adenopathy or may perceive a new ill-defined, typically hypoechoic mass. Doppler may show vascular distortion by the mass or adenopathy.[69]

Other Imaging Modalities

MR angiography (MRA) has been found to be sensitive but not specific in the detection of significant vascular stenosis, nevertheless, normal MRA findings reliably exclude the possibility of significant stenosis. CT and CT angiography (CTA) are excellent at identifying transplant and peritransplant fluid collections, abscess formation, vascular complications, etc. However, due to the need for nephrotoxic contrast and the radiation dose, ultrasound is the preferred screening test, with CT and CTA used for confirmation and problem solving.[70]

Summary

These are very rewarding times in the field of organ transplantation. Advances in organ procurement and preservation; better matching of donors and recipients; refined surgical techniques; availability of new, more effective immunosuppressive agents; and improved post-transplant monitoring of organ recipients have contributed to decreased patient morbidity and improved allograft survival. Although Doppler sonography is only able to make a definitive diagnosis in a small percentage of cases, it is extremely useful as a screening tool in the management of transplant complications. All of this has allowed transplant recipients greater opportunity to return to a more normal lifestyle after surgery.[71,72]

Acknowledgements

Thanks to Dr Luis Fernandez, Department of Surgery, University of Wisconsin for manuscript review, Mercedes Kirk and Jeanne Johnson for manuscript preparation and Mike Ledwidge, RT, RDMS, for image preparation.

REFERENCES

1. Heeger PS, Dinavahi R. Transplant immunology for non-immunologist. *Mt Sinai J Med* 2012;**79**(3):376–87.
2. Klipa D, Mahmud N, Ahsan N. Antibody immunosuppressive therapy in solid organ transplant: Part II. *mAbs* 2010;**2**(6): 607–12.
3. Bestard O, Campistol JM, Morales JM, et al. Advances in immunosuppression for kidney transplantation: new strategies for preserving kidney function and reducing cardiovascular risk. *Nefrologia* 2012;**32**(3):374–84.
4. US Department of Health and Human Services PHS. OPTN/ SRTR Annual Report: Transplant Data 1999–2008. Health Resources and Services Administration; 2009. [cited 2013 March 19]; Available from: *http://optn.transplant.hrsa.gov/ ar2009/survival_rates.htm*.
5. Irshad A, Ackerman SJ, Campbell AS, et al. An overview of renal transplantation: current practice and use of ultrasound. *Semin Ultrasound CT MR* 2009;**30**(4):298–314.
6. Pozniak MA, Zagzebski JA, Scanlan KA. Spectral and color Doppler artifacts. *Radiographics* 1992;**12**(1):35–44.
7. Pozniak MA, Kelcz F, Stratta RJ, et al. Extraneous factors affecting resistive index. *Invest Radiol* 1988;**23**(12):899–904.
8. Cosgrove DO, Chan KE. Renal transplants: what ultrasound can and cannot do. *Ultrasound Q* 2008;**24**(2):77–87.

9. Pozniak MA, Kelcz F, D'Alessandro A, et al. Sonography of renal transplants in dogs: the effect of acute tubular necrosis, cyclosporine nephrotoxicity, and acute rejection on resistive index and renal length. *AJR Am J Roentgenol* 1992;**158**(4):791–7.

10. Tublin ME, Bude RO, Platt JF. Review. The resistive index in renal Doppler sonography: where do we stand? *AJR Am J Roentgenol* 2003;**180**(4):885–92.

11. Ekberg H, Johansson ME. Challenges and considerations in diagnosing the kidney disease in deteriorating graft function. *Transpl Int* 2012;**25**(11):1119–28.

12. Friedewald SM, Molmenti EP, Friedewald JJ, et al. Vascular and nonvascular complications of renal transplants: sonographic evaluation and correlation with other imaging modalities, surgery, and pathology. *J Clin Ultrasound* 2005;**33**(3):127–39.

13. Rivera M, Villacorta J, Jimenez-Alvaro S, et al. Asymptomatic large extracapsular renal pseudoaneurysm following kidney transplant biopsy. *Am J Kidney Dis* 2011;**57**(1):175–8.

14. Minetti EE. Lymphocele after renal transplantation, a medical complication. *J Nephrol* 2011;**24**(6):707–16.

15. Lucewicz A, Isaacs A, Allen RD, et al. Torsion of intraperitoneal kidney transplant. *ANZ J Surg* 2012;**82**(5):299–302.

16. Platt JF, Ellis JH, Rubin JM. Renal transplant pyelocaliectasis: role of duplex Doppler US in evaluation. *Radiology* 1991;**179**(2):425–8.

17. Pozniak MA, Dodd 3rd GD, Kelcz F. Ultrasonographic evaluation of renal transplantation. *Radiol Clin North Am* 1992;**30**(5):1053–66.

18. Jimenez C, Lopez MO, Gonzalez E, et al. Ultrasonography in kidney transplantation: values and new developments. *Transplant Rev (Orlando)* 2009;**23**(4):209–13.

19. Lockhart ME, Robbin ML. Renal vascular imaging: ultrasound and other modalities. *Ultrasound Q* 2007;**23**(4):279–92.

20. Stavros AT, Parker SH, Yakes WF, et al. Segmental stenosis of the renal artery: pattern recognition of tardus and parvus abnormalities with duplex sonography. *Radiology* 1992;**184**(2):487–92.

21. Ponticelli C, Moia M, Montagnino G. Renal allograft thrombosis. *Nephrol Dial Transplant* 2009;**24**(5):1388–93.

22. Hedegard W, Saad WE, Davies MG. Management of vascular and nonvascular complications after renal transplantation. *Tech Vasc Interv Radiol* 2009;**12**(4):240–62.

23. Baxter GM, Morley P, Dall B. Acute renal vein thrombosis in renal allografts: new Doppler ultrasonic findings. *Clin Radiol* 1991;**43**(2):125–7.

24. Kribs SW, Rankin RN. Doppler ultrasonography after renal transplantation: value of reversed diastolic flow in diagnosing renal vein obstruction. *Can Assoc Radiol J* 1993;**44**(6):434–8.

25. McEvoy S, Stunell H, Ramadan T, et al. A review of the imaging and intervention of liver transplant complications. *JBR-BTR* 2010;**93**(5):235–41.

26. Ravindra KV, Guthrie JA, Woodley H, et al. Preoperative vascular imaging in pediatric liver transplantation. *J Pediatr Surg* 2005;**40**(4):643–7.

27. Kluger MD, Memeo R, Laurent A, et al. Survey of adult liver transplantation techniques (SALT): an international study of current practices in deceased donor liver transplantation. *HPB* 2011;**13**(10):692–8.

28. Berrocal T, Parron M, Alvarez-Luque A, et al. Pediatric liver transplantation: a pictorial essay of early and late complications. *Radiographics* 2006;**26**(4):1187–209.

29. Nakamura T, Tanaka K, Kiuchi T, et al. Anatomical variations and surgical strategies in right lobe living donor liver transplantation: lessons from 120 cases. *Transplantation* 2002;**73**(12):1896–903.

30. Sidhu PS, Ellis SM, Karani JB, et al. Hepatic artery stenosis following liver transplantation: significance of the tardus parvus waveform and the role of microbubble contrast media in the detection of a focal stenosis. *Clin Radiol* 2002;**57**(9):789–99.

31. Kaneko J, Sugawara Y, Akamatsu N, et al. Prediction of hepatic artery thrombosis by protocol Doppler ultrasonography in pediatric living donor liver transplantation. *Abdom Imaging* 2004;**29**(5):603–5.

32. Sidhu PS, Shaw AS, Ellis SM, et al. Microbubble ultrasound contrast in the assessment of hepatic artery patency following liver transplantation: role in reducing frequency of hepatic artery arteriography. *Eur Radiol* 2004;**14**(1):21–30.

33. Herold C, Reck T, Ott R, et al. Contrast-enhanced ultrasound improves hepatic vessel visualization after orthotopic liver transplantation. *Abdom Imaging* 2001;**26**(6):597–600.

34. Bekker J, Ploem S, de Jong KP. Early hepatic artery thrombosis after liver transplantation: a systematic review of the incidence, outcome and risk factors. *Am J Transplant* 2009;**9**(4):746–57.

35. Pareja E, Cortes M, Navarro R, et al. Vascular complications after orthotopic liver transplantation: hepatic artery thrombosis. *Transplant Proc* 2010;**42**(8):2970–2.

36. Vivarelli M, Cucchetti A, La Barba G, et al. Ischemic arterial complications after liver transplantation in the adult: multivariate analysis of risk factors. *Arch Surg* 2004;**139**(10):1069–74.

37. Garcia-Criado A, Gilabert R, Salmeron JM, et al. Significance of and contributing factors for a high resistive index on Doppler sonography of the hepatic artery immediately after surgery: prognostic implications for liver transplant recipients. *AJR Am J Roentgenol* 2003;**181**(3):831–8.

38. Stell D, Downey D, Marotta P, et al. Prospective evaluation of the role of quantitative Doppler ultrasound surveillance in liver transplantation. *Liver Transpl* 2004;**10**(9):1183–8.

39. Propeck PA, Scanlan KA. Reversed or absent hepatic arterial diastolic flow in liver transplants shown by duplex sonography: a poor predictor of subsequent hepatic artery thrombosis. *AJR Am J Roentgenol* 1992;**159**(6):1199–201.

40. Doria C, Marino IR. Acute portal vein thrombosis secondary to donor/recipient portal vein diameter mismatch after orthotopic liver transplantation: a case report. *Int Surg* 2003;**88**(4):184–7.

41. Rodriguez-Castro KI, Porte RJ, Nadal E, et al. Management of nonneoplastic portal vein thrombosis in the setting of liver transplantation: a systematic review. *Transplantation* 2012;**94**(11):1145–53.

42. Cheng YF, Chen CL, Huang TL, et al. Risk factors for intraoperative portal vein thrombosis in pediatric living donor liver transplantation. *Clin Transplant* 2004;**18**(4):390–4.

43. Corno V, Torri E, Bertani A, et al. Early portal vein thrombosis after pediatric split liver transplantation with left lateral segment graft. *Transplant Proc* 2005;**37**(2):1141–2.

44. Nishida S, Kadono J, DeFaria W, et al. Gastroduodenal artery steal syndrome during liver transplantation: intraoperative diagnosis with Doppler ultrasound and management. *Transpl Int* 2005;**18**(3):350–3.

45. Tang SS, Shimizu T, Kishimoto R, et al. Analysis of portal venous waveform after living-related liver transplantation with pulsed Doppler ultrasound. *Clin Transplant* 2001;**15**(6):380–7.

46. Salizzoni M, Andorno E, Bossuto E, et al. Piggyback techniques versus classical technique in orthotopic liver transplantation: a review of 75 cases. *Transplant Proc* 1994;**26**(6):3552–3.

47. Darcy MD. Management of venous outflow complications after liver transplantation. *Tech Vasc Interv Radiol* 2007;**10**(3): 240–5.

48. Akamatsu N, Sugawara Y, Kaneko J, et al. Surgical repair for late-onset hepatic venous outflow block after living-donor liver transplantation. *Transplantation* 2004;**77**(11):1768–70.

49. Totsuka E, Hakamada K, Narumi S, et al. Hepatic vein anastomotic stricture after living donor liver transplantation. *Transplant Proc* 2004;**36**(8):2252–4.

50. Lee HJ, Kim KW, Mun HS, et al. Uncommon causes of hepatic congestion in patients after living donor liver transplantation. *AJR Am J Roentgenol* 2009;**193**(3):772–80.

51. Ko EY, Kim TK, Kim PN, et al. Hepatic vein stenosis after living donor liver transplantation: evaluation with Doppler US. *Radiology* 2003;**229**(3):806–10.

52. Jequier S, Jequier JC, Hanquinet S, et al. Orthotopic liver transplants in children: change in hepatic venous Doppler wave pattern as an indicator of acute rejection. *Radiology* 2003;**226**(1):105–12.

53. Baccarani U, Adani GL, Sanna A, et al. Portal vein thrombosis after intraportal hepatocytes transplantation in a liver transplant recipient. *Transpl Int* 2005;**18**(6):750–4.

54. Fitzpatrick E, Mitry RR, Dhawan A. Human hepatocyte transplantation: state of the art. *J Intern Med* 2009;**266**(4):339–57.

55. Nikolaidis P, Amin RS, Hwang CM, et al. Role of sonography in pancreatic transplantation. *Radiographics* 2003;**23**(4): 939–49.

56. Dillman JR, Elsayes KM, Bude RO, et al. Imaging of pancreas transplants: postoperative findings with clinical correlation. *J Comput Assist Tomogr* 2009;**33**(4):609–17. http://dx.doi.org/10.1097/RCT.0b013e3181966988.

57. Foshager MC, Hedlund LJ, Troppmann C, et al. Venous thrombosis of pancreatic transplants: diagnosis by duplex sonography. *AJR Am J Roentgenol* 1997;**169**(5):1269–73.

58. Boggi U, Vistoli F, Signori S, et al. Surveillance and rescue of pancreas grafts. *Transplant Proc* 2005;**37**(6):2644–7.

59. Muthusamy AS, Giangrande PL, Friend PJ. Pancreas allograft thrombosis. *Transplantation* 2010;**90**(7):705–7.

60. Delis S, Dervenis C, Bramis J, et al. Vascular complications of pancreas transplantation. *Pancreas* 2004;**28**(4):413–20.

61. Green BT, Tuttle-Newhall J, Suhocki P, et al. Massive gastrointestinal hemorrhage due to rupture of a donor pancreatic artery pseudoaneurysm in a pancreas transplant patient. *Clin Transplant* 2004;**18**(1):108–11.

62. Buttarelli L, Capocasale E, Marcato C, et al. Embolization of pancreatic allograft arteriovenous fistula with the Amplatzer Vascular Plug 4: case report and literature analysis. *Transplant Proc* 2011;**43**(10):4044–7.

63. Wong JJ, Krebs TL, Klassen DK, et al. Sonographic evaluation of acute pancreatic transplant rejection: morphology–Doppler analysis versus guided percutaneous biopsy. *AJR Am J Roentgenol* 1996;**166**(4):803–7.

64. Nalesnik MA. The diverse pathology of post-transplant lymphoproliferative disorders: the importance of a standardized approach. *Transpl Infect Dis* 2001;**3**(2):88–96.

65. Bates WD, Gray DW, Dada MA, et al. Lymphoproliferative disorders in Oxford renal transplant recipients. *J Clin Pathol* 2003;**56**(6):439–46.

66. Kamdar KY, Rooney CM, Heslop HE. Posttransplant lymphoproliferative disease following liver transplantation. *Curr Opin Org Transplant* 2011;**16**(3):274–80.

67. Vrachliotis TG, Vaswani KK, Davies EA, et al. CT findings in posttransplantation lymphoproliferative disorder of renal transplants. *AJR Am J Roentgenol* 2000;**175**(1):183–8.

68. Meador TL, Krebs TL, Cheong JJ, et al. Imaging features of posttransplantation lymphoproliferative disorder in pancreas transplant recipients. *AJR Am J Roentgenol* 2000;**174**(1):121–4.

69. Scarsbrook AF, Warakaulle DR, Dattani M, et al. Posttransplantation lymphoproliferative disorder: the spectrum of imaging appearances. *Clin Radiol* 2005;**60**(1):47–55.

70. Saad WE, Lin E, Ormanoski M, et al. Noninvasive imaging of liver transplant complications. *Tech Vasc Interv Radiol* 2007;**10**(3): 191–206.

71. Lim KB, Schiano TD. Long-term outcome after liver transplantation. *Mt Sinai J Med* 2012;**79**(2):169–89.

72. Vandermeer FQ, Manning MA, Frazier AA, et al. Imaging of whole-organ pancreas transplants. *Radiographics* 2012;**32**(2):411–35.

Chapter 11

Doppler Imaging of the Prostate

Fred T. Lee, Jr and Fred Lee, Sr

Indications

The most important use of colour Doppler imaging of the prostate remains as an aid in cancer detection. This is particularly relevant in patients in whom cancer is suspected based on prostate specific antigen (PSA) elevation without obvious tumour on grey scale imaging. Other uses for Doppler imaging are largely confined to detection of prostatitis and inflammatory conditions. Controversy continues surrounding diagnosis and treatment of prostate cancer. This is largely attributable to the wide range of biological behaviour found with this disease. Up to 30% of 80-year-old males will have histological evidence of prostate cancer, yet most will die from other causes. Unfortunately, a more aggressive subset remains an important cause of mortality among men, with 33,720 deaths expected in the USA in 2011.[1]

Anatomy

The prostate lies immediately anterior to the rectum and inferior to the bladder. Prostatic zonal anatomy has been extensively described by McNeal.[2] In summary, the prostate is composed of three major zonal areas; the peripheral zone, the central zone and the transition zone (Fig. 11-1).

The peripheral zone is the most posterior, and the central zone is a continuation of the peripheral zone cephalad. The transition zone is the most central area of the prostate, and surrounds the urethra as it courses through the prostate. The anterior fibromuscular stroma lines the prostate anteriorally.

PROSTATE VASCULAR ANATOMY

The prostate is supplied from two arterial sources: the prostatic arteries and the inferior vesical arteries, both arising from the internal iliac system. The prostatic arteries enter the prostate from an anterolateral location on each side, and give off capsular branches as well as urethral branches. Capsular arteries course along the lateral margin of the prostate, and give off numerous perforating branches which penetrate the capsule and supply approximately two-thirds of the total glandular tissue. The areas of penetration into the capsule are commonly referred to as the neurovascular bundles (Fig. 11-2).

The inferior vesical arteries run along the inferior surface of the bladder and also provide urethral branches. In addition to supplying the central portion of the prostate, the inferior vesical arteries also give off branches which supply the bladder base, seminal vesicles and distal ureters (Fig. 11-3).[3,4]

Both the capsular and urethral branches can be visualised with colour Doppler ultrasound. In the absence of inflammation, neoplasm or hypertrophy, the normal prostate is expected to have low-level periurethral and pericapsular flow, with only a low level of flow in the prostatic parenchyma.[5]

Equipment and Technique

Examination of the prostate by ultrasound requires a high-frequency (5–7.5 MHz) end-fire or biplane transrectal transducer. For the purposes of this chapter, conventional colour Doppler and power Doppler are considered simultaneously. For most general applications, an end-fire transducer is favoured due to the ease of switching between axial (coronal) and longitudinal imaging planes, as well as the more favourable angle for transrectal prostatic biopsies. For specialised applications such as I^{131} seed implantation and cryoablation, a true biplane transducer is necessary.

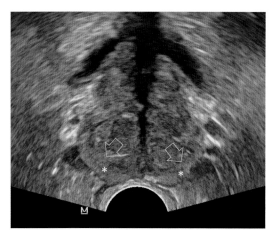

FIGURE 11-1 Axial ultrasound of the prostate in a normal patient. Note peripheral zone (*) separated from the more centrally oriented, periurethral, transition zone by the surgical capsule (open arrows).

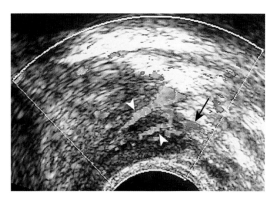

FIGURE 11-2 Axial image of the left neurovascular bundle. Note left neurovascular bundle (arrow) with perforating branches penetrating into the prostate.

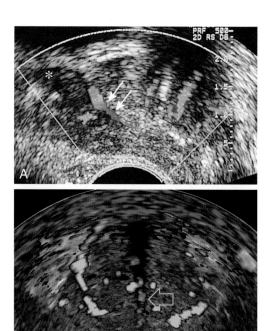

FIGURE 11-3 (A) Sagittal image of the prostate at the level of the seminal vesicle (*) demonstrates periurethral flow (arrows) originating from the inferior vesicle artery. (B) Axial power Doppler image at the level of the mid prostate demonstrates branches of the inferior vesical artery (open arrow) supplying urethra and surgical capsule.

No specific patient preparation is required although some centres will give the patient a pre-examination enema and have them empty their bladder. The patient is generally placed in the left lateral decubitus position, and the knees brought up to the chest. A digital rectal examination is recommended prior to probe insertion to rule out any obstructing pathology and also to allow the examiner to evaluate the prostate by digital examination. The probe is covered with a condom into which coupling gel has been placed, and the probe lubricated and gently inserted into the rectal canal. Examination of the prostate by grey scale imaging

is first performed, and the length, width and height of the gland measured. The prostatic volume is calculated based on the formula for a prolate ellipsoid (length × width × height × 0.523); this allows correlation of the measured PSA with a predicted PSA based on gland volume. Normal prostatic tissue produces approximately 0.3 ng/cc of PSA, whereas cancerous tissue produces approximately 3.0 ng/cc of PSA. Normal levels for polyclonal assays are typically defined as <4.0 ng/mL; unfortunately, up to 20% of prostatic cancers present in patients with 'normal' levels of PSA. A 'predicted' PSA can be generated based on the patient's gland volume × 0.2 for polyclonal assays (or gland volume × 0.1 for monoclonal assays). A level of measured PSA that exceeds predicted PSA increases the suspicion of cancer and increases the positive predictive value of prostatic biopsy.[6]

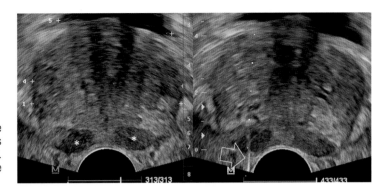

FIGURE 11-4 Bilateral prostate cancer. Axial image of the prostate at mid gland (left) demonstrates bilateral peripheral zone hypoechoic tumours (*). The image on right demonstrates a biopsy needle (open arrow) traversing one of the tumours.

Most prostate cancers (70%) arise in the peripheral zone, with a minority originating in the central (10–15%) and transition zones (10–15%). Because of this, it is very important that the sonographer carefully examine the peripheral zone for signs of tumour. Virtually all prostate cancers will be hypoechoic in relation to normal peripheral zone tissues (Fig. 11-4), although a minority of cribriform carcinomas can demonstrate punctate calcifications.

Tumours in the peripheral zone have ready access to sites of anatomical weakness, including the neurovascular bundles, ejaculatory ducts and apex of the gland. This results in more aggressive clinical behaviour of peripheral zone tumours when compared to other locations. Transition zone tumours tend to behave in a clinically more benign manner because they are distant from sites of anatomical weakness, and thus need to grow quite large before spreading outside of the gland. The main problem with the diagnosis of transition zone tumours is the heterogeneous echotexture of the normal transition zone. Because normal transition zone tissue can be hypoechoic, hyperechoic or contain calcifications or cysts, it is extremely difficult to diagnose subtle changes in echogenicity that may be associated with neoplasia. Therefore, colour Doppler can play a crucial role in the diagnosis of transition zone tumours by identifying areas of abnormal flow.

Colour Doppler of Prostate Cancer

Prostate cancer arises in both the outer (peripheral zone) and central gland (transition zone). Cancers in these two locations have different imaging characteristics and biologic behaviour[7] and thus will be considered separately.

Outer gland (peripheral zone) cancer: Tumours arising in the peripheral zone tend to be isoechoic at grey scale imaging with the background normal prostate (Fig. 11-4). As the tumours enlarge, they become progressively more hypoechoic, and thus become more apparent by ultrasound (Fig. 11-5).

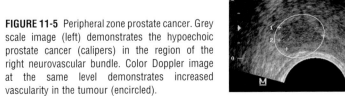
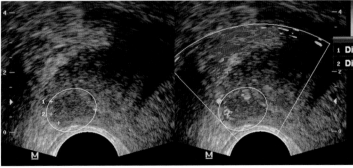

FIGURE 11-5 Peripheral zone prostate cancer. Grey scale image (left) demonstrates the hypoechoic prostate cancer (calipers) in the region of the right neurovascular bundle. Color Doppler image at the same level demonstrates increased vascularity in the tumour (encircled).

Large tumours are usually more de-differentiated with a higher Gleason score. Focal areas of calcification may develop in regions of necrosis. As tumours further increase in size, the risk of extra-capsular extension also increases. Above approximately 1.5 cm in diameter areas of anatomic weakness should be carefully surveyed, including the seminal vesicles, neurovascular bundles, and the apical capsule. Targeted biopsies through these regions can increase the specificity of diagnosis for extra-capsular extension of tumour.[8] As peripheral zone tumours enlarge the degree of microvascular density also increases. In general, these larger tumours are therefore more vascular and demonstrate increased colour Doppler signal.

Inner gland (transition zone) cancer: Transition zone cancers are biologically different to peripheral zone tumours. In general, they are associated with favourable pathologic features, and are less likely to present with early extra-capsular extension. Large-volume transition zone cancers are often associated with low Gleason scores.[7] Cancers that arise in the transition zone are more difficult to detect with ultrasound because of the heterogeneous nature of the background tissue. 'Normal' transition zone tissue is of mixed echogenicity and may contain cysts and calcified foci. Similar to peripheral zone tumours, transition zone cancer is generally hypoechoic and demonstrates increased vascularity at colour Doppler imaging (Fig. 11-6),[7] but because of the heterogeneous background of the transition zone, central cancer can be difficult to detect with grey scale imaging alone.

For a high-risk patient (based on PSA) in whom a peripheral tumour has not been found, a careful examination of the transition zone should be undertaken. For these patients, colour Doppler has been shown to be most useful.[9] Areas of increased colour Doppler signal can be targeted for biopsy with increased positive biopsy rates, but it is controversial as to whether targeted biopsies guided by colour Doppler imaging can replace sextant biopsies.[10–12] Biopsy of areas of increased colour signal when no other sites of cancer have been found can be particularly useful in black males, where the positive predictive value for biopsy based on Doppler findings has been found to be twice that of white males (32.2% vs. 13.5% respectively).[13] There is currently no consensus regarding the use of ultrasound contrast agents in prostate imaging.[14,15] Likewise, spectral Doppler has limited utility in the diagnosis of prostate cancer. While most tumours demonstrate a low resistance waveform (high diastolic flow), this is not a specific finding and does not separate cancer from inflammation.

Colour Doppler of Prostatic Inflammatory Disease

Prostatitis is a difficult condition to diagnose and treat. There are several aetiologies of prostatitis, ranging from bacterial to non-bacterial causes. In the case of bacterial prostatitis, the offending organism is usually *Escherichia coli* or other urinary tract pathogens. Grey scale findings of acute prostatitis include an

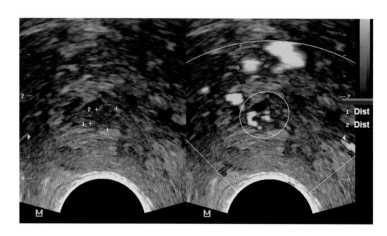

FIGURE 11-6 Transition zone (central gland) prostate cancer. Axial images demonstrate a hypoechoic mass on grey scale ultrasound (calipers) with hypervascularity on power Doppler images (encircled).

hypoechoic rim around the prostate or periurethral areas, and low-level echogenic areas within the prostate.[16] Colour Doppler is useful in cases of diffuse bacterial prostatitis. The severity of the inflammatory reaction is mirrored by focal or diffuse increase in the colour signal in the prostatic parenchyma.[17,18] When focally increased colour signals are seen in cases of prostatitis, there is no reliable non-invasive method to differentiate inflammation from tumour.[17] However, cases of grossly increased flow spread diffusely throughout the gland should be considered prostatitis in the appropriate clinical setting (Fig. 11-7). When the inflammatory process continues to suppuration, a prostatic abscess can develop. On ultrasound, this is seen as a cavity filled with low-level echoes from debris (Fig. 11-8).[19] Colour Doppler may detect increased flow around the rim of the cavity, although this finding is not necessary to make the diagnosis. Cases of bacterial prostatitis are treated by antibiotics, whereas prostatic abscess requires transrectal catheter or transurethral drainage with unroofing of the abscess cavity.

Conclusions

Doppler ultrasound of the prostate contributes significantly to the diagnostic value of sonography in the assessment of prostatic disease. Colour and power Doppler identify areas of abnormal blood flow, which can then be examined more closely with grey scale imaging, or biopsied under ultrasound guidance.

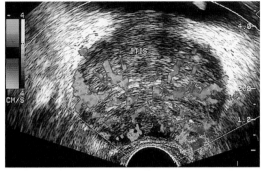

FIGURE 11-7 Prostatitis. Colour Doppler image of diffuse prostatitis demonstrates grossly increased flow throughout the gland.

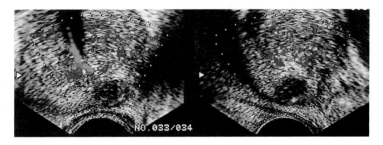

FIGURE 11-8 Prostatic abscess. Markedly hypoechoic lesion with subtle through transmission is present in the peripheral zone of this patient. Note lack of flow in the central portion of this lesion, a finding that would be very unusual for prostate cancer. Drainage confirmed the presence of an abscess.

REFERENCES

1. Siegel R, Ward E, Browley O, et al. Cancer Statistics 2011. *CA Cancer J Clin* 2011;**61**:212–36.
2. McNeal JE. Regional morphology and pathology of the prostate. *Am J Clin Pathol* 1968;**49**:347–57.
3. Flocks RH. The arterial distribution within the prostate gland: its role in transurethral prostatic resection. *J Urol* 1937;**37**:524–48.
4. Clegg EJ. The arterial supply of the human prostate and seminal vesicles. *J Anat* 1955;**89**:209–17.
5. Neumaier CE, Martinoli C, Derchi LE, et al. Normal prostate gland: examination with colour Doppler US. *Radiology* 1995; **196**:453–7.
6. Lee F, Littrup PJ, Loft-Christensen L, et al. Predicted prostate specific antigen results using transrectal ultrasound gland volume: Differentiation of benign prostatic hyperplasia and prostate cancer. *Cancer* 1992;**70**:211–20.
7. Lee F, Siders DB, Torp-Pedersen S, et al. Prostate cancer: Transrectal ultrasound and pathology comparison–A preliminary study of outer gland (peripheral and central zones) and inner gland (transition zone) cancer. *Cancer* 1991; **67**:1132.
8. Lee F, Bahn DK, Siders DB, et al. The role of TRUS-guided biopsies for determination of internal and external spread of prostate cancer. *Semin Urol Oncol* 1998;**16**:129–36.
9. DeCarvalho VS, Soto JA, Guidone PL, et al. Role of colour Doppler in improving the detection of cancer in the isoechoic prostate gland (abstr). *Radiology* 1995;**197**(P):365.
10. Halpern EJ, Frauscher F, Strup SE, et al. Prostate: high-frequency Doppler US imaging for cancer detection. *Radiology* 2002;**225**:71–7.
11. Inahara M, Suzuki H, Nakamachi H, et al. Clinical evaluation of transrectal power Doppler imaging in the detection of prostate cancer. *Int Urol Nephrol* 2004;**36**:175–80.

12. Del Rosso A, Di Pierro ED, Masciovecchio S, et al. Does transrectal colour Doppler ultrasound improve the diagnosis of prostate cancer? *Arch Ital Urol Androl* 2012;**84**:22–5.

13. Littrup PJ, Klein RM, Sparschu RA, et al. Colour Doppler of the prostate: histologic and racial correlations (abstr). *Radiology* 1995;**197**(P):365.

14. Frauscher F, Klauser A, Halpern EJ, et al. Detection of prostate cancer with a microbubble ultrasound contrast agent. *Lancet* 2001;**357**:1849–50.

15. Bogers HA, Sedelaar JP, Beerlage HP, et al. Contrast-enhanced three-dimensional power Doppler angiography of the human prostate: correlation with biopsy outcome. *Urology* 1999; **54**:97–104.

16. Griffiths GJ, Crooks AJR, Roberts EE, et al. Ultrasonic appearances associated with prostatic inflammation: A preliminary study. *Clin Radiol* 1984;**35**:343–5.

17. Patel U, Rickards D. The diagnostic value of colour Doppler flow in the peripheral zone of the prostate, with histological correlation. *Br J Urol* 1994;**74**:590–5.

18. Palmas AS, Coelho MF, Fonseca JF. Colour Doppler ultrasonographic scanning in acute bacterial prostatitis. *Arch Ital Urol Androl* 2010;**82**:271–4.

19. Lee Jr FT, Lee F, Solomon MH, et al. Ultrasonic demonstration of prostatic abscess. *J Ultrasound Med* 1986;**5**:101–2.

Chapter 12

Doppler Ultrasound of the Penis

Myron A. Pozniak

Introduction

Common indications for penile imaging are for evaluation of erectile dysfunction, trauma, priapism, penile carcinoma and Peyronie's disease. Because it is a superficial soft tissue structure, the penis is ideally suited for imaging with ultrasound. The addition of colour and spectral Doppler allows the examiner to delineate vascular anatomy, display dynamic variations in blood flow, measure arterial velocity and infer adequacy of venous drainage. The advantages of Doppler over other imaging modalities are its ease-of-use, patient acceptance, versatility, reproducibility, ready availability, and relatively low cost. By combining imaging with the pharmacologic induction of erection, both anatomic and physiologic abnormalities can be assessed during the flaccid and erect states.

The evaluation of erectile dysfunction (ED) has been the dominant application for penile Doppler, especially in the older population since the prevalence and severity of the disease increases with advancing age.[1] While impotence may be the result of psychogenic, neurogenic or hormonal factors, vascular disease is the most common cause of ED.[2] With the introduction of phosphodiesterase inhibitors [specifically Sildenafil citrate (Viagra©), Verdenafil HCl (Levitra©), and Tadalafil (Cialis©)], the frequency of Doppler studies for ED has significantly decreased.[3] Most centres now prescribe a trial of the phosphodiesterase inhibitors as the initial diagnostic/therapeutic test of ED, with only non-responders being sent on for imaging.

Penile Anatomy and Physiology

The penis contains three longitudinal, cylindrical erectile bodies. Two corpora cavernosa are located in the dorsal two-thirds of the penile shaft, and a single corpora spongiosum is located in the ventral one-third of the shaft. The corpora cavernosa are enclosed by the tunica albuginea, a tough, non-distensible fascial layer. The septum that divides the corpora cavernosa contains fenestrations that create multiple connecting anastomotic channels between the sinusoidal spaces, allowing for free communication across the midline. The dorsal arteries, veins and nerves are situated centrally along the penile dorsum, superficial to the tunica albuginea and deep to Buck's fascia. The urethra is contained within the corpus spongiosium.[4]

On ultrasound, the corpora cavernosa are of uniform hypoechoic echotexture. The tunica can be seen as an echogenic envelope around the corpora. The echogenic walls of the cavernosal arteries can be seen centrally within the corpora. The corpus spongiosum is of higher echogenicity (Fig. 12-1).

ARTERIAL ANATOMY

The internal pudendal artery and its branches are the primary source of arterial supply to the penis. The first three branches are the superficial perineal artery, the bulbar artery and a small urethral artery. The perineal artery is a large and constant branch that, in 80% of cases, has an internal and external branch. The bulbar artery, which supplies the proximal penile shaft, is usually easily identified during angiography because it is associated with a bulbar parenchymal blush in the early arterial phase. The urethral artery, which is of small diameter, arises anterior to the bulbar artery. After these branches, the internal pudendal artery continues as the common penile artery. It then divides into left and right penile arteries, which enter the base of the penis and branch

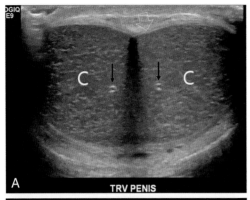

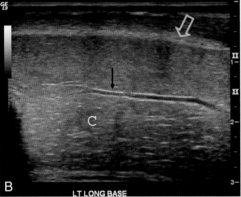

FIGURE 12-1 (A) Transverse and (B) longitudinal ultrasound images of a normal penis. The corpora cavernosa (C) have uniform echogenicity throughout. The echogenic tunica (open arrow) and echogenic walls of the cavernosal artery (arrows) are easily identified.

into a dorsal artery and a cavernosal artery. The dorsal artery extends along the dorsal aspect of the penile shaft towards the glans and terminates at the level of the arterial corona of the glans; it supplies blood primarily to the skin, subcutaneous tissues and glans. Collateral vessels from the dorsal artery often communicate with the cavernosal artery. The cavernosal, or deep penile artery, enters the tunica albuginea proximally and extends the length of the corpus cavernosum. The cavernosal arteries and their helicine branches are the primary source of blood flow to the erectile tissue of the penis. Just as the cavernosal artery supplies blood to the corpus cavernosum, the spongiosal artery supplies the corpus spongiosum[4] (Fig. 12-2).

VENOUS ANATOMY

Venous drainage of the penile erectile tissue (i.e. the sinusoidal spaces) primarily occurs through emissary (efferent) veins which drain the corpus cavernosum, penetrate the tunica albuginea and empty into the circumflex veins; these then drain into the deep dorsal venous system of the penis. The emissary veins may also drain directly into the deep dorsal vein. The superficial dorsal vein drains the distal portion of the corpora cavernosa, as well as the skin and glans. The deep and superficial dorsal veins can be routinely visualised by colour Doppler imaging in the midline of the penile shaft (Figs 12-3 and 12-4). The most proximal portions of the corpora cavernosa are drained by the cavernosal veins directly into the periprostatic venous plexus.[4]

ERECTILE PHYSIOLOGY

When the penis is flaccid, its smooth muscle is in a tonic state, the cavernous sinusoids are collapsed, and the cavernous venules are open.[2] The emissary veins drain the sinusoidal spaces and blood circulates into the dorsal veins. During this state, there is relatively high resistance to blood flow into the penis. Erection starts when an autonomic neurogenic impulse relaxes the cavernosal arterioles and sinusoidal spaces. As erection occurs, there is a marked increase in the volume of arterial inflow into the penis as the cavernous arteries dilate. This is accompanied by relaxation of the smooth muscle of the corpora cavernosa with expansion and elongation of the cavernous sinusoids as they fill with blood. Compression of the cavernous venules between the dilated cavernous sinusoids and the unyielding peripheral tunica albuginea decreases venous outflow. This veno-occlusive mechanism (which depends on neurological stimuli, a sufficient supply of arterial blood, and normal function of the tunica albuginea) maintains sinusoidal distension and rigid erection.

Five stages of erectile physiology have been defined: latent, tumescent, full erection, rigid erection and detumescent. During the latent phase, the diameters of the cavernosal arteries are at their greatest and there is maximum inflow of blood with minimal resistance. During tumescence, the sinusoidal cavities of the corpora cavernosa distend with blood. With full erection, blood flow decreases, as do the diameters of the cavernosal

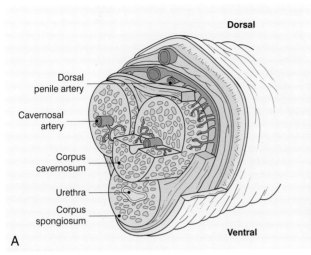
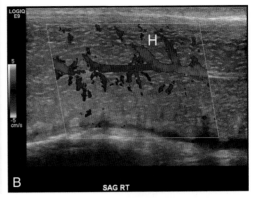

FIGURE 12-2 Normal anatomy. (A) The cavernosal arteries are centrally located in each corpus cavernosus. The urethra courses through the corpus spongiosum. The dorsal penile artery supplies the glands and does not play a direct role in erectile function. (B) Colour Doppler reveals flow in the cavernosal artery and its helicine branches (H).

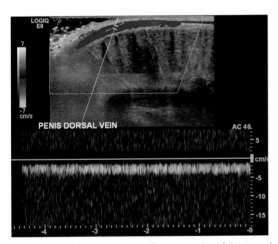

FIGURE 12-3 Colour and spectral Doppler tracing of the normal dorsal penile vein. Note the uniform relatively slow velocity.

Ultrasound Technique

Various techniques for the sonographic examination of the penis have been described with changes over time primarily due to advances in ultrasound technology. A linear transducer operating at 7 MHz or higher frequency should be employed. Slow-flow sensitivity must be optimised. Filters are set at their lowest levels and the Doppler gain is set just below the noise threshold; the pulse repetition frequency is set to the lowest velocity setting possible. All of these settings can then be adjusted if higher than expected velocity distorts the Doppler display.

The evaluation should be performed in a quiet, private setting with the room comfortably warm and darkened, so that the patient is relaxed and not uncomfortable. The scan is performed with the patient lying supine and the penis in the anatomical position (lying superiorly against the anterior abdominal wall). During the examination, the patient may be asked to help keep the penis immobilised by gently holding the corona just under the glans penis and then stretching the shaft along the anterior abdominal wall. Scanning is usually performed on the ventral surface of the penis, but the probe can be placed on the dorsal or

arteries. With a rigid erection, blood inflow (and outflow) ceases and the diameters of the cavernosal arteries are at their narrowest. Detumescence occurs when the trabeculae and arteries contract in response to a release of norepinephrine. During the five stages of erection, different arterial diameters and waveform patterns are normally present on Doppler examination.[5]

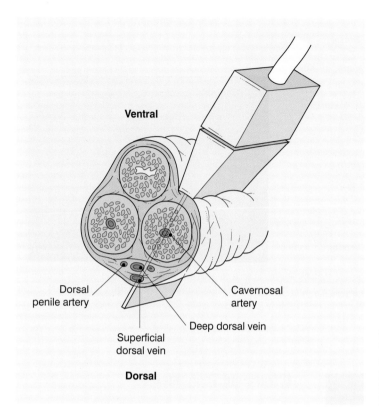

Ventral

Dorsal
penile artery

Cavernosal
artery

Deep dorsal vein

Superficial
dorsal vein

Dorsal

FIGURE   12-4 Ultrasound technique. A linear transducer is placed in a longitudinal plane along the ventral surface of the penis. Since the cavernosal arteries run parallel to the transducer, electronic steering of the Doppler beam is necessary to interrogate flow at an appropriate angle.

lateral surfaces if necessary (Fig. 12-4). Imaging is performed in both the longitudinal and transverse planes from the base of the penis to the glans to visualise anatomical details of the corpora cavernosa, cavernosal arteries and surrounding structures, and also to demonstrate any abnormalities such as fibrosis, scarring, plaques, calcification, haematoma or tumour. The transducer should be applied gently with minimal penile compression. Firm pressure causing vascular compression can resist inflow and affect accuracy of velocity measurement, especially during diastole. The diameter of the arteries and blood flow velocities are measured. Colour Doppler enhances the accuracy of angle correction, which is mandatory for flow velocity determination. In addition, with colour Doppler, blood flow direction can be assessed and the presence of any communications between the cavernosal, dorsal and spongiosal arteries can be detected.[6]

Erectile Dysfunction

The initial report of Doppler sonography combined with pharmacological induction of erection to evaluate vasculogenic impotence was by Lue and associates[7] in the mid-1980s. The use of this study peaked before the introduction of phosphodiesterase inhibitors and has now fallen off significantly. Intra-cavernosal ejection of prostaglandin E1 at a dose of 10 μg into the base of the corpus cavernosum with a 27-gauge needle will result in an erection, even without sexual stimulation. If the response is sub-optimal the initial injection can be supplemented by a further 10 μg after 15 min. If the patient responds with an appropriate erection, then it can be presumed that neurogenic, psychogenic or hormonal issues are the cause of the patient's erectile dysfunction.

The Doppler examination of the cavernosal artery flow profile should be initiated within two minutes of injection. Reassessment is then performed every 2 to 5 minutes depending on the temporal response to the drug, which can vary considerably from patient to patient. Most examinations are finished by 20 minutes. Assessment up to 30 minutes is occasionally required to ensure the maximal pharmacologic effect has been attained. Doppler measurements are most reliable and most easily reproduced when taken at the base of the penis where the penile vessels angle posteriorly toward the perineum. The arterial diameter and waveform of each cavernosal artery is individually assessed. Peak systolic and end-diastolic velocities are measured and recorded. An asymmetric response of the cavernosal arteries during erection or a lack of arterial dilation may suggest the presence of a significant vascular inflow obstruction. The examiner should also carefully search for anatomical penile arterial variants as they may also contribute to vasculogenic impotence.[8]

NORMAL DOPPLER FINDINGS

Prior to injection, during the flaccid state, the systolic waveform is damped and has a monophasic flow profile with a relatively small diastolic component of flow (Fig. 12-5A). Following pharmacological induction of erection, the normal progression of haemodynamic events and the associated Doppler waveform patterns of the cavernosal artery can be classified into several haemodynamic stages. The appearance of the spectral waveform must be correlated with the status of the erection (i.e. flaccid, latent, tumescent, full and rigid).

During the initial latent state, there is a brisk increase in both systolic and diastolic blood flow in the cavernosal artery, and a rounded systolic peak is observed. The flow of blood is antigrade during both systole and diastole, with a pronounced forward diastolic component (Fig. 12-5B). This spectral waveform reflects the low resistance to flow within the sinusoidal spaces. Minimal tumescence normally accompanies this stage. With the increase in blood flow to the corpora cavernosa, intracavernosal pressure becomes increased. As intracavernosal pressure rises, a dichrotic notch appears at end systole and diastolic flow diminishes (Fig. 12-5C). When intracavernosal and diastolic pressures are the same, diastolic flow ceases and there is only systolic blood flow. The systolic envelope narrows and systolic velocity may fluctuate. Increasing tumescence normally occurs during this stage.

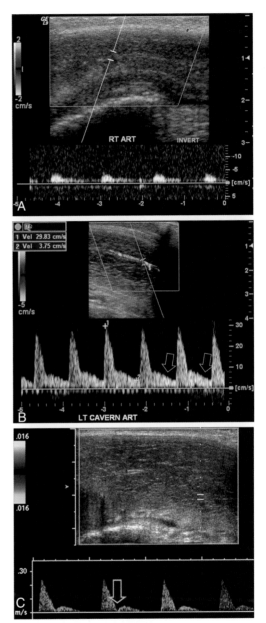

FIGURE 12-5 A sequence of Spectral Doppler tracings illustrating changes in arterial flow dynamics before and after pharmacological induction of erection. (A) Spectral Doppler tracing of the penis flaccid, prior to injection. Flow is weak; velocities are damped. (B) During the initial latent phase of the erectile process brisk flow has developed with systolic velocity approaching 30 cm/s. At this relatively early time after pharmacological enhancement, diastolic flow is still present in the antegrade direction (open arrows). (C) A few minutes later, in the early tumescent phase, systolic flow remains brisk but diastolic velocity has decreased. Note a dicrotic notch is now present in early diastole (open arrow).

Continued

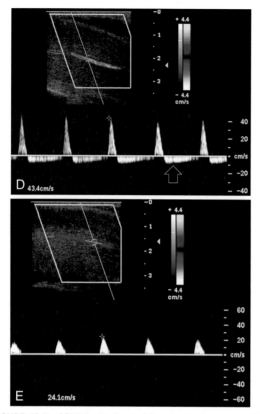

FIGURE 12-5—CONT'D (D) Spectral Doppler tracing approaching rigid erection. The systolic peak has narrowed but velocity remains brisk. Diastolic flow has now reversed as the intracavernosal pressure now exceeds diastolic pressure (open arrow). (E) Spectral Doppler tracing at full rigid erection. Systolic inflow velocities have now decreased as intracavernosal pressure now approximates systolic pressure. No flow is seen during diastole (compared to D).

During full erection, intracavernosal pressure becomes greater than the arterial pressure during diastole because of the veno-occlusive mechanism. Flow reversal is usually seen during diastole and the systolic waveform narrows. During this stage, maximal systolic velocity occurs in the normal patient and strong pulsations are normally seen (Fig. 12-5D). In the rigid phase of erection, intracavernosal pressure approximates arterial systolic pressure, with further narrowing of the systolic envelope, and a decrease in peak systolic velocity (Fig. 12-5E). Both systolic and diastolic flow may cease completely as the pressure in the corporal bodies approaches systolic blood pressure.[5,9–11]

CAVERNOSAL ARTERY DIAMETER

Cavernosal artery diameter should increase as a response to the pharmacologic stimulus, accommodating increased flow. Identification of such dilatation after injection is considered an indicator of appropriate vessel compliance. Various authors suggest a minimal increase of arterial diameter should range between at least 60 to 75%.[7,12] However, obtaining cavernosal arterial diameters is time-consuming and accuracy of measurement is dependent on examiner skill. Poor correlation between the degree of cavernosal artery diameter dilatation and arteriographic confirmation of arterial integrity has been reported therefore, cavernosal artery diameter changes are no longer considered indicative or diagnostic of arterial disease.[13]

ARTERIAL VARIANTS

Variant penile arterial anatomy can be seen in a high percentage of patients suspected of having an arteriogenic cause for their impotence. Communications among the cavernosal, dorsal, and spongiosal arteries are often found along the shaft of the penis (Fig. 12-6). There may be duplication of the cavernosal artery or cross-communication between left and right cavernosal arteries. Rarely, collaterals from the urethral arteries may also be seen. The incidence of communication between dorsal and cavernosal arteries (dorsal–cavernosal perforators) has been reported in as many as 90% of men. 'Spongiosal–cavernosal communications', or 'shunt' vessels, which course from the corpus

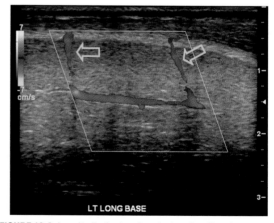

FIGURE 12-6 Longitudinal colour Doppler imaging. Note the presence of two dorsal–cavernosal perforating arteries (open arrows).

spongiosum into the corpus cavernosum are another common variant. Any of these collateral pathways may significantly affect arterial Doppler flow profiles during erection. Although these anatomical variations do not necessarily result in arterial insufficiency, they may cause inaccurate interpretation if they are not appreciated. For example, systolic peak velocities of the cavernosal artery may be significantly lower in men with a full erectile response if arterial collateral communications are present. Careful scanning of the entire penis from the crura to the glans with colour Doppler is essential in identifying these anomalies.[13,14]

Vasculogenic Impotence

DOPPLER FINDINGS OF ARTERIAL INSUFFICIENCY

Peak systolic velocity in the cavernosal arteries after pharmacological injection is considered one of the most important parameters in identifying cases of impotence due to arterial inflow compromise, focal stenosis, occlusion, or collateral steal between arteries (Fig. 12-7). Peak cavernosal artery systolic velocity less than 25 cm/s is considered abnormal. Asymmetric velocities in the side-to-side comparison of peak systolic velocity between cavernosal arteries are considered abnormal if the difference between right and left cavernosal arteries is greater than 10 cm/s.

Underlying arterial disease is assumed in the artery with the lower peak systolic velocity.[15]

Other indicators used to increase the sensitivity of detecting potential arterial inflow compromise include reversal of blood flow during systole, a penile blood flow index and blood flow (or cavernosal artery) acceleration. During rigid erection, reversal of diastolic blood flow is a normal finding; however, reversal of arterial blood flow direction during systole is always considered abnormal and may indicate an underlying vascular abnormality. Systolic flow reversal after pharmacological induction of erection has been observed in patients with significant proximal penile or cavernosal artery stenosis or occlusion with filling of the distal cavernosal artery by collateral flow.[15,16]

VENOUS INCOMPETENCE

In some men, venous incompetence, or failure of the veno-occlusive mechanism, may be the primary cause of vasculogenic impotence. Patients with normal arterial inflow parameters (e.g. peak systolic velocity >25 cm/s) but weak erections will very likely have some degree of venous leakage.[2] Because primary venous leakage is a potentially treatable cause of erectile dysfunction, Doppler examination of the penile venous system may be helpful in identifying these patients who

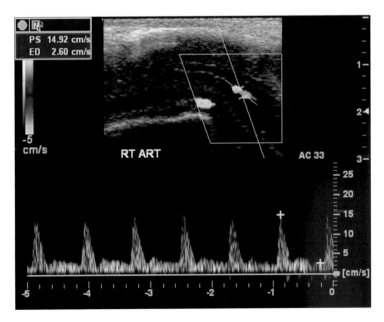

FIGURE 12-7 Spectral Doppler tracing in a patient with arterial insufficiency. Despite appropriate pharmaceutical dose, erectile response was suboptimal. Peak systolic velocity in the cavernosal artery only approximates 15 cm/s. This is well below the accepted normal response.

may benefit from additional invasive studies. If surgical or endovascular therapy is considered for the patient, then cavernosography is generally still required.

In those patients with arterial inflow issues (peak systolic velocity <25 cm/s), however, the veno-occlusive mechanism will not be fully engaged, persistent end-diastolic flow can be expected and venous leak cannot be assessed.

Correlation has been shown between end-diastolic blood flow velocity within the cavernosal arteries and the presence of venous leakage. With a normal erectile response, there should be minimal, if any, flow detected with the cavernosal arteries during the diastolic phase 15–20 min after injection. As previously noted, there should be a decrease and eventual absence or reversal of diastolic flow in the normal spectral Doppler waveform during rigid erection. If there is veno-occlusive dysfunction (venous leak), then this decrease or reversal of diastolic flow will not occur. Persistently high diastolic flow in the cavernosal arteries indicates venous leakage out of the corporal tissue even after maximum peak systolic velocity has been attained (Fig. 12-8). However, just as there are differences of opinion regarding normal and abnormal peak systolic velocity values, various criteria exist as to what constitutes abnormal diastolic velocity. In association with a normal arterial inflow, a persistently high end diastolic velocity of >5 cm/s is considered indicative of a venous leak.[17]

The potential for a false-positive diagnosis of venous leak does exist, especially in young men. The anxiety during a penile ultrasound examination increases sympathetic drive which results in inadequate relaxation of sinusoidal smooth muscle and consequent failure of veno-occlusion. Additional intracavernosal administration of an alpha-adrenergic antagonist such as phentolamine 2 mg, should be considered. Phentolamine blocks the increased sympathetic drive and helps avoid the false-positive diagnosis of venous leak.[18]

Priapism

Priapism is defined as a persistent erection, unrelated to sexual stimulation, lasting longer than four hours. It is classified as either ischaemic or non-ischaemic. Ischaemic priapism can be drug-induced by antihypertensives, cocaine, or psychotropic medications; especially when combined with phosphodiesterase inhibitors. Ischaemic priapism is painful, requiring prompt medical attention. Initially, corporal needle aspiration is performed to decompress the sinusoids and hopefully relieve the venous outflow obstruction. If that fails then surgery is performed for corporal decompression by cavernosal shunting (Fig. 12-9).

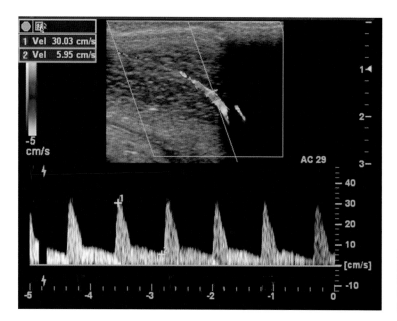

FIGURE 12-8 Spectral Doppler tracing of venous insufficiency. Relatively high-velocity persistent forward flow is seen during diastole (approximating 6 cm/s). This is despite appropriate arterial inflow velocities.

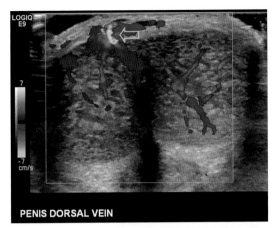

FIGURE 12-9 Transverse color Doppler image of the mid-penis after surgical cavernosal venous shunt. Surgical anastomosis was created between branches of the cavernosal system and dorsal penile vein. Brisk colour flow (open arrow) confirms shunt patency.

If not properly treated, the ischaemic corpora become severely acidotic. Eventually there is degeneration of the tissue, cellular damage and even widespread necrosis. If untreated it will result in irreversible erectile dysfunction and scarring.[19] The Doppler sonographic evaluation of priapism is used to identify the presence of blood flow along the length of the corpora cavernosa. Patients with ischaemic priapism have no blood flow in their cavernosal arteries, whereas those with non-ischaemic priapism have abnormally high-velocity flow. Non-ischaemic priapism is rare and most often due to trauma resulting in a high flow state.[20]

Trauma

Injury to the penis may be the result of blunt or penetrating trauma; or from acute bending of the erect shaft, usually during intercourse. Depending on severity of the insult, subcutaneous or intracorporal haematoma, tunical disruption or urethral tear may occur. The main role of sonography is to exclude albugineal tear because extratunical and cavernosal haematoma can be treated conservatively. Surgery is required, however, when rupture of the tunica albuginea is suspected, especially if the patient reports immediate detumescence associated with a popping sound. Surgical repair of an albugineal tear reduces the risk of post-traumatic curvature, and lowers the incidence of erectile

dysfunction. Colour Doppler sonography can be used to help localise small albugineal tears. By squeezing the penile shaft, a flush of blood can be forced from the cavernosal bodies through the tear.[21]

Following pelvic trauma, Doppler ultrasound is useful for identifying the presence of injury to the penile vasculature.[15] Most non-organic causes of erectile dysfunction in young men are secondary to arterial injury with pelvic fracture. Penile arterial inflow may be compromised by development of a post-traumatic stenosis. Doppler ultrasound can be used to look for a tardus parvus waveform of the affected artery. For patients who experience post-traumatic impotence, Broderick et al.[22] found that a systolic velocity less than 25 cm/s and asymmetric velocities >10 cm/s were helpful parameters in establishing a compromise of penile arterial inflow. In some centres, vascular microsurgery is being performed on the internal pudendal artery to bypass a focal stenosis.

With severe trauma, the cavernosal artery may rupture. This results in unrestricted blood flow into the cavernosal space, creating an arteriosinusoidal, arteriolacunar, or arteriovenous fistula. Since venous outflow is maintained from the cavernosal space, the patient develops only a partial erection that is not acutely painful. Persistent venous outflow prevents complete erection, stasis and hypoxia. This condition is known as high-flow priapism and colour Doppler sonography is very effective in its identification (Fig. 12-10). It shows a characteristic arterial colour blush consistent with extravasation of blood from the lacerated artery. Spectral Doppler displays turbulent high-velocity flow.[15,19,23] In long-standing priapism, this area may appear more circumscribed, mimicking a pseudoaneurysm. Angiographic embolisation of the lacerated artery is currently considered the treatment of choice. It can be performed with an autologous blood clot.[24] Colour Doppler US allows confirmation of successful embolisation by demonstrating disappearance or size reduction of the fistula. If unsuccessful, persistent high-velocity flow in the feeding vessels would be seen.[25]

Peyronie's Disease

Peyronie's disease (induratio penis plastica) is an idiopathic disorder of the connective tissue in which fibrous plaques form in the tunica albuginea with induration of the corpora cavernosa of the penis or a fibrous cavernositis. The incidence increases with age, being less than 2% at 40 years and increasing to over 6% at 70 years. The disease causes penile deviation and affected patients typically complain of pain during erection.[15] Ultrasound imaging can estimate the extent and depth of the plaques, which may be hypo- or hyperechoic and, if longstanding, often contain calcification.

Doppler examination of the penile vasculature is of value to determine if any vascular abnormalities are caused by the fibrous plaques.[26,27] Doppler can differentiate between veno-occlusive dysfunction (considered the primary vascular cause of impotence associated with Peyronie's disease) and arterial

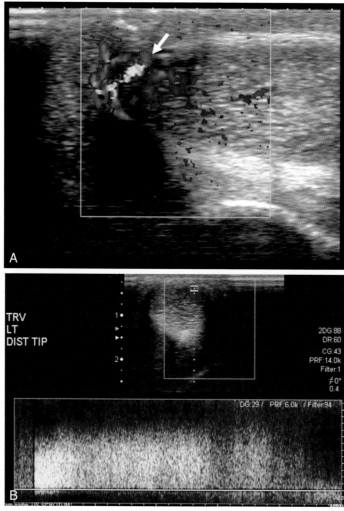

FIGURE 12-10 This patient sustained a penile injury while bull riding 15 days prior to admission. The patient presented with a persistent painless erection. (A) Longitudinal colour Doppler image of the mid-penis. An area of colour flow aliasing within the left corpus cavernosa is the focus of the arterial lacunar fistula (arrow). (B) Corresponding spectral Doppler tracings. There is marked turbulent flow at the site as would be expected with an arterial–lacunar fistula.

Continued

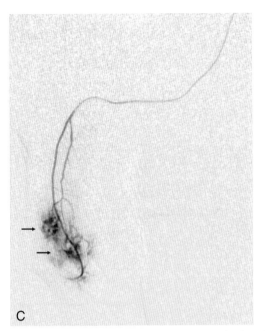

FIGURE 12-10—CONT'D (C) Pre-embolisation arteriography. An early blush (arrows) corresponds to the site of the fistula. This was subsequently successfully embolised. This case is courtesy of Dr Vikram Dogra, University of Rochester Medical Center.

insufficiency.[28] By doing so, Doppler helps establish the correct treatment option for the patient. If Doppler reveals appropriate arterial inflow and an appropriate response to injection, then plaque removal with grafting of bovine pericardium is preferred. However, if Doppler shows abnormal flow profiles or an inadequate response to injection, in addition to the disfigurement, then implantation of a prosthesis should be considered.[29] After surgical intervention Doppler can readily by used for confirmation of success or identification of vascular complications.[30]

Penile Tumours

Penile masses are rare. Diagnostic considerations include haematoma, cavernosal herniation, Peyronie's plaques, penile carcinoma, metastasis, or foreign body. Doppler may show some interesting flow profiles but adds little value to the workup.

Other Imaging Tests

Although arteriography is considered the 'gold standard' for assessing the arteries of the penis, unlike Doppler ultrasound, it only provides anatomical and not functional information. If the Doppler examination suggests the presence of a surgically correctable lesion, many investigators still believe a confirmatory arteriogram (computed tomographic angiography or magnetic resonance angiography) should be performed before surgery is undertaken.

Colour Doppler ultrasound has also proven helpful in evaluating patients with suspected venous incompetence. However, for patients in whom venous surgery is being considered to correct their condition, dynamic infusion cavernosography is necessary since it provides a more complete preoperative picture of the penile vasculature. At many institutions, both cavernosography and cavernosometry are used to determine the presence of veno-occlusive dysfunction and to quantify the degree of venous leakage.

Acknowledgements

Acknowledgements are made to Reginald Bruskewitz, MD; Mike Ledwidge, RDMS, RVT; Jeanne Johnson and Mercedes Kirk.

REFERENCES

1. Corona G, Mannucci E, Mansani R, et al. Aging and pathogenesis of erectile dysfunction. *Int J Impot Res* 2004;**16**(5):395–402.
2. Connolly JA, Borirakchanyavat S, Lue TF. Ultrasound evaluation of the penis for assessment of impotence. *J Clin Ultrasound* 1996;**24**(8):481–6.
3. Weiske WH. Diagnosis of erectile dysfunction – what is still needed today? *Urologe A* 2003;**42**(10):1317–21.
4. *Gray's Anatomy.* Online. Available: http://education.yahoo.com/reference/gray/subjects/subject?id=262.
5. Halls J, Bydawell G, Patel U. Erectile dysfunction: the role of penile Doppler ultrasound in diagnosis. *Abdom Imaging* 2009; **34**(6):712–25. http://dx.doi.org/10.1007/s00261-008-9463-x. Epub 2008 Oct 15.
6. Wilkins CJ, Sriprasad S, Sidhu PS. Colour Doppler ultrasound of the penis. *Clin Radiol* 2003;**58**(7):514–23.
7. Lue TF, Hricak H, Marich KW, et al. Vasculogenic impotence evaluated by high-resolution ultrasonography and pulsed Doppler spectrum analysis. *Radiology* 1985;**155**(3):777–81.
8. Aversa A, Sarteschi LM. The role of penile colour-duplex ultrasound for the evaluation of erectile dysfunction. *J Sex Med* 2007;**4**(5):1437–47. Epub 2007 Jul 21.
9. LeRoy TJ, Broderick GA. Doppler blood flow analysis of erectile function: who, when, and how. *Urol Clin North Am* 2011;**38** (2):147–54. Epub 2011/05/31.

10. Ghanem H, Shamloul R. An evidence-based perspective to commonly performed erectile dysfunction investigations. *J Sex Med* 2008;**5**(7):1582–9.

11. Mihmanli I, Kantarci F. Erectile Dysfunction. *Semin Ultrasound CT MRI* 2007;**28**(4):274–86.

12. Krysiewicz S, Mellinger BC. The role of imaging in the diagnostic evaluation of impotence. *AJR Am J Roentgenol* 1989;**153**(6):1133–9.

13. Jarow JP, Pugh VW, Routh WD, et al. Comparison of penile duplex ultrasonography to pudendal arteriography Variant penile arterial anatomy affects interpretation of duplex ultrasonography. *Invest Radiol* 1993;**28**(9):806–10.

14. Mancini M, Bartolini M, Maggi M, et al. The presence of arterial anatomical variations can affect the results of duplex sonographic evaluation of penile vessels in impotent patients. *J Urol* 1996;**155**(6):1919–23.

15. Herbener TE, Seftel AD, Nehra A, et al. Penile ultrasound. *Semin Urol* 1994;**12**(4):320–32.

16. Altinkilic B, Hauck EW, Weidner W. Evaluation of penile perfusion by colour-coded duplex sonography in the management of erectile dysfunction. *World. J Urol* 2004;**22**(5):361–4. Epub 2004 Jul 20.

17. Bassiouny HS, Levine LA. Penile duplex sonography in the diagnosis of venogenic impotence. *J Vasc Surg* 1991;**13**(1):75–82. discussion 83.

18. Gontero P, Sriprasad S, Wilkins CJ, et al. Phentolamine re-dosing during penile dynamic colour Doppler ultrasound: a practical method to abolish a false diagnosis of venous leakage in patients with erectile dysfunction. *Br J Radiol* 2004;**77**(923):922–6.

19. Sadeghi-Nejad H, Dogra V, Seftel AD, et al. Priapism. *Radiol Clin North Am* 2004;**42**(2):427–43. Epub 2004/05/12.

20. Huang YC, Harraz AM, Shindel AW, et al. Evaluation and management of priapism: 2009 update. *Nat Rev Urol* 2009;**6**(5):262–71. http://dx.doi.org/10.1038/nrurol.2009.50.

21. Bertolotto M, Mucelli RP. Nonpenetrating penile traumas: sonographic and Doppler features. *AJR Am J Roentgenol* 2004;**183**(4):1085–9.

22. Broderick G, McGahan JP, White RD, et al. Colour Doppler US: assessment of post-traumatic impotence. *Radiology* 1990;**177**(suppl):130–4.

23. Hakim LS, Kulaksizoglu H, Mulligan R, et al. Evolving concepts in the diagnosis and treatment of arterial high flow priapism. *J Urol* 1996;**155**(2):541–8.

24. Cantasdemir M, Gulsen F, Solak S, et al. Posttraumatic high-flow priapism in children treated with autologous blood clot embolization: long-term results and review of the literature. *Pediatr Radiol* 2011;**41**(5):627–32. http://dx.doi.org/10.1007/s00247-010-1912-3. Epub 2010 Dec 3.

25. Bertolotto M, Quaia E, Mucelli FP, et al. Colour Doppler imaging of posttraumatic priapism before and after selective embolization. *Radiographics* 2003;**23**(2):495–503.

26. Amin Z, Patel U, Friedman EP, et al. Colour Doppler and duplex ultrasound assessment of Peyronie's disease in impotent men. *Br J Radiol* 1993;**66**(785):398–402.

27. Bertolotto M, de Stefani S, Martinoli C, et al. Colour Doppler appearance of penile cavernosal-spongiosal communications in patients with severe Peyronie's disease. *Eur Radiol* 2002;**12**(10):2525–31. Epub 2002 Apr 30.

28. Levine LA, Coogan CL. Penile vascular assessment using colour duplex sonography in men with Peyronie's disease. *J Urol* 1996;**155**(4):1270–3.

29. Fornara P, Gerbershagen HP. Ultrasound in patients affected with Peyronie's disease. *World. J Urol* 2004;**22**(5):365–7. Epub 2004 Jul 28.

30. Bertolotto M, Serafini G, Savoca G, et al. Colour Doppler US of the postoperative penis: anatomy and surgical complications. *Radiographics* 2005;**25**(3):731–48.

Chapter 13

Doppler Imaging of the Scrotum

Myron A. Pozniak

Introduction

Scrotal sonography was first introduced in the mid-1970s. It remains the imaging modality of choice because it is simple, relatively inexpensive, and quick. Continuing refinements in imaging technology with higher-frequency transducers, and increased Doppler sensitivity have greatly enhanced perception of testicular anatomy and pathology. The haemodynamic information acquired with Doppler adds to the imaging findings; frequently reinforcing and often clinching the diagnosis. In this era, a thorough ultrasound evaluation of the scrotum must include Doppler.

Indications

The two clinical conditions that most commonly warrant an ultrasound examination with Doppler are evaluation of acute scrotal pain and a palpable scrotal mass. Differentiating an acute inflammatory process from testicular torsion is now the domain of colour Doppler. Differentiating a mass as intratesticular versus extratesticular can be accomplished by imaging alone, but colour Doppler adds valuable haemodynamic information and helps to further characterise the abnormality. Other common indications for use of scrotal Doppler include evaluation of trauma and infertility.

Testicular Anatomy

The normal adult testis is an egg-shaped gland which is approximately 3–5 cm in length and 2–4 cm in width and thickness with a volume of 4 cm^3. Testicular size varies with age and stage of sexual development. The surface of the testicle is covered by the tunica albuginea, a thin, dense, inelastic fibrous capsule. Just within the tunica albuginea is the tunica vasculosa, through which the branches of the testicular artery course before entering into the gland (Fig. 13-1). Numerous thin septations (septula) arise from the tunica albuginea and create 250–400 cone-shaped lobules containing the seminiferous tubules (Fig. 13-2). These tortuous tubules course towards the mediastinum of the testis (Fig. 13-3) and progressively merge to form larger ducts known as tubuli recti. These, in turn, join with each other to form a network of epithelium-lined spaces embedded in the fibrostroma of the mediastinum called the rete testis. These continue as 10–15 efferent ductules which pass into the head of the epididymis.

The epididymis is a comma-shaped structure that runs along the posterolateral aspect of the testis (Fig. 13-4). The head of the epididymis is located next to the upper pole of the testis and receives the efferent ductules. The ductules eventually converge through the body and tail and form the vas deferens which continues on in the spermatic cord. Along with the vas, the cord also contains the testicular artery, cremasteric artery, differential artery, the pampiniform plexus of veins, the genitofemoral nerve and lymphatic channels.

The testis and epididymis are enveloped by the tunica vaginalis, a fascial structure composed of an outer parietal layer and an inner visceral layer which surrounds the entire gland, except along the posterior aspect where the vessels and nerves enter. The extent to which the tunica vaginalis envelops the testis directly correlates with the risk for developing testicular torsion. The potential space between the parietal and visceral layers normally contains a small amount of lubricating fluid, but a larger volume of fluid in this space represents a hydrocele.

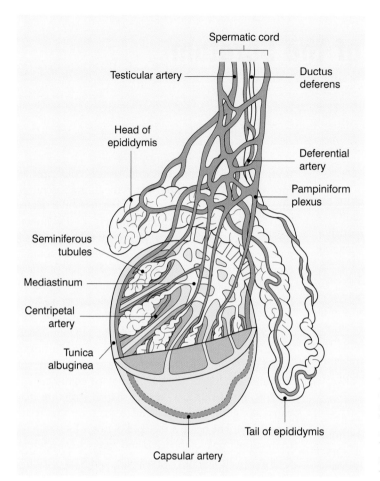

FIGURE 13-1 The testicular artery supplies flow to the epididymis and the testicle. As the testicular artery courses through the spermatic cord, it is surrounded by the pampiniform plexus of veins. The capsular artery, a branch of the testicular artery, courses just beneath the tunica albuginea. The centripetal arteries are branches of the capsular artery and course between the septa supplying the testicular parenchyma.

TESTICULAR ARTERIAL ANATOMY

The right and left testicular arteries originate from the aorta just below the renal arteries. They course through the deep inguinal ring to enter the spermatic cord, accompanied by the cremasteric and deferential arteries, which supply the soft tissues of the scrotum, epididymis and vas deferens. The testicular artery penetrates the tunica albuginea along the posterior aspect of the testis and gives off capsular branches which course through the tunica vasculosa. These capsular branches then give rise to the centripetal arteries which carry blood from the capsular surface, centrally towards the mediastinum along the septula (Figs 13-5 and 13-6). Branches of the centripetal arteries then course backward towards the capsular surface; these are known as recurrent rami. In about 50% of testes,

a more robust artery can be seen passing directly from the testicular artery at the mediastinum into the parenchyma, known as the transtesticular artery (Fig. 13-7). It is occasionally accompanied by a vein. Small anastomoses do exist between the testicular artery, cremasteric, and differential arteries. Branches of the pudendal artery may also supply the scrotal wall.

TESTICULAR VENOUS ANATOMY

Testicular venous outflow courses mostly through the mediastinum testis, into the spermatic cord, and eventually up through the inguinal canal. As the veins exit the scrotum through the spermatic cord, they form a web-like network that surrounds the testicular artery, known as the pampiniform plexus (Fig. 13-8). This plexus functions as a heat exchange mechanism,

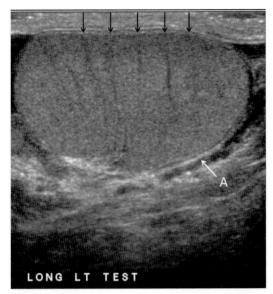

FIGURE 13-2 Longitudinal view of a normal testicle. The testicle is of relatively uniform echogenicity. On this high-resolution image, the testicular septa can be perceived as fine lines dividing the parenchyma into the individual lobules (black arrows). Note the echogenic tunica albuginea surrounding the testicle (A).

pulling warmth away from the testicular arterial inflow, thereby helping to maintain spermatogenesis at a lower, more optimal temperature.

On the left side, the testicular vein usually drains into the left renal vein; on the right side, drainage is directly into the inferior vena cava just below the right renal vein. The testicular veins normally have valves that prevent retrograde flow of venous blood to the scrotum, but if they are absent or become incompetent; this predisposes to development of a varicocele. This results in compromise of the heat exchange mechanism and, therefore, is a frequent cause of infertility.[1]

Technique

Prior to any ultrasound examination, the testes should be examined with a gloved hand, especially if the sonographic study is being conducted to evaluate a palpable mass. The examination is performed with the patient in the supine position. A towel is placed under the scrotum for support. If the testis is tender, the patient may be asked to hold it in a position which would facilitate the exam. This is particularly useful for the evaluation of a small mass. The patient should be asked to

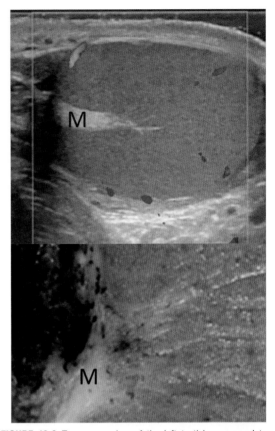

FIGURE 13-3 Transverse view of the left testicle compared to a specimen in the region of the mediastinum testis. The mediastinum testis is an echogenic fibrous structure. It is the point of confluence of the efferent ductules and the septa. Note its triangular echogenic appearance on the ultrasound (M) and how well it correlates with the dense white fibrous stroma on the specimen.

hold it between thumb and forefinger, and the ultrasound transducer is then gently placed upon it. Some men may have a vigorous cremasteric response during the examination resulting in the testis being drawn upward and puckering the scrotal wall. To avoid shadowing from trapped air, copious amounts of gel need to be worked into the scrotal skin folds. Imaging with the patient standing upright, or while performing a Valsalva manoeuvre, is useful for evaluating the testicular venous system, in particular for determining valvular competence in patients with suspect varicocele, or for improving detection of an inguinal hernia.

A high-frequency (10 MHz or greater) linear-array transducer is used for both greyscale and Doppler

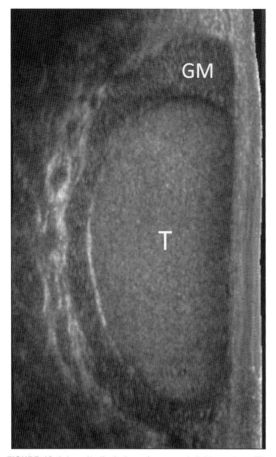

FIGURE 13-4 Longitudinal view of a normal right scrotum. The slightly hypoechoic epididymis wraps as a comma shape around the testis (T). The larger more prominent area is known as the globus major or the head of the epididymis (GM).

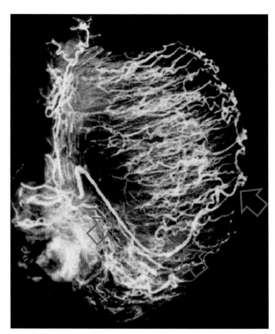

FIGURE 13-5 Microangiogram of the testicle. A prominent capsular branch (open arrows) courses from the testicular artery under the capsular surface. Centripetal arterial branches emanate from it and pass into the lobules of the testicle. Image courtesy of Dr. Thomas Winter.

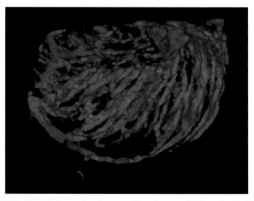

FIGURE 13-6 3-D rendered power Doppler acquisition of a testicle. With very sensitive Doppler settings, the network of centripetal arteries is seen fanning across this normal testicle.

imaging, with direct contact scanning on the scrotal skin. Examination is performed in both the longitudinal and transverse planes for each testis to allow assessment of any differences in size and echogenicity between the two sides. The split screen mode is useful for side-to-side comparison. Oblique imaging of the epididymis and spermatic cord should also be performed. Any extratesticular masses or fluid collections should be noted as well.

DOPPLER TECHNIQUE

Ultrasound examination of the scrotum is not complete without the application of colour Doppler. The procedure is a mandatory part of the imaging evaluation to confirm the presence (or absence) of uniform, symmetric vascular perfusion of the testes and epididymides (Fig. 13-9). The settings for colour Doppler scanning must be optimised for low-volume and low-velocity flow. If colour noise is excessive at low-flow settings

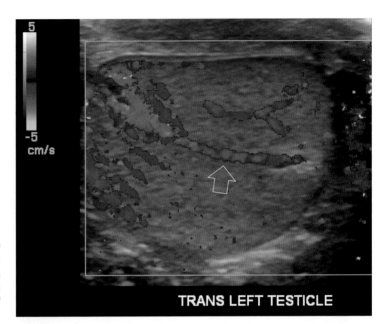

TRANS LEFT TESTICLE

FIGURE 13-7 Longitudinal colour Doppler image of a testicle. A transtesticular artery (open arrow) can be seen coursing obliquely through the testicle along the mediastinum. It is a branch of the testicular artery, but is seen in less than half of normal cases.

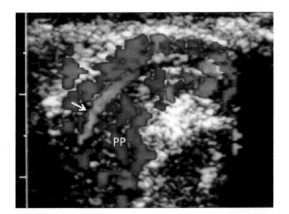

FIGURE 13-8 The pampiniform plexus of veins (PP) is a web-like collection of vessels surround the testicular artery (arrow) as it passes through the spermatic cord.

and interferes with the examination, colour artefact can be decreased by properly adjusting gain and pulse repetition frequency settings. Temporal resolution can be improved by minimising the overall image size and zooming in to the area of interest. Additionally decreasing depth, limiting the number of focal zones and limiting the size of the colour box will also improve temporal resolution. Use of appropriate technical parameters should assure demonstration of intratesticular vascularity in all normal adult patients. In the prepubertal age group, intratesticular flow volume is less and therefore more difficult to identify. The application of power Doppler may be helpful. Spectral Doppler can assess arterial and venous waveforms and quantify velocities (Fig. 13-10), but its application in the scrotum is relatively limited, except for a few conditions such as partial torsion or extreme swelling secondary to inflammation predisposing to ischaemia. In those cases spectral Doppler can best identify the high resistance to arterial inflow caused by venous outflow compromise or parenchymal congestion.

Doppler sensitivity varies greatly between ultrasound systems and software levels. Therefore, the examiner must be familiar with normal flow perception on their equipment. A good 'rule of thumb' is to examine the contralateral side (provided it is normal) to establish a colour flow baseline which can then be used as the standard by which to judge the abnormal testis or epididymis. When comparing flow between sides, be sure to set imaging parameters to the non-affected side; then, without changing any settings, image the affected side. Some advanced ultrasound machines can adjust imaging parameters automatically as depth and position of colour box changes with scanning. If possible, override this software feature to avoid misperception of asymmetric colour flow.

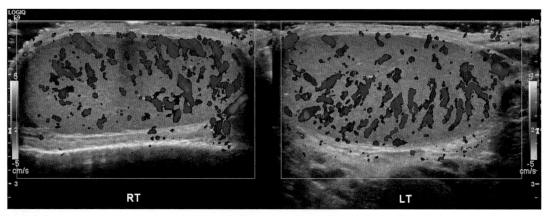

FIGURE 13-9 Transverse colour Doppler ultrasound image of both testicles using a split screen format. Note the symmetry of echotexture and the uniformity and symmetry of colour flow.

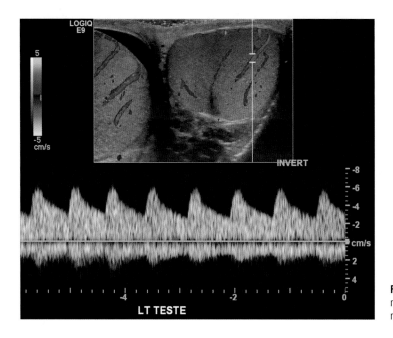

FIGURE 13-10 Spectral Doppler waveform of a normal left testicular artery. The resistive index is normal (approx. 60%).

NORMAL ULTRASOUND AND DOPPLER FINDINGS

A normal ultrasound examination of the scrotum reveals uniform, homogeneous echogenicity throughout both testes. The epididymis is usually isoechoic or slightly hypoechoic compared with the testes. The size and echogenicity of testes and epididymides should be relatively the same bilaterally.

Colour Doppler should reveal bilaterally symmetric and relatively uniform flow through both testes and epididymides (Fig. 13-9). A fan-like array of the centripetal arteries should be present through the testicles (Fig. 13-6). Spectral Doppler tracings of testicular arterial inflow demonstrate relatively low resistance (Fig. 13-10); this is in contrast to the cremasteric and deferential arteries which have relatively high resistance to flow. The normal testicular artery resistive indices in adults range from 0.46 to 0.78, with a mean of 0.64. Similar findings are reported in the intratesticular arteries of postpubescent boys, with resistive indices ranging from 0.48 to 0.75 (mean, 0.62). In prepubertal boys, however, resistance is higher to the point that diastolic arterial flow may not be detectable. Supratesticular arteries to the vas deferens or cremaster muscle, on the other hand, have higher impedance with low-diastolic flow and resistive indices ranging from 0.63 and 1.0, with a mean of 0.84.

Pulsed Doppler is relatively insensitive in detecting arterial flow in prepubescent patients. In contrast, power Doppler has been shown to reveal arterial flow in 92% of testes in pre-pubescent patients, while colour Doppler demonstrates flow in 83% of cases. In postpubescent patients, both Doppler imaging techniques demonstrated flow in 100% of cases.[2,3]

Venous flow velocities in the epididymides may fluctuate with respiration. Cardiac periodicity rarely manifests at the level of the scrotum.

Acute Scrotal Pain

INFLAMMATORY DISEASE

Acute epididymo-orchitis is the most common cause of acute scrotal pain in men over the age of 20, accounting for up to 80% of cases, but it is frequently clinically indistinguishable from spermatic cord torsion. Patients usually present with an acutely painful, tender, swollen scrotum, with associated erythema, urinary tract symptoms, fever and leukocytosis. Sometimes, however, the signs and symptoms may be less distinct, making clinical differentiation between infection and torsion extremely difficult. The process typically first manifests in the epididymis and then ascends to affect the testicle, but isolated epididymitis, orchitis, or even focal orchitis can be encountered.

The cause of the infection varies with age.[4] In adult patients less than 35 years of age, *Chlamydia trachomatis* and *Neisseria gonorrhoeae* (sexually transmitted organisms) are the most common agents. In prepubertal boys and in men over 35 years of age, the disease is most frequently caused by *Escherichia coli* and *Proteus mirabilis*. Cytomegalovirus is the most common agent in the immunocompromised patient. In most normal paediatric patients, a bacterial pathogen is not isolated and the inflammation is presumed to be viral in nature.

Those patients who have an underlying urogenital congenital anomaly are prone to infection from Gram-negative bacteria.[5]

The sonographic appearance of epididymo-orchitis varies depending on the stage of the process. The sensitivity of greyscale sonography for detecting epididymo-orchitis is reported to be about 80%. In the early, acute stage, the epididymis and/or testicle will be enlarged and hypoechoic. With the onset of tissue breakdown and haemorrhage, the echogenicity begins to increase. There may be reactive thickening of the scrotal wall. A hydrocele may be present and it may contain debris. If allowed to progress, microabscesses may develop and the appearance becomes more complex and variable. Further progression can lead to frank intra- or extratesticular abscess, ischaemia and eventually necrosis. Scarring associated with chronic orchitis typically results in a small hyperechoic testis.[6] The diagnosis of infection and inflammation typically hinges on the identification of hyperaemia by colour Doppler – an asymmetric appearance with more robust flow (an increased number and prominence of discernible vessels) in association with an enlarged, painful, hypoechoic epididymis and/or testis (Fig. 13-11). Several studies have demonstrated sensitivity and specificity for the diagnosis of scrotal inflammatory disease by colour Doppler sonography approximating 100%. Early in the inflammatory process, vasodilatation and hyperemia results in a low-resistance flow pattern on spectral Doppler (Fig. 13-12).[7]

In cases of severe epididymitis, periepididymal swelling may obstruct testicular venous outflow, leading to testicular ischaemia or infarction. An enlarged, heterogeneous testicle with reduced or absent colour flow and a contiguous abnormal epididymis may be seen on greyscale imaging (Fig. 13-13). Hyperaemia of the epididymis helps to differentiate testicular ischaemia following inflammation from that caused by torsion. A high-resistance waveform, along with decreased or reversed diastolic flow, may be seen on the spectral Doppler tracing and suggests venous infarction[8] (Fig. 13-14).

If left untreated, the process may progress to abscess formation (Fig. 13-15), which usually manifests as an enlarged testicle with a complex, septated collection of fluid/debris and tissue of mixed echogenicity. It may be difficult to distinguish from a testicular

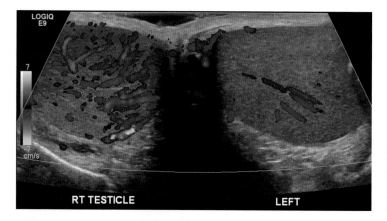

FIGURE 13-11 Transverse colour Doppler image of the scrotum including both testicles. This paediatric patient presented with right scrotal pain. Colour Doppler reveals marked hyperaemia of the right testicle and obvious asymmetry in perfusion. The diagnosis is right orchitis.

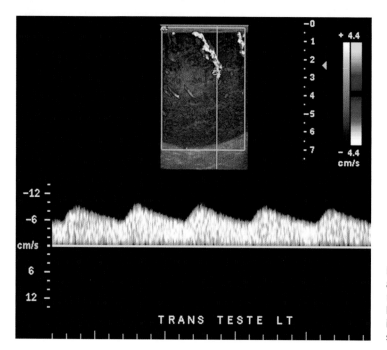

FIGURE 13-12 Spectral Doppler tracing obtained in an area of focal orchitis. Flow during diastole is relatively brisk, resulting in a resistive index of less than 50%. This is seen relatively early in the inflammatory process before the accumulation of significant oedema and/or pus.

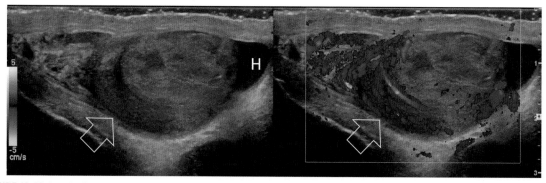

FIGURE 13-13 Longitudinal greyscale and colour Doppler image of the right scrotum. The patient presented with severe pain. The epididymis is oedematous, swollen and markedly hyperaemic (open arrows). Note almost complete absence of flow within the testicle. This is indicative of venous outflow compromise. Note the reactive hydrocele (H) and scrotal wall thickening.

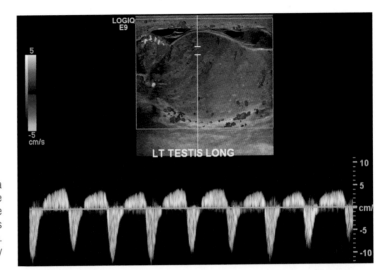

FIGURE 13-14 Colour and spectral Doppler of a severely inflamed left epididymis and testicle. The testicle is markedly enlarged and swollen. The echotexture is irregular. Flow during diastole is reversed resulting in a resistive index of >100%. These findings indicate a severe inflammatory process with the venous outflow occlusion.

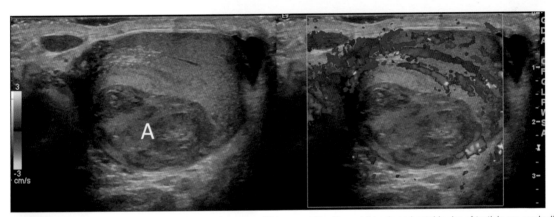

FIGURE 13-15 Greyscale and colour Doppler image of severe epididymoorchitis. The epididymis and outside rim of testicle are markedly hyperaemic. No flow is seen in the central part of the testicle. Note the areas of tissue breakdown and liquification consistent with intratesticular abscess (A).

neoplasm, as both can present as complex cystic/solid masses. Older abscesses may have radiating echogenic septa separating hypoechoic spaces. Increased blood flow around the abscess cavity and no internal flow is present on colour Doppler. Surgical exploration may be necessary to rule out the presence of a tumour and débride the abscess.

Occasionally, testicular inflammation may be focal, even rounded, with areas of decreased echogenicity and swelling. Hyperaemia concentrated in the abnormal, tender area may suggest inflammation over neoplasm, but there is overlap in this appearance with neoplasm, especially lymphoma (Fig. 13-16).

An inflammatory process may be isolated to the spermatic cord. This is most often associated with a recent viral illness. The patient typically presents with a nagging ache that is difficult to localise within the scrotum. Imaging reveals an enlarged and oedematous and hyperaemic spermatic cord. (Fig. 13-17).

TORSION

Torsion is divided into two types – extravaginal which occurs exclusively in newborns and intravaginal. Extravaginal torsion occurs outside the tunica vaginalis when the testes are not yet fixed and are free to rotate.[9] The testis is typically necrotic at birth. Ultrasound

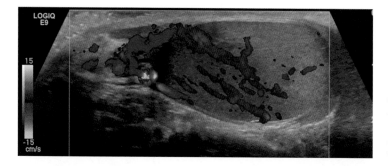

FIGURE 13-16 Longitudinal colour Doppler image of a testicle. This patient complained of severe scrotal tenderness. Note the asymmetric appearance of this testicle. The upper pole is hypoechoic and hypervascular. The lower pole has normal echogenicity and significantly less flow. The diagnosis was focal orchitis with associated epididymitis.

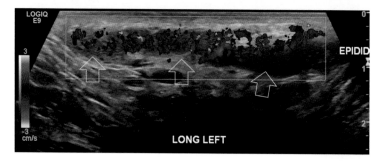

FIGURE 13-17 Longitudinal image along the spermatic cord. Note the enlargement, hypoechoic echotexture and striking hyperaemia of the spermatic cord (open arrows). The patient was recovering from a viral upper respiratory illness. This represents a viral corditis.

reveals an enlarged heterogeneous testis, a reactive hydrocele, skin thickening and no colour Doppler flow in the testis or spermatic cord. Intravaginal torsion occurs most frequent in adolescent boys. A bell-clapper deformity, in which the tunica vaginalis completely encircles the epididymis, distal spermatic cord, and testis, is the key predisposing factor. This deformity is usually bilateral and leaves the testis free to swing and rotate within the tunica vaginalis (Fig. 13-18).

The diagnosis of spermatic cord torsion must be established quickly to allow for prompt surgical intervention, since obstruction of blood flow may result in the loss of testicular viability within a few hours (typically four) of onset of symptoms. Clinical history and physical findings, however, overlap with those of inflammatory disease to such a degree that even an experienced urologist may have difficulty in differentiating the two conditions. Symptoms and signs include sudden pain in the scrotum, lower abdomen or inguinal area (frequently accompanied by nausea, vomiting and low-grade fever), a tender testicle with a transverse orientation, and a swollen, erythematous hemiscrotum. The false-positive rate of nearly 50% for clinical diagnosis of testicular torsion often results in unnecessary surgical exploration.[10]

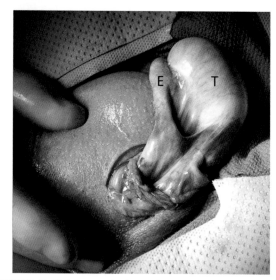

FIGURE 13-18 Intraoperative image during testicular torsion repair. The testicle (T) and epididymis (E) have been delivered through a small incision. Note the great degree of mobility because of the Bell Clapper deformity.

Greyscale sonography by itself has a low sensitivity and specificity when evaluating patients for suspected torsion. Findings will depend on the length of time that torsion has been present. During the first few hours, testicular appearance is normal, but after about 4–6 h, as the veins are obstructed, there is vascular engorgement and the testis becomes enlarged and oedematous, with a hypoechoic appearance as compared to the contralateral testicle. After 24 h, vascular congestion, haemorrhage and infarction will cause the testis to appear heterogeneous. The epididymis may also be enlarged and hypoechoic because of prolonged vascular stasis.

The application of colour Doppler to the diagnosis of torsion increases sensitivity in adults to 90–100% with a high specificity. Unlike greyscale imaging, colour and spectral Doppler are almost always abnormal even during the early stages of torsion. Instrument settings should be optimised on the normal side to identify low-velocity flow before ascertaining that there is indeed decreased blood flow on the symptomatic side. If arterial flow cannot be detected in the symptomatic testicle but can in the contralateral testicle, the diagnosis of torsion is effectively established. The characteristic finding of ischaemia is a completely avascular testicle (Fig. 13-19). In the late stages of torsion, colour Doppler may reveal an increase in peritesticular blood flow because of inflammation in the surrounding soft tissues of the scrotum.

Evaluation of the small testicles of prepubescent boys, however, can be very difficult because of inherently low-velocity blood flow. In addition, if the patient has intermittent torsion, and by the time the patient arrives for the ultrasound examination the torsion spontaneously resolves, flow may appear normal on colour Doppler. Since absence of flow is demonstrated only if torsion is present at the time of sonographic examination, differentiating between normal testicles and testicles with intermittent torsion may be difficult to accomplish.

With full torsion (greater than 360°) the addition of spectral Doppler does little other than to confirm the obvious fact that there is no flow. It should identify very high resistance in the spermatic artery within the cord above the level of the twist. With partial torsion (between 180° and 360°) however, the spermatic cord twists only enough to occlude the venous outflow. Because the artery has a thicker wall, patency is maintained. The resultant spectral Doppler tracing reveals a high-resistance arterial waveform within the cord and the testicle (Fig. 13-20).[11,12]

If the spermatic cord spontaneously untwists prior to the ultrasound examination, colour Doppler will likely reveal diffuse, reactive hyperaemia. Although this finding will mimic epididymo-orchitis, resolution of acute scrotal pain concurrent with increased blood flow is highly indicative of spontaneous detorsion. Colour Doppler ultrasound can also be used to monitor non-surgical detorsion of the testicle as the testis is manually rotated; if this manoeuvre is successful, blood flow is re-established to the testicle and can be detected on Doppler. This non-surgical approach, however, is only considered a temporising measure. It is not a substitute for surgical intervention, which is still necessary to correct the underlying anatomical deformity that predisposes to torsion.

Direct evaluation of the spermatic cord on its long axis may reveal a snail-shell-shaped mass at the point of the twist (Fig. 13-21). Running the transducer along the affected cord in the transverse projection may show a vortex-like spin of the cord ending at the point of obstruction.

The use of echo-enhancing agents has been studied for improving imaging of small testicles with low-velocity and low-volume flow. In an animal study by Brown et al.[13] the authors examined induced testicular torsion with greyscale imaging, colour Doppler, power Doppler and spectral Doppler analysis. Injection of

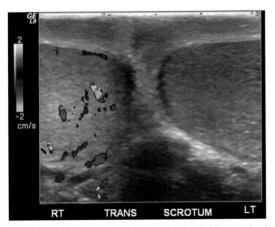

FIGURE 13-19 A five-year-old boy presented with left scrotal pain. This colour Doppler image, optimised for low-flow sensitivity, clearly shows asymmetric perfusion. Some flow is detected on the right whereas there is absolutely no flow seen on the left. The diagnosis was left testicular torsion and the patient was immediately transferred to the operating room.

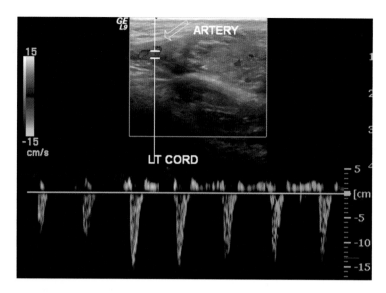

FIGURE 13-20 Longitudinal view of left spermatic cord near the testicle. This young man complained of intermittent left scrotal pain. The colour Doppler image shows only a few small foci of blood flow within the testicle. A spectral Doppler tracing of the epididymal artery (open arrow) shows reversed flow in diastole. These findings support the diagnosis of partial torsion with occluded venous outflow.

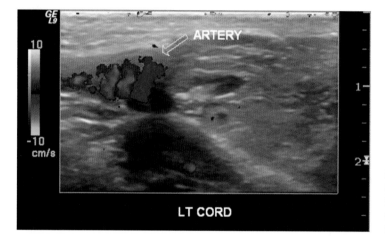

FIGURE 13-21 A longitudinal view of the left scrotum. In the region of the junction of the cord with the epididymis, colour Doppler reveals a "snail shell" appearance of the vasculature (open arrow), the result of a twisting torsion.

contrast media did not enhance greyscale images, but visualisation of all vessels in both normal and rotated testicles was significantly improved with both colour and power Doppler. Asymmetry of blood flow was more obvious. The authors concluded that diagnosis of testicular ischaemia could be made with greater confidence using an intravenous ultrasound contrast agent because of improved demonstration of altered perfusion patterns.

Hand-held continuous-wave Doppler has no role in the evaluation of testicular torsion because of its inability to provide range-gated information. Normal or increased blood flow within the scrotal wall detected by the continuous wave beam may lead the examiner to incorrectly conclude that intratesticular flow is preserved.

Although testicular torsion may be accurately diagnosed by sonography, this does not guarantee successful surgical salvage. Success depends on a timely diagnosis and the duration of ischaemia. Indeed, the more obvious the ultrasound diagnosis, the less likely the chance of salvage. The testicle devoid of colour flow but with an appropriate ultrasound appearance is much more likely to be salvaged at surgery. The testicle that presents with irregular echotexture is likely necrotic and needs to be removed (Fig. 13-22).[14,15]

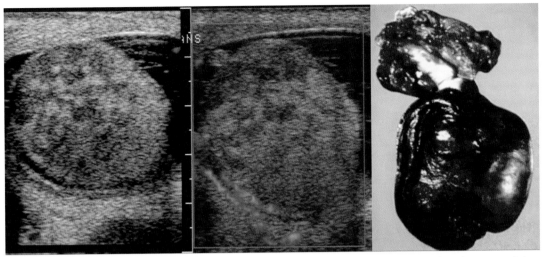

FIGURE 13-22 Transverse imaging view, power Doppler view, and resected specimen of a testicle. Grossly irregular echotexture and absence of flow on power Doppler indicate that this is a severely compromised testicle with torsion. A completely necrotic testicle was identified at surgery.

TORSION OF THE APPENDIX TESTIS

The appendix testis is a Müllerian duct remnant that is attached to the upper pole of the testis. Doppler ultrasound is rarely able to identify flow within the structure. Newer, more sensitive equipment can occasionally reveal the presence of flow within a tender appendix testis (Fig. 13-23). Patients who develop torsion of the appendix testis usually present with acute scrotal pain. Physical examination reveals a small firm, palpable, tender nodule. Ultrasound evaluation

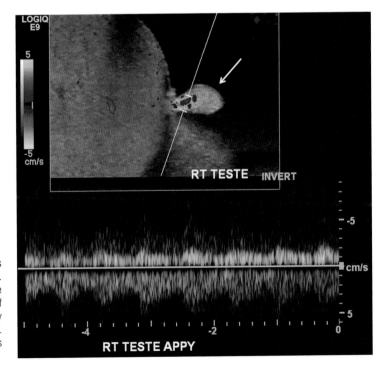

FIGURE 13-23 A longitudinal view of the left testes at the area of maximum tenderness in this patient. The appendix testis (arrow) was conspicuous as the focus of pain. Note the hyperaemia at the base of this structure. It is quite rare to actually identify colour Doppler flow in the appendix testis. Presumably this was torsion/detorsion of this appendix which resulted in focal hyperaemia.

usually reveals a hyperechoic rounded structure attached to the testicle with a reactive hydrocele. The patient will usually confirm an increase in pain when the transducer is over the appendix testis, and that typically clinches the diagnosis. Colour Doppler may reveal increased flow around the twisted testicular appendage but more importantly it rules out testicular torsion or an acute inflammatory process. After torsion and necrosis the appendix testis may slough and become calcified, in which case it becomes known as a scrotal pearl. Twinkle artifact may be present on colour Doppler and should not be confused for true flow (Fig. 13-24).

TRAUMA

Testicular trauma typically results from an athletic injury, a direct blow or a straddle injury. Clinical examination of a traumatised, tender testicle can be difficult because of pain and swelling; however, ultrasound can visualise and confirm testicular integrity, or identify the presence of haematoma, haematocele, or rupture. Colour Doppler sonography provides excellent delineation of blood flow throughout the testis, differentiating hyperaemic, contused regions from devascularised or ischaemic areas (Fig. 13-25).

In the case of testicular rupture, sonographic identification is extremely important because prompt diagnosis and quick surgical intervention are required to successfully correct the condition. If surgery is

performed within 72 h of the trauma, approximately 80% of ruptured testes can be salvaged. If rupture is present, ultrasound may demonstrate a disrupted tunica albuginea; a heterogeneous testicle with asymmetric, poorly defined margins; thickening of the wall of the scrotum; and/or a large haematocele. Perception of blood flow will be diminished or absent on colour or spectral Doppler examination (Fig. 13-26).

Unlike rupture, intratesticular fracture, small haematomas and haematoceles do not require surgery if the tunica albuginea has not been interrupted and Doppler imaging shows normal blood flow to the testicle. Sonographic findings associated with a testicular fracture include a linear hypoechoic band crossing the parenchyma of the testicle, a smooth well-defined testicular outline, an intact tunica albuginea, and often an associated haematocele. Normal Doppler signals indicate unimpaired blood flow and viable testicular tissue. If Doppler signals are absent, ischaemia is very likely and surgical intervention is called for. Acute haematomas are usually hyperechoic relative to adjacent testicular parenchyma. Older haematomas may have both hyper- and hypoechoic areas, and there may be associated thickening of the scrotal wall. On colour Doppler, the septa of haematomas are avascular. Acute haematoceles are relatively uniform and echogenic. As they mature, proteinaceous septations develop and again are nonvascular on colour Doppler.[16,17]

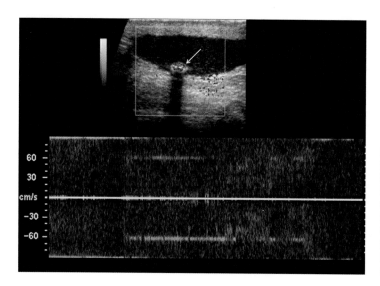

FIGURE 13-24 Power and spectral Doppler image at the base of the right scrotum, distant from the testicle itself. An echogenic structure with acoustic shadowing is layering dependently (arrow). Power Doppler reveals colour emanating from this structure indicating frequency shift, however, the spectral Doppler waveform is completely disorganised. This is consistent with twinkle artifact produced when the Doppler beam interacts with crystalline material, in this case a calcified left scrotal pearl.

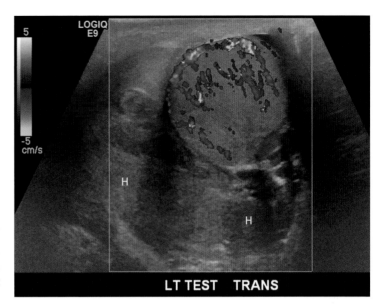

FIGURE 13-25 Transverse view of the left testicle in a patient with acute trauma. Scrotal swelling and tenderness prevented adequate physical examination. Imaging reveals a large echogenic collection within the tunica vaginalis consistent with an acute haematoma (H). The testicle is hyperaemic, however, integrity is maintained and flow is present throughout.

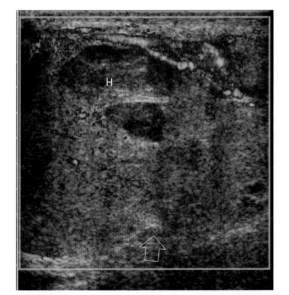

FIGURE 13-26 Longitudinal power Doppler image of a traumatised testicle. There is hyperaemia in the epididymis. Some flow is present in the upper portion of the testicle, but none in the inferior pole. There is a fracture through the mid-testicle with a large haematoma (H). A break of the tunica albuginea is seen in the mid-testicle with disruption of the normal rounded contour (open arrow). This testicular rupture was repaired surgically.

Scrotal Mass

TESTICULAR NEOPLASM

Patients with testicular neoplasms usually present with a palpable scrotal mass or a dull aching sensation. For palpable scrotal masses, ultrasound is widely considered the imaging modality of choice. The principal role of ultrasound is to distinguish intra- from extratesticular lesions, because the majority of extratesticular masses are benign, whereas intratesticular masses are considered malignant until proven otherwise.[18] Ultrasound can easily differentiate solid from cystic masses and confirm their intra- or extratesticular location. The main role of ultrasound is to identify those masses which require additional assessment and possible surgical intervention.

On greyscale images, testicular neoplasms usually appear as a discrete mass whose echo pattern differs from that of the normal testis. Most neoplasms have hypoechoic components although heterogeneity of echotexture is frequently observed (particularly with larger and non-seminomatous germ cell tumours). Sonographic differentiation of seminoma, embryonal cell carcinoma, teratoma and choriocarcinoma can be difficult, especially since 40–60% of testicular neoplasms have mixed histological elements.

Seminomas are the most common single-cell-type testicular tumour in adult males (40–50%). The 'classic' ultrasound appearance of seminomas has been described as a well-defined, uniformly hypoechoic lesion, with no evidence of calcification, haemorrhage, or cystic areas.[19] But the larger the lesion, the less likely it maintains the classic appearance (Fig. 13-27).

Teratomas generally are very heterogeneous with well-defined margins. Dense echogenic foci caused by calcification, cartilage, immature bone, fibrosis, and non-calcified fibrous tissue are interspersed with areas of haemorrhage, cysts and necrosis.[20] Choriocarcinomas and embryonal cell tumours generally appear as small masses with haemorrhage and associated calcification.

The ultrasound appearance of mixed germ cell tumours is that of a heterogeneous, small mass with poorly defined margins, anechoic areas due to cystic necrosis, and echogenic foci of haemorrhage. If the tumour invades the tunica, the normal contour of the testicle may be distorted.[8] Testicular neoplasms have mixed histological components in 40–60% of cases, with the most common combination being that of teratoma and embryonal carcinoma (teratocarcinoma). Ultrasound findings of mixed tumours will vary, depending on which cell lines are dominant and if there are no particular ultrasound findings that permit differentiation for possible preoperative planning.

Testicular carcinoid is extremely rare and usually presents as painless testicular enlargement or as a discrete mass. The tumour may be primary, associated with teratoma or metastatic. Primary testicular carcinoid is believed to arise from pluripotential germ cells or from the development of a simplified teratoma without other teratomatous elements. Very few (<3%) have associated carcinoid syndrome.[21] On ultrasound testicular carcinoid appears as a solid well-defined hypoechoic intratesticular mass with or without dense calcification. On Doppler it has increased vascularity similar to seminoma[22] (Fig. 13-28).

Metastatic disease to the testicle is rare with prostate and kidney being the more common primary sites. Metastases are more common over the age of 50 and are typically hypoechoic. Colour Doppler enhances perception by typically revealing displacement of the normal vascular architecture around the expanding mass.

If a testicular mass is suspected of being a neoplasm, the rest of the scrotum should be examined carefully to exclude any invasion of the tunica albuginea or epididymis. Hydroceles are often associated with testicular neoplasm and that makes them more difficult to palpate. Because a hypoechoic appearance has also been reported with other testicular conditions (e.g. epididymo-orchitis, trauma, spermatic cord torsion, sarcoid), the additional extratesticular findings may help in the differential diagnosis.

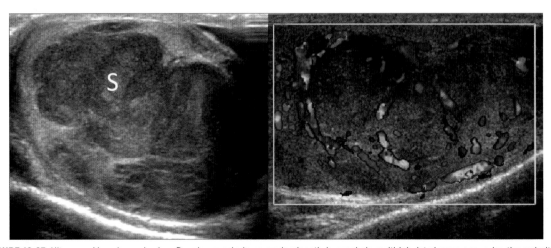

FIGURE 13-27 Ultrasound imaging and colour Doppler reveal a large predominantly hypoechoic multi-lobulated mass occupying the majority of this testicle (S). On colour Doppler, note how the vasculature is displaced around the expansile mass. A seminoma was surgically removed by orchiectomy.

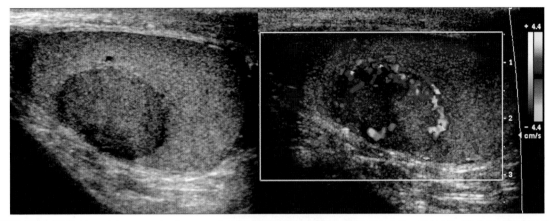

FIGURE 13-28 (A) Right scrotal sonography shows a well-defined solid mass without calcification in the right testis. (B) Colour Doppler shows the hypervascularity of this right testicular mass; a proven carcinoid tumour of the testicle. Case courtesy of Kyoung-Sik Cho, MD, Asan Medical Center, University of Ulsan, College of Medicine.

Colour Doppler and spectral Doppler sonography are considered to be of minimal benefit in the evaluation and characterisation of adult testicular masses and the diagnosis of testicular neoplasm. This is because vascularity of these lesions is extremely variable Small lesions tend to be hypovascular while larger lesions tend toward hypervascular compared with normal testicular parenchyma (Fig. 13-29).

An infiltrative neoplasm of the testicle, such as leukaemia or lymphoma, typically presents as an enlarged hypoechoic area on greyscale imaging. Colour Doppler often demonstrates hyperaemia in the neoplasm. Since these are infiltrative tumours, the underlying vascular architecture is often preserved (Fig. 13-30), with an appearance quite similar to inflammation. The absence of pain, however, should make one lean towards infiltrative tumour and away from orchitis.

BENIGN TESTICULAR LESIONS

Benign intratesticular masses are rare, but recognition is important to avoid unnecessary biopsy, or worse orchiectomy. Almost all intratesticular cystic lesions are benign. The list includes cysts of the tunica albuginea, simple intratesticular cysts, epidermoid cyst (Fig. 13-31), tubular ectasia of the rete testis (Fig. 13-32), and intratesticular spermatocele. Colour Doppler ultrasound helps in confirming the benign nature of these since no alterations in blood flow are demonstrated.[23]

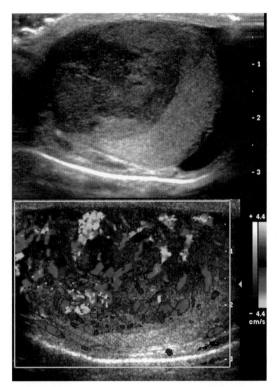

FIGURE 13-29 Greyscale and colour Doppler longitudinal images of the left testis being evaluated for a palpable mass. A large hypoechoic mass occupies the majority of the testicle. Colour Doppler shows vigorous flow throughout this lesion. Note however that the normal fan-shaped distribution has been replaced by neovascularity. This was a surgically proven embryonal carcinoma of the testis.

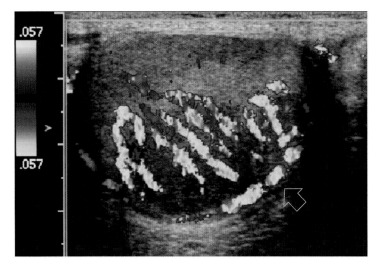

FIGURE 13-30 Longitudinal colour Doppler image of a 59-year-old male with a palpable scrotal mass. Overlying a hypoechoic mass colour Doppler reveals hyperaemia of the capsular artery (open arrow) and centripetal arteries without much anatomical distortion. Colour imaging alone would have suggested an inflammatory process, but the patient is absolutely asymptomatic and therefore lymphoma was entertained and proven at surgery.

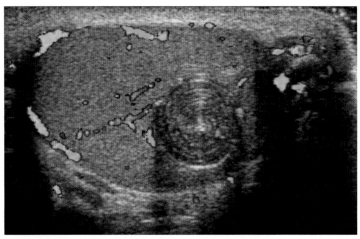

FIGURE 13-31 Colour Doppler image of the testicle reveals a rounded lesion. Note the circumferential rings mimicking an onion. This is a unique feature of epidermoid cysts. Note the absence of any flow within the lesion or at its periphery. Image courtesy of Dr. Jason Wagner.

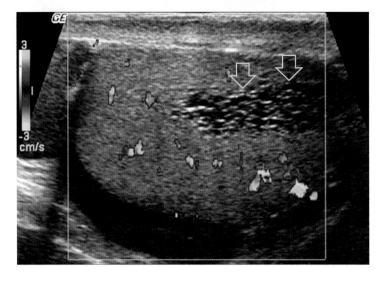

FIGURE 13-32 Colour Doppler image focused on the region of the mediastinum testis. A collection of small tubules is present (open arrows). The absence of colour flow confirms that they are dilated rete testis – prominent efferent ductules commonly associated with a spermatocele.

Bilateral, eccentrically located, intratesticular adrenal rest tumours may be seen in patients with congenital adrenal hyperplasia and primary adrenal insufficiency. In most cases, they are hypoechoic oblong lesions peripherally located close to the mediastinum.[24] They are bilateral in 83–100% of cases.[25] They may undergo extensive fibrosis and eventually become hyperechoic with acoustic shadowing. Vascularity on colour Doppler is variable relative to the normal testicle. Vessels may be seen entering from the adjacent testis without change in course or calibre (Fig. 13-33). Some lesions may exhibit a spoke-like pattern of converging vessels. There are two theories for the origin of these lesions. One says they originate from hilar pluripotential cells, which proliferate as a result of the elevated level of adrenocorticotropic hormone. The other says they originate from aberrant adrenal cortical tissue that adheres to the testes and descends during prenatal life.[26] Whatever the origin, these should be recognised as benign lesions and first treated with adrenal suppression with dexamethasone.

VARICOCELE

Varicoceles are present in approximately 15% of men. Incompetent or absent valves in the internal testicular veins predispose to stasis or retrograde blood flow, resulting in dilatation of the pampiniform plexus. This is the cause of the majority of varicoceles. Varicoceles occur more commonly on the left; this is attributed to the longer course of the gonadal vein and its direct drainage into the left renal vein. Varicoceles are important clinically because of their association with infertility. Diagnosis of varicoceles is important, because treatment improves sperm quality in over half of cases.[27]

On ultrasound a varicocele is seen to consist of dilated (>2 mm diameter), serpiginous channels in the head of the epididymis and spermatic cord. Colour Doppler has been shown to be very accurate in detecting varicocele.[1] At rest and with normal respiration, colour will saturate the tubules at intervals related to respiratory pressure fluctuations. With more vigorous respiration, to-and-fro movement of blood may manifest as alternating colour in the same vessel, changing direction between inspiration and expiration. Colour Doppler identification of varicocele is enhanced by having the patient perform a Valsalva manoeuvre or by having the patient stand up. This increases the abdominal pressure and results in the reversal of blood flow into the pampiniform plexus, thereby causing further distension. When the Valsalva manoeuvre is performed, a brief burst of reversed flow is common (Fig. 13-34). This is due to the expulsion of the venous blood in the gonadal vein of the pelvis below the lowest competent valve. As soon as this volume of blood is expressed, then flow usually stops, waiting for the scrotal venous pressure to rise above that generated by the Valsalva. When the pressure is released as the

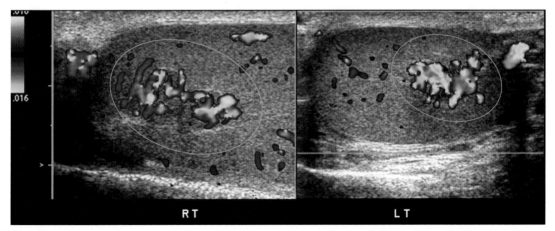

FIGURE 13-33 Colour Doppler images of both right and left testicles show several hyperaemic foci (encircled). Since the patient has a known history of congenital adrenal hyperplasia, these are presumed to represent benign rests of adrenal tissue. Biopsy should not be required. Imaging follow-up can be performed to prove stability.

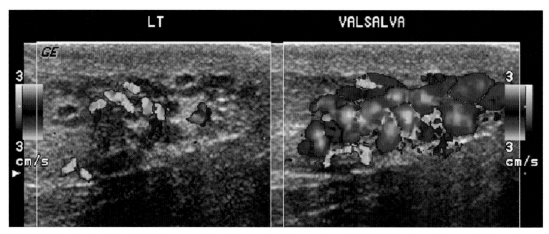

FIGURE 13-34 Longitudinal view of the left spermatic cord in a patient being evaluated for infertility. A serpiginous collection of vessels is present. With Valsalva manoeuvre, note the marked engorgement and increased flow.

patient relaxes, the direction of blood flow reverts to normal. With valvular incompetence however, when the Valsalva manoeuvre is performed, there is constant reversal of flow. The venous outflow from the left kidney finds the left gonadal vein as the path of least resistance. With the release of Valsalva flow reverts back to the normal direction (Fig. 13-35).

Whenever a varicocele is identified, obstruction by a retroperitoneal mass, such as a left renal malignancy invading the renal vein should be considered. A brief scan of the upper abdomen should be performed to assess for this possibility.

Varicoceles can extend into the testicle. They manifest as dilated intratesticular veins (greater than 2 mm) with a positive response to the Valsalva manoeuvre. Incidence is estimated at less than 1%. Typically these are associated with testicular atrophy (Fig. 13-36).[28]

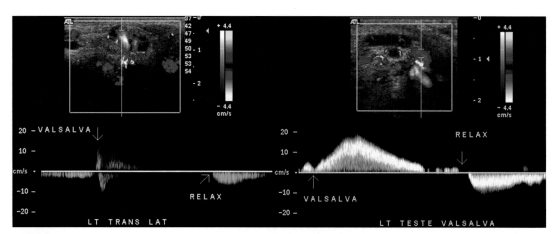

FIGURE 13-35 Spectral Doppler tracings of the left spermatic cord in two patients with a known varicocele. The tracings were obtained as a Valsalva manoeuvre was initiated, maintained, and released. The first patient has a brief reversal of flow at the start of Valsalva as blood below the distal-most valve is forced downward. Then because of valve competency and high central pressure, venous flow becomes stagnant. Upon relaxation of the Valsalva, flow surges forward again. When the second patient initiates Valsalva flow reversal persists for a prolonged time as renal venous outflow is shunted down the gonadal vein because of the high central pressure and incompetent valves of the gonadal vein. As pressure builds within the venous plexus of the scrotum, reverse flow progressively slows until the point of relaxation at which time flow surges forward.

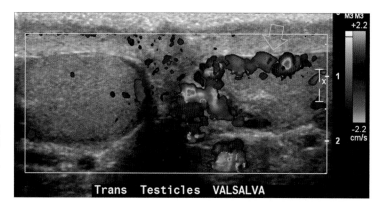

FIGURE 13-36 Transverse colour Doppler image at the level of the mid-testes. A varicocele is present within the left cord. Large dilated vessels are seen extending into the testicle (open arrow). Flow within the veins of the intratesticular varicocele has a similar response to the Valsalva manoeuvre.

After successful surgical varicocelelectomy colour Doppler ultrasound can confirm a decrease in the diameter of the pampiniform plexus of veins.[29]

Other Imaging Procedures

Computed tomography (CT) is primarily used for staging and follow-up of testicular tumour metastatic to the retroperitoneum or elsewhere. Magnetic resonance imaging (MRI), because of its high cost and limited availability, is reserved for problem solving of difficult cases. MRI has been shown to be diagnostic and cost-effective following equivocal scrotal ultrasound, however, even in an aggressive MRI environment only a small percentage of scrotal sonograms required the addition of MRI. Currently, other than in select paediatric cases and in the evaluation of cryptorchidism, MRI has not been found to hold significant advantage over ultrasound in the evaluation of the scrotum; but the modality continues to evolve.[30]

Although scintigraphy continues to be a dependable means of imaging testicular blood flow, it lacks sonography's ability to provide anatomical information, as well as perfusion status, and it exposes the patient to radiation. Therefore, nuclear scintigraphy should be reserved for those situations when the sensitivity of colour Doppler for low-velocity, low-volume testicular arterial flow is not satisfactory and there are questions regarding the findings (e.g. in the small testicles of prepubescent patients) or when the examiner has limited proficiency with colour Doppler evaluation.

Conclusions

The scrotal contents are ideally situated for examination by ultrasound. Their superficial location allows the use of high-frequency transducers and yields very high-resolution images of the testes and associated structures. The addition of haemodynamic information by spectral and colour Doppler allows the examiner to make a very specific diagnosis with a high degree of confidence in several very important disease states. Thoughtful fusion of the anatomical and physiological findings will allow many problems to be clarified and managed without the need for further imaging or intervention.

REFERENCES

1. Petros JA, Andriole GL, Middleton WD, et al. Correlation of testicular colour Doppler ultrasonography, physical examination and venography in the detection of left varicoceles in men with infertility. *J Urol* 1991;**145**(4):785–8.
2. Paltiel HJ, Rupich RC, Babcock DS. Maturational changes in arterial impedance of the normal testis in boys: Doppler sonographic study. *AJR Am J Roentgenol* 1994;**163**(5):1189–93.
3. Luker GD, Siegel MJ. Scrotal US in pediatric patients: comparison of power and standard colour Doppler US. *Radiology* 1996;**198**(2):381–5.
4. Hermansen MC, Chusid MJ, Sty JR. Bacterial epididymoorchitis in children and adolescents. *Clin Pediatr (Phila)* 1980;**19**(12):812–15.
5. Basekim CC, Kizilkaya E, Pekkafali Z, et al. Mumps epididymoorchitis: sonography and colour Doppler sonographic findings. *Abdom Imaging* 2000;**25**(3):322–5.
6. Cook JL, Dewbury K. The changes seen on high-resolution ultrasound in orchitis. *Clin Radiol* 2000;**55**(1):13–18.
7. Farriol VG, Comella XP, Agromayor EG, et al. Gray-scale and power Doppler sonographic appearances of acute inflammatory diseases of the scrotum. *J Clin Ultrasound* 2000;**28**(2):67–72.
8. Lee JC, Bhatt S, Dogra VS. Imaging of the epididymis. *Ultrasound Q* 2008;**24**(1):3–16.

9. Backhouse KM. Embryology of testicular descent and maldescent. *Urol Clin North Am* 1982;**9**(3):315–25.

10. Dubinsky TJ, Chen P, Maklad N. Colour-flow and power Doppler imaging of the testes. *World J Urol* 1998;**16**(1):35–40.

11. Dogra VS, Sessions A, Mevorach RA, et al. Reversal of diastolic plateau in partial testicular torsion. *J Clin Ultrasound* 2001;**29**(2):105–8.

12. Lin EP, Bhatt S, Rubens DJ, et al. Testicular torsion: twists and turns. *Semin Ultrasound CT MR* 2007;**28**(4):317–28. Epub 2007/09/19.

13. Brown JM, Taylor KJ, Alderman JL, et al. Contrast-enhanced ultrasonographic visualization of gonadal torsion. *J Ultrasound Med* 1997;**16**(5):309–16.

14. Middleton WD, Middleton MA, Dierks M, et al. Sonographic prediction of viability in testicular torsion: preliminary observations. *J Ultrasound Med* 1997;**16**(1):23–7.

15. Prando D. Torsion of the spermatic cord: the main gray-scale and Doppler sonographic signs. *Abdom Imaging* 2009;**34**(5):648–61.

16. Deurdulian C, Mittelstaedt CA, Chong WK, et al. US of acute scrotal trauma: optimal technique, imaging findings, and management. *Radiographics* 2007;**27**(2):357–69.

17. Bhatt S, Dogra VS. Role of US in testicular and scrotal trauma. *Radiographics* 2008;**28**(6):1617–29.

18. Ulbright T, Roth L. Testicular and paratesticular tumours. In: Sternberg SS, editor. *Diagnostic surgical pathology.* 3rd ed. Philadelphia: Saunders; 1999. p. 1973–2033.

19. Cotran R, Kumar P, Collins T. The male genital tract. In: Robbins SL, editor. *Pathologic basis of disease.* 6th ed. Philadelphia: Saunders; 1999. p. 1011–34.

20. Woodward PJ, Sohaey R, O'Donoghue MJ, et al. Tumours and tumour-like lesions of the testis: radiologic-pathologic correlation. *Radiographics* 2002;**22**(1):189–216.

21. Zavala-Pompa A, Ro JY, el-Naggar A, et al. Primary carcinoid tumour of testis. Immunohistochemical, ultrastructural, and DNA flow cytometric study of three cases with a review of the literature. *Cancer* 1993;**72**(5):1726–32.

22. Kim B. Scrotum. In: Kim SH, editor. *Radiology Illustrated: Uroradiology.* Philadelphia: WB Saunders; 2003. p. 625–64.

23. Dogra VS, Gottlieb RH, Rubens DJ, et al. Benign intratesticular cystic lesions: US features. *Radiographics* 2001;**21**:Spec No: S273–81.

24. Dogra VS, Gottlieb RH, Oka M, et al. Sonography of the scrotum. *Radiology* 2003;**227**(1):18–36.

25. Proto G, Di Donna A, Grimaldi F, et al. Bilateral testicular adrenal rest tissue in congenital adrenal hyperplasia: US and MR features. *J Endocrinol Invest* 2001;**24**(7):529–31.

26. Stikkelbroeck NM, Otten BJ, Pasic A, et al. High prevalence of testicular adrenal rest tumours, impaired spermatogenesis, and Leydig cell failure in adolescent and adult males with congenital adrenal hyperplasia. *J Clin Endocrinol Metab* 2001;**86**(12):5721–8.

27. Pierik FH, Dohle GR, van Muiswinkel JM, et al. Is routine scrotal ultrasound advantageous in infertile men? *J Urol* 1999;**162**(5):1618–20.

28. Tetreau R, Julian P, Lyonnet D, et al. Intratesticular varicocele: an easy diagnosis but unclear physiopathologic characteristics. *J Ultrasound Med* 2007;**26**(12):1767–73.

29. El-Haggar S, Nassef S, Gadalla A, et al. Ultrasonographic parameters of the spermatic veins at the inguinal and scrotal levels in varicocele diagnosis and post-operative repair. 3. *Andrologia* 2012;**44**:210–13.

30. Choyke PL. Dynamic contrast-enhanced MR imaging of the scrotum: reality check. *Radiology* 2000;**217**(1):14–15.

Chapter 14

Doppler Ultrasound of the Female Pelvis

Michael J. Weston

Introduction

Ultrasound is integral to modern gynaecological practice. This has been recognised by bodies such as the Royal College of Obstetricians and Gynaecologists, who have made ultrasound part of the core requirements in their training modules. Assisted conception units have long been aware of the value of ultrasound. Monitoring of ovaries during stimulated cycles, egg retrieval and assessing the early development of the implanted gestation are but a few of the techniques that could not be done without ultrasound assessment. Transvaginal ultrasound has allowed much more detailed inspection of gynaecological physiological and pathological processes by being able to place a high-frequency transducer next to the organ(s) of interest. However, using the greyscale appearances of the changing ovaries and endometrium through the menstrual cycle only takes one so far. Doppler techniques allow the blood flow in these organs to be assessed. For instance, it has been shown that reduced perfusion of the sub-endometrial myometrium is associated with subfertility. Furthermore, most pathological processes involve alteration of the normal vascular pattern. These changes need to be distinguished from the physiological neo-vascularisation that occurs in the ovary around the developing follicle with each menstrual cycle. Hitherto, our ability to distinguish the disordered vascularity of a malignant process from the increased flow seen in benign tumours, physiological changes and inflammatory conditions has been poor. Recent research has concentrated on overall flow quantification using three-dimensional (3D) power Doppler but there are many conditions in which the use of more conventional Doppler techniques is better known and more widely researched. Contrast-enhanced ultrasound (CEUS) is also beginning to find niche roles within gynaecological practice; for instance, the use of ultrasound contrast agents in assessing tubal patency is well known. This chapter will set out the current state of knowledge on the application of Doppler techniques in these various gynaecological conditions.

Anatomy

Correct identification of the pelvic vessels is essential for accurate Doppler assessment and interpretation. Gynaecological applications place emphasis on the uterine and ovarian vessels but the relationship of the other major arteries and veins in the pelvis is also important. Gynaecological masses may compromise the iliac veins or, alternatively, iliac artery pathology, such as an aneurysm may mimic an adnexal mass unless correctly identified.

The iliac artery arises at the aortic bifurcation and courses inferiorly and laterally to emerge at the groin as the common femoral artery. The approximate surface markings for this course are given by a line from the umbilicus to the point of maximum pulsation in each groin. The common and external iliac veins run posterior and medial to their accompanying artery. The paired artery and vein often form a lateral boundary to the ovaries (Fig. 14-1). The internal iliac artery arises medially from the common iliac artery approximately 4 cm from the aortic bifurcation. The internal iliac artery divides into anterior and posterior branches; the uterine artery arises from the anterior branch. The uterine artery runs in the base of the broad ligament medially to the cervix, where it gives branches to the upper vagina and cervix. It ascends in the broad ligament giving off branches to the myometrium until it reaches the cornual region. Here

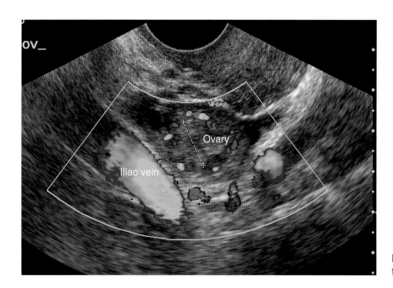

FIGURE 14-1 Vessels lateral to ovary – these help the operator locate the ovary.

it turns laterally to supply the fallopian tube and ovaries and anastomoses with branches from the ovarian artery. The uterine vein mirrors the artery's course and eventually drains into the internal iliac vein.

The ovarian artery arises from the aorta just below the renal arteries. It runs in the retroperitoneum behind the paracolic gutter, crossing the ureter and psoas muscle. At the pelvic brim it enters the suspensory ligament of the ovary and runs to the lateral end of the broad ligament below the fallopian tube. Branches supply the ovary and fallopian tube as well as anastomosing with uterine artery branches. Consequently, the ovary has a dual blood supply. Ovarian veins arise from a venous plexus in the mesovarium and suspensory ligament, they accompany the ovarian artery, draining into the renal vein on the left and the IVC on the right.

Technique

An empty bladder may improve the geometry for assessing uterine artery flow by transabdominal scan. Transvaginal scanning has made many pelvic vessels much more readily accessible for study, particularly improving visualisation of the ovarian artery.

The area of interest is first identified on greyscale ultrasound. Initial interrogation with colour Doppler often uses quite a large colour box. The size of the box should be altered to suit the size of the area of interest. A smaller colour box allows better frame rates

and pulse repetition rates, which in turn improve detection of flow. It may be necessary to move a small colour box around over the area of interest and it may be necessary to alter machine settings to look for high and low flow velocities. Flexibility of approach and familiarity with the machine controls will improve the accuracy of the Doppler information.

The following generalisations apply:

Filtration. A low filtration setting is needed, particularly when assessing pelvic venous disease and perfusion of tissues.

Persistence. A moderate degree of colour persistence is usually best.

Velocity range. Velocity ranges should be chosen to suit the vessel being investigated. Blood flow in most pelvic veins is up to 10 cm/s, whereas most arteries have peak systolic velocities of 10–50 cm/s.

Spectral Doppler – angle of insonation and sample volume. The angle of insonation should be as small as possible, ideally less than 60°, but the shape of the pelvis may limit the positioning of the probe with either transabdominal or transvaginal approaches. Resistance and pulsatility indices are angle independent but measurement of peak velocity requires accurate angle correction.

The genital vessels are generally small, so a small spectral sample volume should be used to better fit the vessels.

Volume flow. Machines capable of 3D volume scanning are usually also capable of 3D colour power Doppler scanning. The colour box size is chosen to encompass the structure of interest. The resulting data volume can then be interrogated, either on or off line, to yield a number of perfusion indices. Potential indices are: vascularisation index (VI), which is the percentage number of colour voxels in the region of interest; or the vascularisation flow index (VFI) – the mean colour value of all the voxels in the region of interest.

Sample volume artefacts. The vessels being interrogated are often small so the spectral Doppler sample volume may encompass other structures that confuse the spectral trace. If both arterial and venous components are included it may confuse the operator about the true diastolic flow.

Twinkling artefact. Colour and power Doppler may produce signals even in the absence of flow. This may be because too much gain is applied but it may be because of bowel wall motion, or reverberation artefact behind calcification or tiny cysts. Some have used this artefact to better detect small calcifications (most usually in looking for renal calculi).

Applications

MENSTRUAL DISORDERS

Dysfunctional uterine bleeding is one of the most common gynaecological complaints. Many cases will have an underlying hormonal cause but in up to half of these cases ultrasound may reveal an underlying structural defect – the most frequent being submucosal fibroids, adenomyosis or endometrial polyps. The Doppler characteristics of each of these will be discussed later. However, Doppler also has a more general role to play in these cases as it has been shown that women with pain on menstruation have increased myometrial vascularisation during the early menstrual phase,[1] and that those with irregular bleeding are also more likely to show increased perfusion of uterine and sub-endometrial blood vessels (Fig. 14-2).[2] The pathophysiology underlying these observations is not yet fully understood. Endometrial ablation is a recognised treatment of dysfunctional bleeding but measurement of the Doppler indices in the uterine arteries does not help determine who will show a good

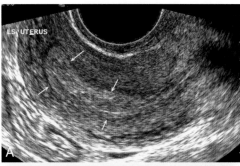

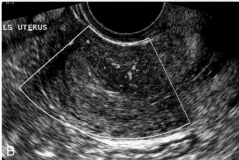

FIGURE 14-2 Myometrial vascularisation. (A) Greyscale ultrasound showing secretory phase endometrium (arrows) in a woman with heavy periods. (B) Colour Doppler in the same patient reveals increased myometrial vascularity.

response to ablation; although assessment one year after ablation helps predict the duration of amenorrhoea or eumenorrhoea.[3]

FERTILITY

Normal Cycle

The normal menstrual cycle starts on day one with bleeding heralding the shedding of the endometrium. Ultrasound shows the endometrium reduces to a minimum basal layer and it may occasionally show blood and clot in the cavity. The endometrium then enters the proliferative phase, displaying a distinct trilaminar appearance. As the time of ovulation approaches, the basal endometrium becomes more echogenic; this echogenicity spreading towards the central echogenic line until, in the secretory phase after ovulation, the whole width of the endometrium becomes of equal increased echogenicity (Fig. 14-3). During the proliferative phase, the ovary shows enlargement of a few of the antral follicles, until one becomes dominant (Fig. 14-4). This continues to enlarge until it is about

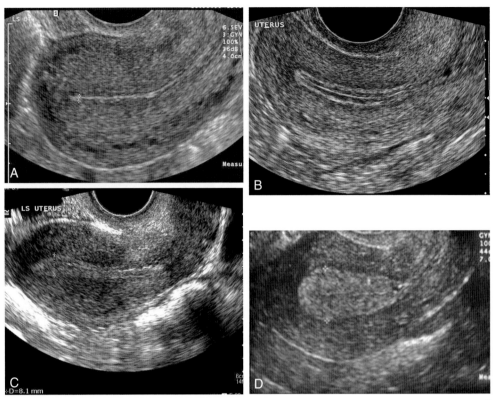

FIGURE 14-3 Normal appearances of cyclical endometrium. (A) Menstrual phase showing the endometrium as a thin line; (B) follicular/proliferative phase showing a trilaminar appearance of the endometrium; (C) periovulatory phase showing the echogenicity of the basal layer of endometrium has extended to the midline echo; (D) luteal/secretory phase showing thickened uniform echogenicity.

2.5 cm in diameter at which point the follicle ruptures and ovulation occurs (usually around day 14). The follicle then forms the corpus luteum during the secretory phase. 3D power Doppler has been used to measure the vascular flow index during the normal cycle; the vascular indices in the dominant ovary and the dominant follicle/corpus luteum show an increase in the proliferative phase such that they are 1.7 times greater than in the basal state. After ovulation there is a continued rise in the vascularity with the corpus luteal flow peaking about 7 days after ovulation with an index three times greater than in the basal state. The contralateral, non-dominant ovary in that cycle shows no changes in blood flow.[4] Hormonally suppressed ovaries show a low vascular flow index throughout the cycle.[5] The resistance index (RI) of the corpus luteum measured by TV colour and spectral Doppler shows that the pre-ovulatory follicle has a high RI, which decreases greatly on ovulation as the corpus luteum is formed. The increased vascularity around the corpus luteum has been likened to a ring of fire (Fig. 14-5). The RI decreases further in the early luteal (secretory) phase but then increases in the late luteal phase. This late increase does not occur if pregnancy has become established, as the RI remains at the low midluteal level until 7 weeks of pregnancy.[6] Fertility specialists can use the peri-ovulatory follicular volume and subfollicular vascularisation as predictors of successful pregnancy in intra-uterine insemination techniques – too large a follicle is likely to be anovulatory.[7] Furthermore, in oocyte retrieval techniques, it has been suggested pregnancy rates are higher in those whose embryo transfer cohort contains at least one embryo from a highly vascular follicle[8] (Box 14-1).

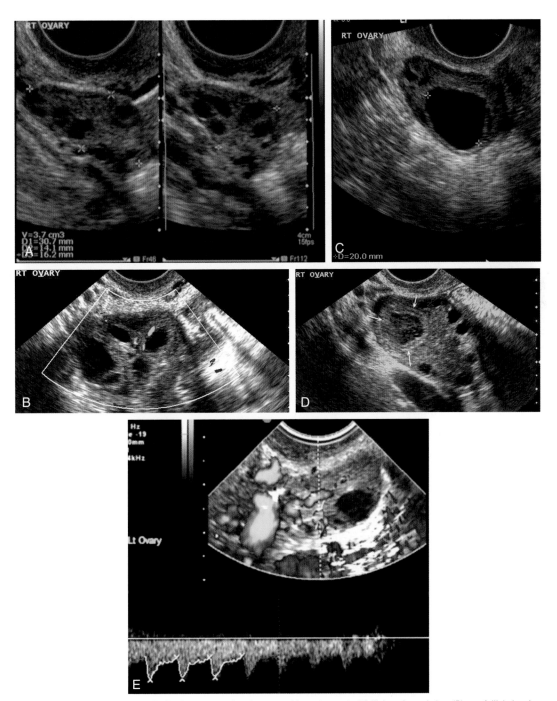

FIGURE 14-4 Normal ovarian cycle. (A) Early phase ovary showing several immature antral follicles of equal size; (B) one follicle has increased flow around it and will start to grow; (C) mid-cycle showing a dominant follicle of 2 cm diameter; (D) post-ovulation ovary with a corpus luteum; (E) spectral trace of 'active' ovary showing low-resistance flow with good diastolic flow.

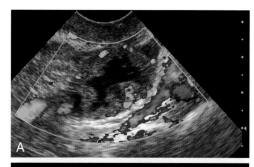

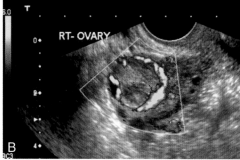

FIGURE 14-5 Corpus luteum showing a 'ring of fire' of increased colour Doppler flow around it (A) and another with a ring of power Doppler flow (B).

BOX 14-1 THE NORMAL MENSTRUAL CYCLE

- Day 1 is the first day of menstrual blood loss
- The proliferative or follicular phase is the first half of the cycle leading up to ovulation
- The secretory or luteal phase is the second half of the cycle after ovulation
- Vascularity of the dominant ovary increases from the mid-follicular phase up to the mid-luteal phase
- Impedance to flow in the dominant ovary decreases from the mid-follicular phase to the mid-luteal phase
- Late luteal phase shows a decrease in vascularity and an increase in impedance – unless pregnancy has developed
- The presence of this variation correlates with fertility

There is also cyclical variation in the supplying ovarian and uterine arteries. An increase in volume flow and a reduction in the RI occur in the luteal (secretory) phase compared with the follicular (proliferative) phase. It is the presence of this variation that appears to correlate with fertility rather than any absolute value. Normal ranges of values are given in Table 14-1. The

TABLE 14-1 Variation in Doppler Indices in the Uterine and Ovarian Arteries during the Menstrual Cycle

	RI OVA	PI OVA	VEL OVA (cm/s)	PI UTA
Early follicular	0.65–0.7	1.8–2.2	20	1.67 ± 0.22
Late follicular/ ovulation	0.55–0.6	1.0–1.3	40	1.89 ± 0.4
Luteal	0.6–0.65	1.3–1.8		2.23 ± 0.67
Non-conception	0.6–0.7	1.8–2.2		3.85 ± 1.1
Postmenopausal	0.6–1.0	1.3–4.0		1.8–3.8

RI = resistance index; PI = pulsatility index; OVA = ovarian artery; VEL = velocity; UTA = uterine artery.

pre-pubertal uterine artery has a high impedance pattern with absent diastolic flow. The change to a lower impedance pattern and the development of diastolic flow indicates the onset of the menarche.

Ovarian Reserve

The age at which some women seek to start a family has been increasing. Fertility units in particular, need to determine the ovarian reserve to help evaluate if an in vitro fertilisation (IVF) cycle is likely to be successful. Commonly, an antral follicle count of less than four, or an ovarian volume of <3 cc measured in the first few days of a menstrual cycle, are associated with non-pregnancy or IVF cycle cancellation.[9] More recently, it has been suggested that assessing the basal ovarian stromal blood flow may help.[10] Being unable to detect any stromal flow in at least one ovary is not just a technical issue but it is more probably related to low ovarian reserve (Fig. 14-6).

Post-menopausal ovaries typically have no detectable flow, or only high-impedance flow with no diastolic flow in the ovarian arteries. The same is true of the post-menopausal uterine artery, in which diastolic flow is also absent.

Tubal Patency and Colour Doppler

The use of ultrasound contrast agent instilled directly into the uterine cavity to assess patency of the Fallopian tubes has become an accepted precursor to other tests of tubal patency, such as hysterosalpingography, or laparoscopy and dye injection. Intriguingly, loss

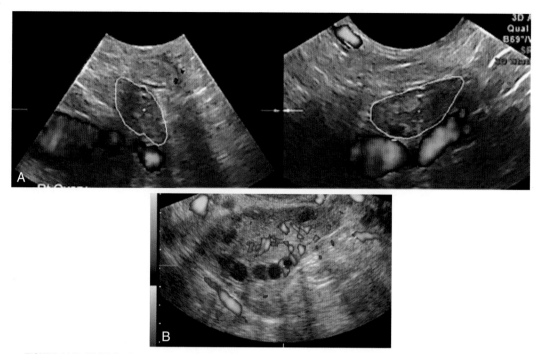

FIGURE 14-6 (A) Minimal or no stromal flow in a post-menopausal ovary; compared with a pre-menopausal ovary (B).

of sub-endometrial flow on colour Doppler can also indicate tubal blockage,[11] although the mechanism for this is not fully understood.

DISEASES OF THE UTERINE BODY

Fibroids

Fibroid vascularity is very variable. The attenuation of sound by some fibroids may make any assessment of vascularity impossible. Detection of flow into a fibroid may help confirm its nature; for instance, demonstrating a vascular connection between the uterus and the fibroid may help distinguish a sub-serosal or pedunculated fibroid from an adnexal mass. Likewise, differentiation of an endometrial polyp from a sub-mucosal fibroid (Fig. 14-7) may be helped by finding more than one feeding vessel as polyps should have only a single vessel (Box 14-2).

Fibroids are often a cause of dysfunctional uterine bleeding. Fibroids are hormonally driven, being more common during menstrual years and tending to regress after the menopause. Visibly vascular fibroids are thought more likely to respond to hormonal

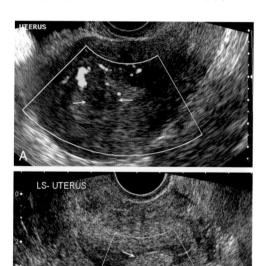

FIGURE 14-7 (A) A submucosal fibroid (arrows) with predominantly reduced echoity and more than one feeding vessel; compare (B) an endometrial polyp (arrows) with a generally increased echoity and only one feeding vessel.

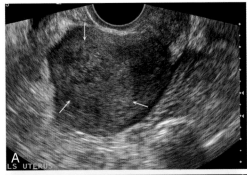

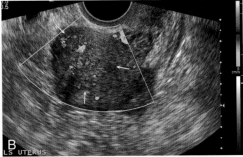

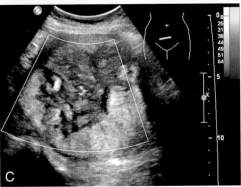

FIGURE 14-8 A highly vascular fibroid (A) on greyscale and (B) on colour Doppler. Vascularity does not predict sarcomatous change, nor does complexity of appearance and necrosis. (C) A complex fibroid with necrosis that turned out to be a lipoleiomyoma.

manipulation in the suppression of heavy bleeding. Uterine artery embolisation is an alternative to surgery for fibroid-related bleeding, although magnetic resonance imaging is better than ultrasound at assessing suitability and response. A new technique of transvaginal Doppler ultrasound-guided uterine artery occlusion using a temporary clamp has been proposed as a further alternative with some good results in pilot studies.[12]

Nearly all sarcomatous fibroids are diagnosed incidentally on histology following fibroid removal for other reasons.[13] It has long been a goal to detect some vascular feature that would allow diagnosis of a leiomyosarcoma; factors such as the larger a lesion, the more peripheral and central vascularity that is found and lower impedance values have all been put forward as predictive of sarcoma (Fig. 14-8). None has been found useful in practice. Currently, the use of 3D ultrasound and finding increased vascular density have been linked to higher cellular activity scores[14] but the imaging diagnosis of sarcoma remains elusive. The most useful sign remains rapid growth on sequential scans.

Endometrial Cancer

Ultrasound is used to measure the endometrial thickness in women presenting with postmenopausal bleeding. It is used for its negative predictive value as those with a bi-layer thickness of 4 mm or less are extremely unlikely to have cancer and so do not need biopsy or hysteroscopy. However, this still leaves many women with an endometrial thickness of over 4 mm who have unnecessary biopsy as most will still not have cancer. The challenge is to define some combination of endometrial thickness and vascular change that will be more predictive. It has been shown that women with endometrial cancer have lower impedance values in the uterine arteries, as well as in myometrial and endometrial vessels[15] but that these changes are not distinct enough to allow prospective diagnosis. Valentin and her group have shown that using power Doppler on ordinary 2D transvaginal ultrasound to define a vascularity index (percentage of

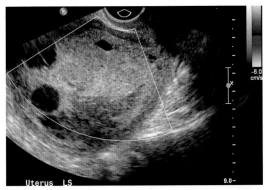

FIGURE **14-9** Endometrial cancer – the image shows a much thickened complex-appearing endometrium that was proven to be cancer. The lack of vascularity clearly does not exclude malignant change.

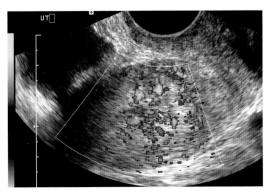

FIGURE **14-10** Invasive endometrial cancer and colour power Doppler shows increased vascularity throughout this post-menopausal uterus. This is associated with a higher grade of tumour and greater depth of invasion into myometrium than those with less vascularity.

the endometrial area on the most vascularised imaging section that contains power Doppler signal) and combining this with the endometrial thickness can improve the positive predictive value for cancer (Fig. 14-9).[16] This contradicts some of their earlier work but is more in accord with other researchers using 3D power Doppler. As yet, these models need to be clinically validated (Box 14-3).

The depth of invasion of endometrial cancer into the myometrium and the histological grade of the tumour affect prognosis. The more advanced tumours are likely to have a mixed or low echogenicity on greyscale ultrasound and are more likely to have greater vascularity, using either 3D or 2D techniques, together with a higher colour score, lower impedance and a greater number of visible feeding vessels (Fig. 14-10).[17,18] In practice, most centres will use postoperative histology to guide therapy.

BOX 14-3 ENDOMETRIAL CANCER

- Endometrial thickness of 4 mm or less is used as a negative predictor of endometrial cancer
- Vascularity of the endometrium may help predict which women with post-menopausal bleeding and a thickened endometrium need biopsy – this is not yet proven
- Greater depth of myometrial invasion by tumour is associated with greater vascularity and lower impedance
- Initial endometrial biopsy followed by histology of the hysterectomy specimen remain the gold standard

Endometritis

This is usually a clinical diagnosis and there may be no signs on ultrasound. Inflammation of the endometrium may occur post-partum, following instrumentation, or as part of a wider pelvic inflammatory disorder. There are no specific ultrasound signs but finding fluid or debris in the endometrial cavity in someone with appropriate clinical features may help. Doppler features, if any, are of increased endometrial vascularity and reduced impedance (Fig. 14-11). Some authors believe that uterine artery RI showing an increase back to normal higher levels of impedance is a marker of response to treatment.[19]

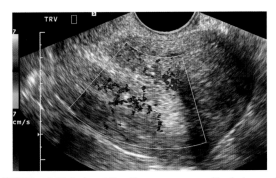

FIGURE **14-11** Endometritis. There are no specific features of endometritis on ultrasound and the diagnosis relies on clinical factors. However, increased vascularity, as in this example, may be demonstrated.

Tamoxifen

Tamoxifen is used in the maintenance treatment of breast cancer. It also has an oestrogenic effect on the endometrium and is associated with increased endometrial thickness and higher rates of hyperplasia, polyp formation and endometrial cancer. There is an increase in uterine artery blood flow and a decrease in impedance with the use of tamoxifen, but nothing specific that allows the diagnosis of endometrial cancer.

Hormone Replacement Therapy

The use of hormone replacement therapy does not alter the normal high-impedance post-menopausal uterine blood flow. It may make fibroids become more vascular.

Retained Products of Conception

Retained products of conception (RPOC) may occur after normal delivery or after spontaneous or induced miscarriage. It can be very difficult to determine if the material seen in the endometrial cavity is true RPOC, or just blood clot. It has been shown that no clinical or greyscale sonographic feature predicts the disorder when compared against the histology of the removed contents.[20] However, there is recent recognition that some RPOC are associated with marked focal hypervascularity (Fig. 14-12). This seems to be a much more common finding in women who have had an induced termination of pregnancy.[21] It is important to realise that these findings do not represent arterio-venous malformations (AVM) and that the great majority of them will resolve with expectant management.[22,23] Ultrasound can be used to monitor the involution of the hyper-vascularity and βHCG should be checked to exclude the possibility of underlying molar change as this may also show hyper-vascularity. True, acquired uterine AVM are usually caused by curettage, show similar focal hyper-vascularity and are likely to require further treatment such as embolisation (Fig. 14-13). Consequently, it is important to be aware of the clinical circumstances when interpreting the Doppler findings. Conversely, women with an incomplete miscarriage have a better rate of spontaneous passage of the products if the suspected products are avascular[24] (Box 14-4).

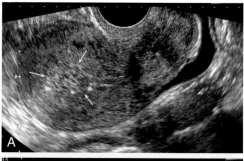

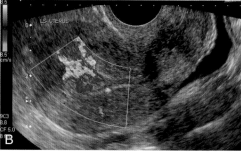

FIGURE 14-12 Longitudinal views of a uterus following miscarriage. (A) Greyscale image showing tissue of increased echogenicity in the endometrial cavity likely to be retained products of conception. (B) There is greatly increased vascularity in the underlying myometrium implying that these are adherent, vascularised products of conception.

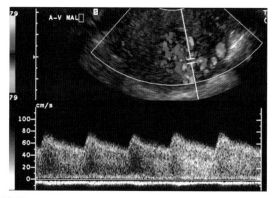

FIGURE 14-13 Spectral trace of increased vascularity in a uterus following curettage. There is low impedance flow. Arterio-venous malformations are commoner after curettage.

Trophoblastic Disease

Gestational trophoblastic disease is diagnosed on histology and response to treatment is usually monitored with βHCG assays.

Contrast-enhanced colour Doppler ultrasound shows that invasive moles and choriocarcinomas show a marked increase in uterine and tumour vascularity following enhancement, whereas non-invasive moles do not show any intra-tumoral blood flow.[25] Use of contrast-enhanced ultrasound may permit the detection of small invasive moles within the myometrium (Fig. 14-14).

Power Doppler has been used to monitor response to chemotherapy with methotrexate and loss of vascularity in a tumour nodule may be an independent marker that predicts response even when βHCG values appear to have plateaued.[26]

CERVICAL CANCER

Cervical cancer is diagnosed clinically, either following a screening smear or following symptoms such as post-coital bleeding. Staging for a long time has been based on clinical examination, often under anaesthetic. More recently, magnetic resonance imaging has become the accepted imaging test for staging when available. Ultrasound has generally had little role to play in the past, except for the incidental diagnosis of relatively large tumours. However, Doppler ultrasound has been found by some to show promise in assessing prognostic risk factors.

Cervical tumours show vascularity (Fig. 14-15) whereas the normal cervical stroma does not. Prolapsing cervical polyps can be identified on colour Doppler by virtue of their vascularity and their feeding vessels (Fig. 14-16). Both squamous cell carcinomas (SCC) and adenocarcinomas (AC) are vascular and cannot be distinguished on Doppler criteria, though SCC are more likely to be hypo-echoic and AC iso-echoic compared to normal cervical stroma.[27] It is postulated that the more abundant the tumour vascularisation, the more likely it is that the tumour will be larger, have deeper invasion, lymphovascular space invasion and nodal metastases.[28] Others have not found so strong a correlation, confining themselves to saying that tumour vascularity on 3D power Doppler correlates with cervical volume but not with other markers of worse prognosis.[29] This work has not yet found a practical application.

The development of thrombo-embolic events, which may be diagnosed on Doppler ultrasound or on computed tomography, is associated with tumour progression in women on follow-up for stage IIIB cervical cancer[30] and indicates a poorer prognosis.

OVARIAN DISEASE

Cancer

There has been considerable research effort put into defining ultrasound characteristics that will detect early

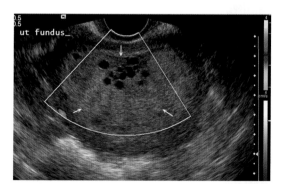

FIGURE 14-14 Molar pregnancy proven on histology. The uterine cavity is distended by uniformly echogenic tissue containing an area of small cysts. Non-invasive moles do not show increased vascularity.

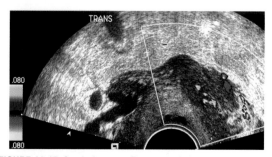

FIGURE 14-15 Cervical cancer. Transvaginal view of tumour on the ectocervix. Note that the tumour is vascular.

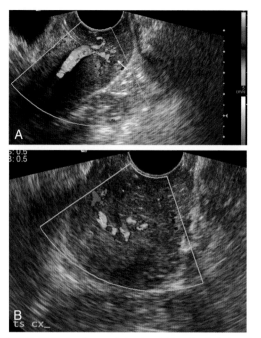

FIGURE 14-16 Prolapsing cervical polyp. (A) Longitudinal view of the cervix showing vessels running through the cervical canal to the polyp (arrow); (B) transverse view through the cervix showing the polyp is vascularised.

ovarian cancer and distinguish benign from malignant adnexal masses. Most such programmes use greyscale features such as size, echogenicity, septations, nodularity and solid components, as well as Doppler indices of vascularity, to give a risk of malignancy. When combined with clinical features of age, menopausal status and tumour markers such as CA-125, or tumour-specific growth factor, they can achieve reasonable accuracy.[31,32] There are several such indexes or logistic regression programmes to help in the diagnosis but so far, it is known that an experienced observer can outperform these.[33] There will always be a small subset of adnexal masses thought appropriate for surgery that will not be characterisable by ultrasound.

Normal physiological processes in women of menstrual years will produce follicular cysts, neovascularisation and low-impedance flows. The challenge for Doppler ultrasound is to separate these normal events from the abnormal flow patterns seen in pathological lesions. Initially, it was thought that malignant tumours showed lower impedance values on RI and PI than benign processes (Fig. 14-17). However, although there is a trend towards this, the indices are not a useful prospective clinical tool. Interest of late has focused on the pattern of colour/power Doppler

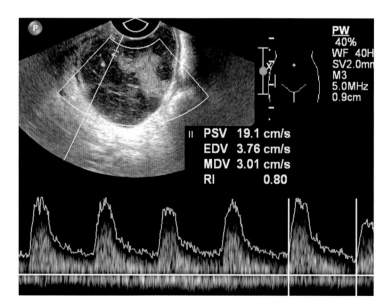

FIGURE 14-17 Ovarian cancer. A typical appearance of an ovarian cancer with a mixed cystic and solid lesion. There is visible colour flow within the tumour and the spectral trace shows diastolic flow. However, the resistance index (RI) of 0.8 falls outside the range that used to be used to predict malignancy. The use of spectral indices has fallen into disuse in the diagnosis of ovarian cancer because of this.

spread in the tumour and the amount of vascularity. Not everyone has found 3D power Doppler to be helpful, Ohel et al.[34] found no significant differences between benign and malignant ovaries on any of the indices of vascularity and perfusion. Alcazar and his group have been strong advocates for the use of Doppler in ovarian masses. Their work[35] shows that finding colour Doppler flow within any solid portion or excrescence in a tumour increases the likelihood of the lesion being malignant and that this increases the diagnostic accuracy over the greyscale findings (Fig. 14-18). The impact of this finding depends on the clinical presentation;[36] colour Doppler performs best in those being investigated for symptoms of cancer; it is less effective in those with benign symptoms and is outperformed by greyscale findings in asymptomatic women. Some corroboration is offered by work looking at the development of malignancy within endometriotic cysts. Finding a vascularised solid nodule within a cyst otherwise thought to be

due to endometriosis is a marker of malignant change (Fig. 14-19; Box 14-5).[37]

The use of Doppler to look for vascularised solid nodules in tumours mirrors the work done on the use of gadolinium enhancement in magnetic resonance imaging; both techniques are assessing vascularity of the lesion. Most centres will use an imaging algorithm that starts with ultrasound. Doppler is used to help solve problems, even though meta-analyses[38] indicate that this may not improve sensitivity or specificity. Those masses thought to be benign are followed-up with ultrasound, those thought to be definitely malignant are staged with CT and those which are indeterminate, are further categorised using MRI.

Screening for Ovarian Cancer

Most women with ovarian cancer present with advanced stage disease. Ideally, by screening women, it is hoped to identify ovarian cancer at an earlier stage at a time when treatment will be curative. There have been several large studies undertaken looking at tumour markers, ultrasound and Doppler. The main problem is the large number of false-positive scans in the screened population. So far, it can be said that the use of transvaginal ultrasound, as opposed to just transabdominal ultrasound, decreases the number of lesions that need to be operated on for the detection of each cancer. Some believe that the use of Doppler further decreases the number of false positives, although this is not proven. Likewise, refining the screened population, either with family history or tumour markers, has the same effect but at the expense of missing some tumours. Despite all the screening effort, there are still interval cancers that arise between screening rounds. Consequently, although the research effort continues, screening for ovarian cancer in the normal population has not yet been shown to be worthwhile.

Ovarian Torsion

Ovarian torsion (Box 14-6) is one of the causes of acute pelvic pain. It is more common in children and young adults and may be associated with vomiting. It is often associated with an underlying lesion such as a cyst or dermoid. Diagnosis is made more difficult because the ovary may tort and detort spontaneously; because of this, patterns of Doppler flow can be very variable.

Affected children may present with intermittent abdominal pain and tenderness.[39] Some believe all

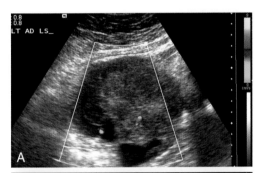

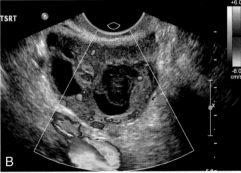

FIGURE 14-18 Ovarian cancer. (A) The solid component of the ovarian lesion contains colour flow indicating that this is a malignant lesion. (B) A large abnormal post-menopausal ovary. The presence of the colour flow increases the predictive value for cancer. Both of these lesions were proven to be cancers.

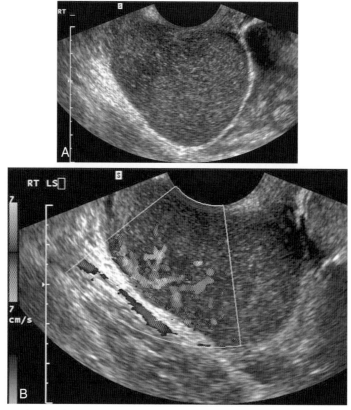

FIGURE 14-19 (A) Initial grey-scale view of an adnexal mass mimicking the features of an endometrioma. However, the use of colour Doppler (B) clearly shows that this is a solid malignant lesion (monochrome image of a colour Doppler study).

BOX 14-5 OVARIAN CANCER

- Indices of vascular impedance are unhelpful in diagnosing malignancy
- Vascularisation of solid nodules is predictive
- Risk of Malignancy Indices are helpful, but experienced observers can usually outperform them
- Some lesions will remain uncharacterisable by ultrasound
- MRI is used as a problem-solving tool

BOX 14-6 OVARIAN TORSION

- More common in children and young adults
- Look for free fluid and underlying ovarian cyst or dermoid
- Vascularity often abnormal but may be increased or decreased
- Check venous flow, absence is very suggestive
- The whirlpool sign adds specificity
- Absence of signs does not exclude the diagnosis

children will show an abnormal flow pattern in the affected ovary, either with reduced overall vascularity and a greater impedance in the supplying vessel or, if recent de-torsion has occurred, with increased vascularity and low impedance when compared to the pain-free side (Fig. 14-20).

Adults may show similar signs of abnormal blood flow and free fluid in about three quarters of those

with torsion. Absence of any signs does not exclude the diagnosis.[40] Indeed, some authors find that using Doppler does not add to the accuracy of the pre-operative diagnosis in women with acute pain.[41]

Additional signs should be sought. The 'whirlpool' sign[42] of vessels spiralling round each other or the ovary can be seen with greyscale ultrasound, or with

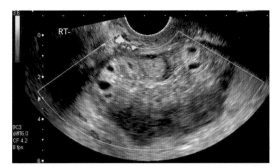

FIGURE 14-20 Ovarian torsion. The ovary is greatly enlarged, the follicles stand out within a small halo and there is absence of detectable blood flow on power Doppler. These are typical features of torsion.

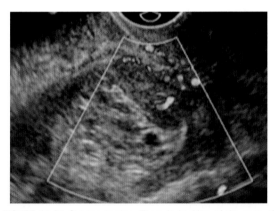

FIGURE 14-21 Ovarian torsion. There is beaking of the cornual region of the uterus with the impression of a twist or whirlpool of adjacent flow.

Doppler (Fig. 14-21); although if there is torsion, there may be no flow in the vessels. This sign adds specificity to the ultrasound diagnosis of torsion. The flow pattern in the draining ovarian veins[43] is also worth interrogating as it has been reported that absent flow, or abnormality in the venous flow may be the only sign of torsion.

OTHER ADNEXAL LESIONS
Sepsis

The majority of inflammatory conditions will be associated with clinical signs of sepsis and it is these clinical signs and symptoms that are essential for diagnosis of these inflammatory disorders. Most inflammatory conditions will show increased blood flow, particularly

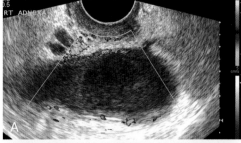

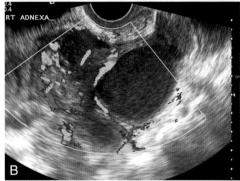

FIGURE 14-22 Pyosalpinx. (A) A dilated fallopian tube filled with pus and with increased vascularity in the walls. (B) A more complex tubo-ovarian abscess with several loculations and increased vascularity. The diagnosis is really made from the clinical features and the increased vascularity is merely confirmatory.

in circumferential vessels draped around the cystic component (pus) of a tubo-ovarian abscess (Fig. 14-22). Sepsis may provoke thrombosis of the iliac or gonadal veins (Fig. 14-23). More chronic forms of sepsis, such as pelvic actinomycosis associated with long-term intra-uterine device use, do not have any specific Doppler features.

Endometriosis

Endometriomas are classically detected as, 'an adnexal mass in a pre-menopausal patient with ground-glass echogenicity of the cyst fluid, one to four locules and no solid parts with detectable blood flow'.[44] Ground-glass cysts in post-menopausal women are more likely to be malignant, as are any lesions that have vascularised solid parts. However, women who present with pelvic pain from their endometrioma are likely to show increased vascularisation around the endometriotic cyst.[45]

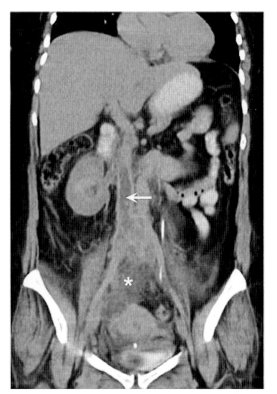

FIGURE 14-23 Coronal CT scan showing inflammatory changes in the pelvis (*) and a thrombus extending up the inferior vena cava (arrow).

Hydrosalpinx

The main value of Doppler ultrasound in hydrosalpinx is in confirming that the tubular adnexal fluid-containing structure is not a blood vessel.

Ectopic Pregnancy

Ultrasound, particularly transvaginal ultrasound, plays a vital role in the diagnosis of ectopic pregnancy (Box 14-7). Women presenting with pain and bleeding

BOX 14-7 ECTOPIC PREGNANCY

- Pregnancy of unknown location – a useful concept encompassing ectopic pregnancy
- Doppler ultrasound may show trophoblastic flow and increase detection of the ectopic sac
- Beware confusing a vascular corpus luteum with an ectopic
- Conservative treatment can be guided by Doppler monitoring of the trophoblast vascularity

in early pregnancy require ultrasound to establish the site and viability of any gestation. Scans should not be done prior to 6 weeks menstrual age as these have a high rate of being non-diagnostic and may lead to erroneous over-diagnosis of ectopic pregnancy. No-one has suffered tubal rupture from ectopic pregnancy prior to 6 weeks menstrual age. After 6 weeks, failing to find a gestation sac in the presence of a positive pregnancy test leads to the concept of a 'pregnancy of unknown location'. This includes a pregnancy in the right place but too small to see, a recently miscarried pregnancy and ectopic pregnancy. Transvaginal ultrasound has a high sensitivity for locating an ectopic pregnancy based on the greyscale signs of an adnexal mass, echogenic ring (doughnut) sign (Fig. 14-24), or echogenic free fluid. Some authors believe that the addition of colour or power Doppler to look for the increased flow in the trophoblast improves the detection

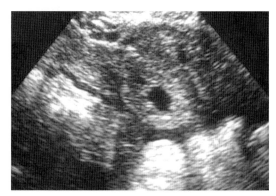

FIGURE 14-24 Ectopic pregnancy. The classic appearance of a tubal ectopic with an echogenic ring and an echo-poor centre (doughnut sign).

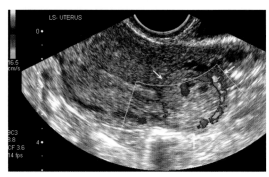

FIGURE 14-25 Ectopic pregnancy. A cornual ectopic pregnancy shows increased vascularity around the trophoblast (arrow) and hence is probably still growing.

rate of the ectopic gestation (Fig. 14-25). There is the potential pitfall of mistaking the 'ring-of-fire' produced by increased blood flow around a corpus luteum for an ectopic. Uterine artery blood flow indices do not allow distinction of a normally sited pregnancy from an ectopic. Once an ectopic pregnancy has been located, treatment depends on its size and whether or not the pregnancy is dead. Not all will need surgery. Conservative treatment with methotrexate can be guided by Doppler assessment of whether there is active trophoblast or not.

PELVIC CONGESTION SYNDROME

It has long been accepted that testicular vein incompetence is a cause of scrotal varicocele and pain in men. It has been much less accepted that a similar syndrome in women of chronic pelvic pain, dyspareunia and pelvic varices might exist. The finding of dilated pelvic veins on ultrasound is relatively commonplace. The more numerous they are and the greater the diameter, usually over 4 mm, the more likely there is to be evidence of reflux on venous Doppler during Valsalva manoeuvre. Reversed flow velocities of over 2 cm/s are thought to be significant. Confirmation of these findings comes from studies of trans-femoral catheter ovarian vein venography and embolisation[46,47] to bring resolution of the symptoms.

NON-GYNAE PATHOLOGY

Iliac and Uterine Artery Aneurysm/Lymphocysts

Iliac artery aneurysms should be readily identified by their communication with the main vessels and by the presence of blood flow within them, which is often swirling in nature. If thrombosed, they may present more of a diagnostic challenge in the differentiation from an adnexal cystic mass but mural calcification and the relationship to the iliac vessels should provide the answer (Fig. 14-26).

Uterine artery pseudoaneurysms are secondary to operative interventions, usually during delivery (commonly Caesarean section).[48] Doppler ultrasound will show an intrauterine cystic mass that has high-speed internal flow. Reported cases have been treated with trans-catheter embolisation.

Lymphocysts are common after pelvic lymphadenectomy for gynaecological cancer.[49] They may appear

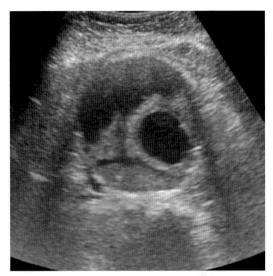

FIGURE 14-26 A large iliac aneurysm demonstrating how the intramural thrombus can produce complex appearances and mimic an adnexal mass for the unwary.

about 2 weeks after operation and can persist for up to a year. Most are asymptomatic. Ultrasound detects them as cystic structures on the pelvic side walls and Doppler is used to confirm that they are not vascular.

Deep Vein Thrombus

Deep vein thrombus (DVT) is usually detected by ultrasound of the lower limb veins. Pelvic and transvaginal sonography may be used to assess the cranial extent of any clot into the iliac veins. Typically, in acute thrombosis, the vein will be swollen by the presence of echo-poor clot and Doppler will either show complete cessation of flow, or flow around the margins of the clot. Chronic thrombosis is more likely to show the vein to be reduced in calibre, with clot of increased echogenicity and flow in re-canalised channels through the clot. DVT remains a leading cause of maternal mortality during pregnancy and the post-partum period.[50]

Bowel Masses

Ultrasound is not the primary imaging modality to detect bowel masses but such masses may be seen serendipitously during pelvic ultrasound for other causes. Bowel wall thickening and mural hypervascularity are non-specific markers of inflammatory

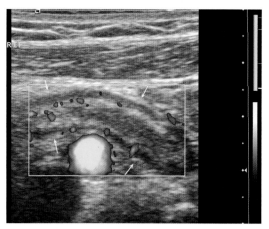

FIGURE 14-27 Longitudinal view of an inflamed appendix demonstrating vascularity in the wall.

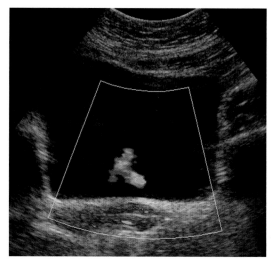

FIGURE 14-28 Ureteric jets demonstrated by colour Doppler entering the bladder.

conditions, including diverticular disease, appendicitis (Fig. 14-27), Crohn's disease and infective colitis. Indeed, in women, transvaginal ultrasound done for pelvic pain may increase the detection rate of appendicitis, as a proportion of appendixes will lie low in the pelvis.

Ureteric Jets

The passage of urine into the bladder from the ureteric orifices is marked by intermittent jets of urine secondary to ureteric peristalsis, rather than a continuous trickle. These jets can be seen on greyscale ultrasound but are more readily visible using colour Doppler (Fig. 14-28). Injuries to the ureter are a known complication of gynaecological surgery. Finding normal ureteric jets in the postoperative period is a good way of excluding ureteral injury, or occlusion.[51]

Pelvic organ prolapse is associated with an alteration in ureteric jets. Longer-duration, lower-velocity jets are present when there is associated bladder outlet obstruction and hydronephrosis.[52]

Summary

Doppler ultrasound in gynaecology has progressed over recent years. There has been a move away from measuring indices of flow impedance and a change to assessing the distribution of vascularity, the proportion of the lesion it takes up and the overall blood flow.

Many areas remain controversial and unproven. The distinction of benign from malignant disease with Doppler remains elusive. However, there are clearly useful roles in fertility medicine, ectopic pregnancies and ovarian torsion. There will undoubtedly be further developments to come.

REFERENCES

1. Royo P, Alcazar JL. Three-dimensional power Doppler assessment of uterine vascularization in women with primary dysmenorrhea. *J Ultrasound Med* 2008;**27**(7):1003–10.
2. Hussein M. Transvaginal Doppler sonography for evaluation of irregular uterine bleeding with DMPA. *Arch Gynecol Obstet* 2011;**283**(6):1325–8.
3. Kuzel D, Toth D, Fucikoa Z, et al. Uterine arteries Doppler velocimetry provides 3-years follow up endometrial ablation outcome. *Prague Med Rep* 2008;**109**(2–3):166–74.
4. Jokubkiene L, Sladkevicius P, Rovas L, et al. Assessment of changes in volume and vascularity of the ovaries during the normal menstrual cycle using three-dimensional power Doppler ultrasound. *Hum Reprod* 2006;**21**(10):2661–8.
5. Hope JM, Long K, Kudla M, et al. Three-dimensional power Doppler angiography of cyclic ovarian blood flow. *J Ultrasound Med* 2009;**28**(8):1043–52.
6. Tamura H, Takasaki A, Taniguchi K, et al. Changes in blood-flow impedance of the human corpus luteum throughout the luteal phase and during early pregnancy. *Fertil Steril* 2008;**90**(6):2334–9.
7. Engels V, Sanfrutos L, Perez-Medina T, et al. Periovulatory follicular volume and vascularization determined by 3D and power Doppler sonography as pregnancy predictors in intrauterine insemination cycles. *J Clin Ultrasound* 2011;**39**(5):243–7.

8. Robson SJ, Barry M, Norman RJ. Power Doppler assessment of follicle vascularity at the time of oocyte retrieval in in-vitro fertilization cycles. *Fertil Steril* 2008;**90**(6):2179–82.

9. Gibreel A, Maheshwari A, Bhattacharya S, et al. Ultrasound tests of ovarian reserve; a systematic review of accuracy in predicting fertility outcomes. *Hum Fertil (Camb)* 2009;**12**(2):95–106.

10. Younis JS, Haddad S, Matilsky M, et al. Undetectable basal ovarian stromal blood flow in infertile women is related to low ovarian reserve. *Gynecol Endocrinol* 2007;**23**(5):284–9.

11. Demir B, Kocak M, Beydilli G, et al. Diagnostic accuracy and efficacy of color Doppler mapping for tubal patency. *J Obstet Gynaecol Res* 2011;**37**(7):782–6.

12. Vilos GA, Vilos EC, Abu-Rafea B, et al. Transvaginal Doppler-guided uterine artery occlusion for the treatment of symptomatic fibroids: summary results from two pilot studies. *J Obstet Gynaecol Can* 2010;**32**(2):149–54.

13. Wu TI, Yen TC, Lai CH. Clinical presentation and diagnosis of uterine sarcoma, including imaging. *Best Pract Res Clin Obstet Gynaecol* 2011;**25**(6):681–9.

14. Minsart AF, Ntoutoume Sima F, Vandenhoute K, et al. Does three-dimensional ultrasound predict histopathologic findings of uterine fibroids? A preliminary study. *Ultrasound Obstet Gynecol* 2012;**40**(6):714–20.

15. Bezircioglu I, Baloglu A, Cetinkaya B, et al. The diagnostic value of Doppler ultrasonography in distinguishing endometrial malignancies in women with postmenopausal bleeding. *Arch Gynecol Obstet* 2012;**285**(5):1369–74.

16. Opolskiene G, Sladkevicius P, Valentin L. Prediction of endometrial malignancy in women with postmenopausal bleeding and sonographic endometrial thickness ≥4.5 mm. *Ultrasound Obstet Gynecol* 2011;**37**(2):232–40.

17. Galvan R, Merce L, Jurado M, et al. Three–dimensional power Doppler angiography in endometrial cancer: correlation with tumor characteristics. *Ultrasound Obstet Gynecol* 2010;**35**(6):723–9.

18. Epstein E, Van Holsbeke C, Mascilini F, et al. Gray-scale and color Doppler ultrasound characteristics of endometrial cancer in relation to stage, grade and tumor size. *Ultrasound Obstet Gynecol* 2011;**38**(5):586–93.

19. Ozbay K, Deveci S. Relationships between transvaginal colour Doppler findings, infectious parameters and visual analogue scale scores in patients with mild acute pelvic inflammatory disease. *Eur J Obstet Gynecol Reprod Biol* 2011;**156**(1):105–8.

20. Levin I, Almog B, Ata B, et al. Clinical and sonographic findings in suspected retained trophoblast after pregnancy do not predict the disorder. *J Minim Invasive Gynecol* 2010;**17**(1):66–9.

21. Mungen E, Dundar O, Babacan A. Postabortion Doppler evaluation of the uterus: incidence and causes of myometrial hypervascularity. *J Ultrasound Med* 2009;**28**(8):1053–60.

22. Mulic-Lutvica A, Eurenius K, Axelsson O. Uterine artery Doppler ultrasound in postpartum women with retained placental tissue. *Acta Obstet Gynecol Scand* 2009;**88**(6):724–8.

23. Kitahara T, Sato Y, Kakui K, et al. Management of retained products of conception with marked vascularity. *J Obstet Gynaecol Res* 2011;**37**(5):458–64.

24. Casikar I, Lu C, Oates J, et al. The use of power Doppler colour scoring to predict successful expectant management in women with an incomplete miscarriage. *Hum Reprod* 2012;**27**(3):669–75.

25. Emoto M, Sadamori R, Hachisuga T, et al. Clinical usefulness of contrast-enhanced color Doppler ultrasonography in invasive and noninvasive gestational trophoblastic diseases: a preliminary study. *J Reprod Med* 2011;**56**(5–6):224–34.

26. Cavoretto P, Gentile C, Mangili G, et al. Transvaginal ultrasound predicts delayed response to chemotherapy and drug resistance in stage I low-risk trophoblastic neoplasia. *Ultrasound Obstet Gynecol* 2012;**40**(1):99–105.

27. Epstein E, Di Legge A, Masback A, et al. Sonographic characteristics of squamous cell cancer and adenocarcinoma of the uterine cervix. *Ultrasound Obstet Gynecol* 2010;**36**(4):512–16.

28. Jurado M, Galvan R, Martinez-Monge R, et al. Neoangiogenesis in early cervical cancer: correlation between color Doppler findings and risk factors. A prospective observational study. *World J Surg Oncol* 2008 Nov 25;**6**:126.

29. Belitsos P, Papoutsis D, Rodolakis A, et al. Use of three-dimensional power Doppler ultrasound for the study of cervical cancer and precancerous lesions. *Ultrasound Obstet Gynecol* 2012;**40**(5):576–81.

30. Renni MJ, Russomano FB, Mathias LF, et al. Thromboembolic event as a prognostic factor for the survival of patients with stage IIIB cervical cancer. *Int J Gynecol Cancer* 2011;**21**(4):706–10.

31. Wang LM, Song H, Song X, et al. An improved risk of malignancy index in diagnosis of adnexal mass. *Chin Med J (Engl)* 2012;**125**(3):533–5.

32. Rossi A, Braghin C, Soldano F, et al. A proposal for a new scoring system to evaluate pelvic masses: Pelvic Masses Score (PMS). *Eur J Obstet Gynecol Reprod Biol* 2011;**157**(1):84–8.

33. Valentin L, Ameye L, Savelli L, et al. Adnexal masses difficult to classify as benign or malignant using subjective assessment of gray-scale and Doppler ultrasound findings: logistic regression models do not help. *Ultrasound Obstet Gynecol* 2011;**38**(4):456–65.

34. Ohel I, Sheiner E, Aricha-Tamir B, et al. Three-dimensional power Doppler ultrasound in ovarian cancer and its correlation with histology. *Arch Gynecol Obstet* 2010;**281**(5):919–25.

35. Guerriero S, Alcazar JL, Ajossa S, et al. Transvaginal Doppler imaging in the detection of ovarian cancer in a large study population. *Int J Gynecol Cancer* 2010;**20**(5):781–6.

36. Alcazar JL, Guerriero S, Laparte C, et al. Contribution of power Doppler blood flow mapping to gray-scale ultrasound for predicting malignancy of adnexal masses in symptomatic and asymptomatic women. *Eur J Obstet Gynecol Reprod Biol* 2011;**155**(1):99–105.

37. Testa AC, Timmerman D, Van Holsbeke C, et al. Ovarian cancer arising in endometrioid cysts: ultrasound findings. *Ultrasound Obstet Gynecol* 2011;**38**(1):99–106.

38. Dodge JE, Covens AL, Lacchetti C, et al. The Gynecology Cancer Disease Site Group. Preoperative identification of a suspicious adnexal mass: a systematic review and meta-analysis. *Gynecol Oncol* 2012;**126**(1):157–66.

39. Tsafrir Z, Azem F, Hasson J, et al. Risk factors, symptoms, and treatment of ovarian torsion in children: the twelve-year experience of one center. *J Minim Invasive Gynecol* 2012;**19**(1):29–33.

40. Mashiach R, Melamed N, Gilad N, et al. Sonographic diagnosis of ovarian torsion: accuracy and predictive factors. *J Ultrasound Med* 2011;**30**(9):1205–10.

41. Peled Y, Ben-Haroush A, Eitan R, et al. The accuracy of the preoperative diagnosis in women undergoing emergent gynecological laparoscopy for acute abdominal pain. *Arch Gynecol Obstet* 2011;**284**(6):1439–42.

42. Valsky DV, Esh-Broder E, Cohen SM, et al. Added value of the gray-scale whirlpool sign in the diagnosis of adnexal torsion. *Ultrasound Obstet Gynecol* 2010;**36**(5):630–4.

43. Nizar K, Deutsch M, Filmer S, et al. Doppler studies of the ovarian venous blood flow in the diagnosis of adnexal torsion. *J Clin Ultrasound* 2009;**37**(8):436–9.

44. Van Holsbeke C, Van Calster B, Guerriero S, et al. Endometriomas: their ultrasound characteristics. *Ultrasound Obstet Gynecol* 2010;**35**(6):730–40.

45. Alcazar JL, Garcia-Manero M. Ovarian endometrioma vascularization in women with pelvic pain. *Fertil Steril* 2007;**87**(6):1271–6.

46. Tropeano G, Di Stasi C, Amoroso S, et al. Ovarian vein incompetence: a potential cause of chronic pelvic pain in women. *Eur J Obstet Gynecol Reprod Biol* 2008;**139**(2):215–21.

47. Tinelli A, Prudenzano R, Torsello M, et al. Suprapubic percutaneous sclero-embolization of symptomatic female pelvic varicocele under local anesthesia. *Eur Rev Med Pharmacol Sci* 2012;**16**(1):111–17.

48. Isono W, Tsutsumi R, Wada-Hiraike O, et al. Uterine artery pseudoaneurysm after Caesarean section: case report and literature review. *J Minim Invasive Gynecol* 2010;**17**(6):687–91.

49. Tam KF, Lam KW, Chan KK, et al. Natural history of pelvic lymphocysts as observed by ultrasonography after bilateral pelvic lymphadenectomy. *Ultrasound Obstet Gynecol* 2008;**32**(1):87–90.

50. Brown HL, Hiett AK. Deep vein thrombosis and pulmonary embolism in pregnancy: diagnosis, complications, and management. *Clin Obstet Gynecol* 2010;**53**(2):345–59.

51. Lojindarat S, Suwikrom S, Puangsa-art S. Postoperative color Doppler sonography of the ureteral jets to detect ureteral patency in laparoscopic hysterectomy. *J Med Assoc Thai* 2011;**94**(10):1169–74.

52. Lo TS, Long CY, Lin YH, et al. Doppler ureteric jet in urogenital prolapse. *Int Urogynecol J* 2012;**23**(1):49–56.

Chapter 15

Clinical Applications of Doppler Ultrasound in Obstetrics

Imogen Montague

The circulatory changes that occur during pregnancy involve modification of vascular structure within the uterus (spiral arteries), the development of a neocirculation (the placenta and the fetus), a redistribution of blood flow and alteration in circulating blood volume such that the placenta in the third trimester receives 20% of the total maternal circulation and maternal blood volume increases by a similar value. Certain disease processes and certain complications of pregnancy are at least in part mediated by a microvascular abnormality. Thus, for example, impaired trophoblast migration of the spiral arteries is a major component in pre-eclampsia. As a result Doppler studies are now essential tools in the detection of complications of pregnancy, detection and characterisation of certain fetal abnormalities, as well as detection and management of maternal disease.

The Uteroplacental Circulation

The uterine artery is a branch of the anterior division of the internal iliac artery, and divides further into four arcuate arteries, each of which divides into more than 25 spiral arteries. There are therefore between 100 and 200 spiral arteries which enter the intervillus space. During early pregnancy, trophoblast cells invade this space and disrupt the wall of the spiral arteries as part of the process of placental formation. There are two separate waves of invasion. Between implantation and 10 weeks, the trophoblastic invasion is limited to the decidual layer. From about 14 weeks until 22 weeks, the invasion extends as far as the spiral arteries. This invasion of the spiral arteries affects the resistance to blood flow within

the spiral arteries and thereby in the arcuate and main uterine arteries (Fig. 15-1).[1]

METHOD OF EXAMINATION

The complexity of the uteroplacental circulation makes accurate identification of the vessel under study difficult with either continuous wave or duplex Doppler ultrasound. Originally flow velocity waveforms were obtained using these modalities by angling the transducer towards the cervix on either side of the lower quadrant of the uterus.[2,3] However the uterine arteries are more accurately identified using colour Doppler, which is now the recommended technique to study this artery. The region lateral to the lower uterus is examined and the external iliac artery and the adjacent vein are identified. The uterine artery crosses the external iliac artery on its course from the internal iliac artery to the body of the uterus. It is important to angle the transducer to improve the angle of insonation whilst maintaining vessel identification on colour Doppler. Spectral waveforms are obtained by placing the pulsed Doppler range gate within the vessel at this point (Fig. 15-2A).[4] The spectral waveform from the normal uteroplacental system is unidirectional, of low pulsatility, and demonstrates frequencies throughout the cardiac cycle (Fig. 15-2B). This is a result of the trophoblastic invasion of the spiral arteries; end-diastolic frequencies increase to a maximum at 24–26 weeks of gestation (see Fig. 15-7).[5]

It is possible to calculate several indices to quantify blood flow; however, the most commonly used in the uterine artery is the resistance index (RI) (see Fig. 15-7A). After 26 weeks of gestation the normal range of the resistance index is between 0.45 and

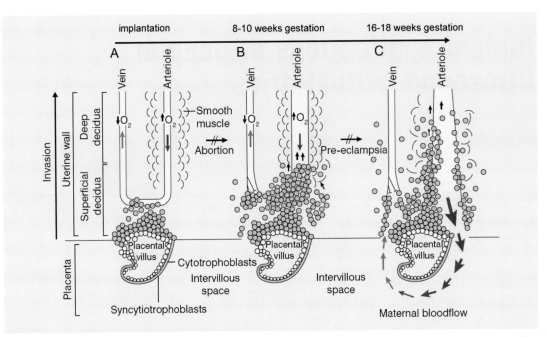

FIGURE 15-1 Endovascular trophoblast invasion into the endometrium occurs in two waves: (A) shows the situation shortly after implantation; (B) at 8–10 weeks the decidual segments of the spiral arteries are invaded; (C) at 16–18 weeks the myometrial segments are invaded. This results in low resistance to blood flow on the maternal side of the placental bed in a normal pregnancy.

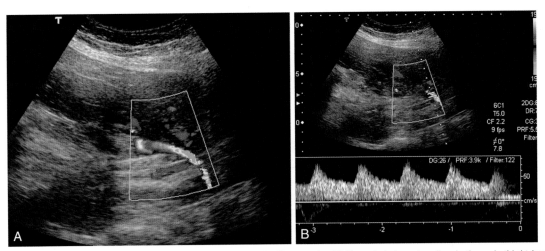

FIGURE 15-2 (A) Course of the left uterine artery as it crosses over the iliac vessels. (B) Normal uterine artery flow in the early third trimester demonstrating high diastolic flow.

0.58. Decreased end-diastolic flow with a consequently raised resistance index above 0.58 is considered abnormal, as is a notch in early diastole in either uterine artery, suggesting failure of trophoblastic invasion of the spiral arteries (Fig. 15-3).[6,7]

PROBLEMS AND PITFALLS

A comparative histological study of third-trimester placental biopsy at caesarean section[8] has demonstrated that the uterine artery flow impedance reflects

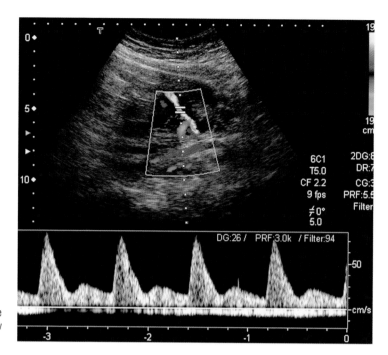

FIGURE 15-3 Uterine artery waveform in intrauterine growth retardation demonstrating low diastolic flow and an early diastolic notch.

impaired trophoblast migration. Nonetheless, there are a number of reasons for caution. Impedance to flow varies throughout the uteroplacental circulation, with the lowest value seen in the arcuate vessels on the placental side of the uterus and the highest value seen in the uterine arteries on the non-placental side of the uterus.[9] The physiological variations and anatomical complexities of the uteroplacental vascular tree make it difficult to obtain accurate and reproducible measurements using continuous wave Doppler, with interobserver variations ranging from 3.9 to 17%.[10,11] In later pregnancy, between 37 and 40 weeks, maternal position may also alter flow patterns, with the umbilical artery resistance being higher in the supine position than in the decubitus.[12] Furthermore, variations in uterine activity (Fig. 15-4), maternal heart rate

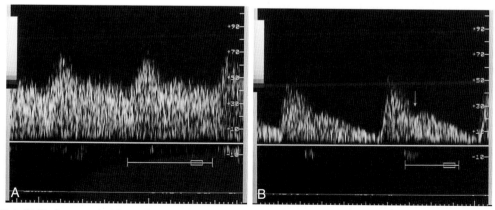

FIGURE 15-4 (A) Uterine artery in labour. Blood flow characteristics in the uterine artery between contractions are normal. (B) During a contraction the overall flow velocity in the uterine artery is reduced. However, the diastolic velocity is reduced further than the peak systolic velocity and there is an early diastolic notch (arrow).

and exercise also significantly alter the waveform.[13,14] The examination should therefore be performed with the mother resting and only during a period of uterine inactivity. The effect of exercise is more marked in complicated pregnancies, but there are no data evaluating the effect of exercise to improve sensitivity or specificity of Doppler in predicting fetal outcome. The time of day, or recent eating by the mother do not appear to have an effect on the uterine artery flow.[14,15] Most of the antihypertensive drugs appear to have no effect on fetomaternal blood flow.[16] However, nifedipine appears to produce a reduction in umbilical artery resistance, and this has therefore been suggested as a better drug to use during pregnancy.[17] The effect of smoking on blood flow has been somewhat controversial with researchers reporting either no effect or a significant effect from smoking a cigarette.[18,19] However, because of the dispute and the potential for cigarette smoking to alter flow patterns in chronic smokers, this author advocates that patients should not smoke for at least 1 hour prior to a Doppler study.

PATHOLOGY

Although superficially attractive, the use of uterine artery Doppler, even in primiparous mothers where the risk of hypertensive complications is greater, is neither sensitive nor specific in the detection of pre-eclampsia, or small-for-gestational-age infants.[20] This is typical for results seen in low- and moderate-risk pregnancies. The routine use of uterine artery Doppler studies to screen low-risk populations for subsequent development of pre-eclampsia and intrauterine growth retardation (IUGR) has a poor positive predictive value. Furthermore, screening can only be useful if there is an intervention available which will improve the outcome, and treatment options for both conditions are limited with, currently, no proven interventions to prevent either pre-eclampsia or IUGR. Therefore, in low-risk populations, using uterine artery Doppler studies as a screening tool is not recommended by national authorities, such as the National Institute for Health and Clinical Excellence (NICE) in England and Wales.[21]

However, in a high-risk population, the presence of abnormalities in the uterine artery studies beyond 24 weeks of gestation may indicate the need for more intensive maternal and fetal surveillance to allow early identification of IUGR or pre-eclamptic toxaemia. This screening technique could potentially be used to rationalise patient care pathways dependent upon their uterine artery Doppler studies.

COEXISTENT MATERNAL DISEASE

Uterine artery Doppler appears to be of significantly greater utility when there is pre-existing maternal disease. In chronic renal disease, for example, an abnormal artery waveform predicts pre-eclampsia and IUGR with a high degree of accuracy. Only 8% of patients with negative Doppler findings in one study developed complications of pregnancy.[22] By contrast, although the resistance index is increased in the uterine arteries of diabetics with a morphological vasculopathy, there is no relationship with short- or long-term diabetic control and it is not a good predictor of diabetes-related fetal morbidity; presumably because these changes are reflecting the risk of acidosis as a result of hypoxia rather than metabolic acidosis.[23,24] In patients with pre-existing, essential hypertension, uterine artery Doppler appears to be useful in defining groups of patients who are at risk of developing complications. If the systolic blood pressure is greater than 140 mmHg, then resistance indices in both uterine arteries is increased. If the systolic blood pressure is less than 140 mmHg, three separate groups may be identified: those with (a) bilateral or (b) unilateral abnormalities of the waveform within the uterine arteries; and (c) those with an entirely normal uterine artery flow. The prognosis appears to be related to the degree of abnormality of uterine artery flow. In systemic lupus erythematosus, one study suggests that an abnormal uterine artery Doppler will identify all those pregnancies with an adverse outcome.[25]

Doppler Examination of the Fetoplacental Circulation

The placenta rather than the lungs is the organ of gaseous exchange in the fetus. Two umbilical arteries convey deoxygenated blood from the fetus to the placenta, and one umbilical vein returns oxygenated blood from the placenta to the fetal inferior vena cava. The umbilical arteries take origin from the fetal internal iliac arteries coursing alongside the lateral walls of the bladder in the urachus to the umbilical insertion. The umbilical vein courses posteriorly and cephalad in the falciform ligament to join the left branch of the portal vein. The oxygenated blood is then shunted through the liver to the inferior vena cava by the ductus venosus. Colour Doppler confers some advantages in the evaluation of the umbilical artery over duplex Doppler alone. Identification of a free loop of umbilical cord and the umbilical artery on colour Doppler allows unambiguous sampling of the correct vessel at the most appropriate angle to get the best waveform. Spectral waveforms are obtained by placing the pulsed Doppler range gate within the vessel. Research studies

correlating abnormal umbilical artery Doppler findings to prenatal outcome relate to sampling of a free loop of umbilical cord. In clinical use, Doppler waveforms must therefore be recorded from a free loop of the cord. However in situations where there is oligohydramnios, and particularly in twin pregnancies with a 'stuck twin', sampling flow from the umbilical arteries within the fetal abdomen as they course alongside the bladder may be the only option to achieve satisfactory Doppler signals (Fig 15-5).

Doppler waveforms within the umbilical artery change with gestational age in a similar fashion to those

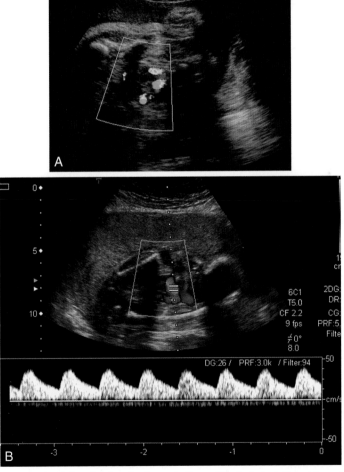

FIGURE 15-5 (A) Relative oligohydramnios. Colour flow Doppler demonstrating umbilical arteries in the pelvis on either side of an empty bladder. (B) Relative oligohydramnios sampling from the umbilical artery within the pelvis demonstrates normal umbilical artery flow patterns.

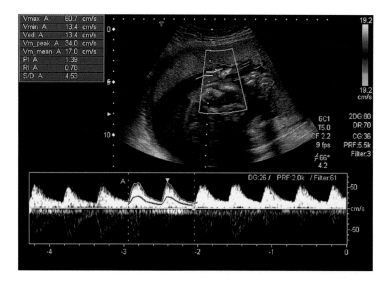

Vmax A	60.7	cm/s
Vmin A	13.4	cm/s
Ved A	13.4	cm/s
Vm_peak A	34.0	cm/s
Vm_mean A	17.0	cm/s
PI A	1.39	
RI A	0.78	
S/D A	4.53	

FIGURE 15-6 Umbilical artery waveform at 26 weeks gestation. Note the PI of 1.39 which is just above the mean value for this gestation.

of the uterine artery (Fig. 15-6). Resistance and pulsatility indices demonstrate a gradual reduction with increase in gestational age. Normal values of the pulsatility index are shown in Figure 15.7.

PROBLEMS AND PITFALLS

Variations in fetal heart rate[26] and the presence of fetal breathing movement[27] may significantly alter the arterial waveforms, although within the physiological range of 120–160 beats per minute it is not necessary to correct indices for fetal heart rate.[28] Nonetheless, it is important to examine umbilical artery waveforms during a period of fetal inactivity and in the absence of fetal breathing; duplex and colour Doppler ultrasound are of value in enabling the waveform to be sampled rapidly and accurately. Measurement of three consecutive cardiac cycles reduces the coefficient of variation of measurements to less than 5%.[29]

All Doppler devices have inherent filtration which removes low-frequency noise and vessel wall movement artefact. On most current machines the high-pass filter can be varied, but it is important not to set this higher than 100 Hz and preferably lower than 50 Hz, if a false impression of absent diastolic flow is not to be created.

PATHOLOGY AND APPLICATIONS

(See Tables 15-1–15-3.)

Intrauterine Growth Retardation

Normal waveforms from the umbilical artery are unidirectional and demonstrate forward flow throughout the cardiac cycle. Decreased end-diastolic flow (Fig. 15-8) and consequently raised Doppler indices are considered abnormal and are thought to reflect increased placental resistance caused by damage to placental tertiary villi.[30] In more extreme cases, end-diastolic flow may be absent (Fig. 15-9) or even reversed (Fig.15-10).

Reduction in end-diastolic flow velocities within the umbilical artery waveform is thought to occur as a result of reduced tertiary villi formation and therefore could be an indicator of placental dysfunction, IUGR and fetal distress. In spite of the attraction of the hypothesis that Doppler would provide an early indicator of failure of the tertiary villus, it has not proved to be of value as a primary screening tool in low-risk pregnancies for IUGR. However, in high-risk pregnancies, particularly those in which there is pregnancy-induced hypertension, or which have other clinical or sonographic evidence of fetal growth retardation, the umbilical artery waveform is a good indicator of fetal compromise. Progressive reduction in the diastolic component of umbilical artery flow mirrors the risk and severity of potential fetal compromise.[31,32] Furthermore, not only may fetuses at increased risk be identified and managed more intensively but high-risk pregnancies, such as those

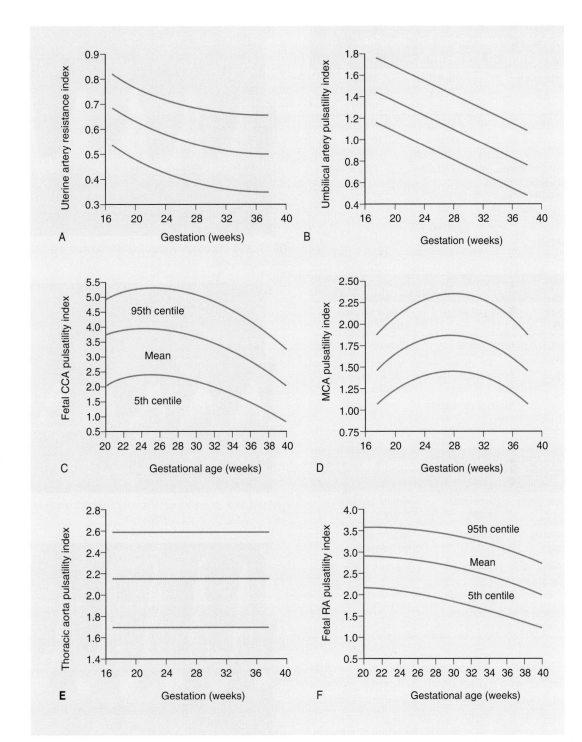

FIGURE 15-7 Normal values during pregnancy for (A) uterine artery resistance index (RI), and (B) umbilical artery pulsatility index (PI). Fetal common carotid artery (CCA) PI (C) falls steeply after 32 weeks gestation, mirrored by the middle cerebral artery (MCA) PI (D). Normal values are also shown for the fetal descending thoracic aorta PI (E) and renal artery (RA) PI (F). (Reproduced with permission from Pearce, References ranges and sources of variation for indices of pulsed Doppler flow velocity waveforms from the uteroplacental and fetal circulation, British J Obstet Gynaecol, 1988; 95(3): 248–256.)

TABLE 15-1 Indications for Doppler Examination in Pregnancy		
Uterine artery	**Umbilical artery**	**Middle cerebral artery**
High risk screening	Intrauterine growth retardation	Intrauterine growth retardation
Pre-existing disease, e.g. renal disease, systemic lupus erythematosus	Post dates	Fetal anaemia
Previous IUGR	Fetal abnormality	
Trophoblastic disease		

TABLE 15-2 Features of Abnormality		
Uterine artery	**Umbilical artery**	**Middle cerebral artery**
Raised indices	Raised indices	Decreased indices
Notch	Absent end-diastolic flow	Raised maximum velocities
	Reversed end-diastolic flow	

TABLE 15-3 Factors Contributing to Abnormal Flow		
Uterine artery	**Umbilical artery**	**Middle cerebral artery**
Pre-existing disease	Fetal activity	Direct cerebral compression
Exercise	Breathing	
Uterine activity	Cord compression	
Antihypertensives ?Cigarettes	?Cigarettes	

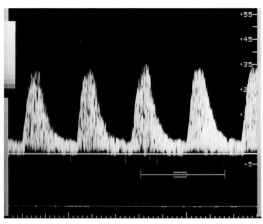

FIGURE 15-8 In intrauterine growth retardation there is reduction of end-diastolic flow.

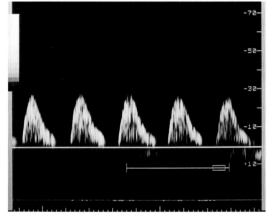

FIGURE 15-9 Severe intrauterine growth retardation with absent end-diastolic flow in the umbilical artery.

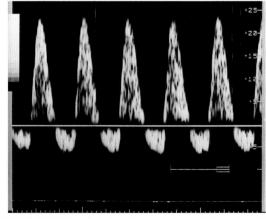

FIGURE 15-10 Reversed diastolic flow in the umbilical artery. This implies a fetus at risk of significant morbidity/mortality.

with established IUGR or pregnancy-induced hypertension but with normal umbilical artery waveforms appear to carry no greater risk of fetal morbidity or fetal loss than a normal pregnancy. The corrected perinatal mortality rate is reduced when the results of umbilical artery Doppler are made available to clinicians, who are then able to act with more appropriate and timely intervention.[33] The finding of absent or reversed end-diastolic flow in a pregnancy with established IUGR is an indication for the serious consideration of early delivery.[34] However in late third trimester, as the umbilical artery pulsatility index normally decreases (Fig. 15-7B), using absent or reversed end diastolic flow in the umbilical artery is not sensitive for predicting poor outcome. This is because the flow in the umbilical vessels nearer term becomes so large it is very difficult for placental pathology to result in absent or reversed flows and the sonographer can be falsely reassured by positive flows although there may be progressive placental pathology. Fetuses with evidence of cerebral redistribution and adverse neurological sequelae can have umbilical artery PI values still within the normal range.[35]

Post Dates Pregnancy

The management of a post dates pregnancy is extremely difficult. No single parameter has been established that will confidently predict outcome and, although there has been some enthusiasm for a role for Doppler in the assessment of post dates pregnancy, there is not universal agreement about its value.[36] In this author's view, therefore, umbilical artery Doppler should be looked upon as one of the factors that may contribute to the monitoring of post dates pregnancies. Absence or reversal of diastolic flow is an indication for immediate delivery and in this situation, an operative delivery may need to be considered.

Twin and Higher-Order Pregnancy

In uncomplicated multiple pregnancy, there is the same progressive decrease in placental resistance as is seen in singleton pregnancies, with a consequent fall in indices with increasing gestational age. Doppler appears to be of no value in predicting adverse outcomes in unselected pregnancies.[37] However, in pregnancies with discordant growth patterns, Doppler analysis of the umbilical arteries appears to be a useful adjunct to serial growth measurements, allowing recognition of high-risk twin pregnancies which require more intense surveillance[38] (Fig. 15-11).

In twin-to-twin transfusion syndrome, the shared circulation has the result that Doppler waveforms in the umbilical arteries of both twins are similar. Doppler studies of these vessels appear to be of no predictive or management value in this condition, although colour and power Doppler may allow documentation of placental anastomoses and consequent guidance of laser ablation.

In triplet and higher-order pregnancies Doppler studies of the umbilical vessels are valuable for the serial surveillance of fetal well-being. Discordant growth with early placental failure becomes more common as the

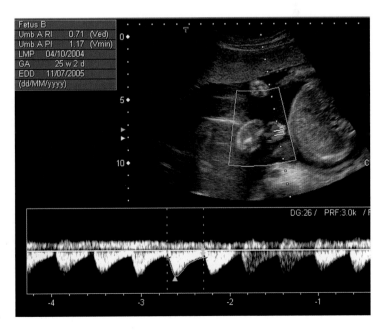

FIGURE 15-11 Umbilical Doppler in twin pregnancy.

total number of fetuses of a given pregnancy increases. Clinical challenges arise with the management of severe preterm fetal compromise in one or more fetus where preterm delivery of that fetus is indicated, but this may compromise well-grown co-fetuses, who can be iatrogenically damaged by preterm intervention. Use of colour Doppler to identify the intra-abdominal segments, or abdominal wall insertion of the umbilical artery is sometimes necessary to be confident of appropriate cord sampling in multiple pregnancy.

Diabetes

Both pre-existing vascular disease and hypertensive disorders of pregnancy are common in mothers with diabetes. In these cases, the value of an abnormal umbilical artery Doppler signal has the same significance in identification of uteroplacental insufficiency as in the non-diabetic population. However, diabetic pregnancies are also at risk of metabolic complications and Doppler flow patterns will not detect these complications, it is therefore vital that a normal umbilical artery flow does not give either the clinician or the mother false reassurance.[22]

Fetal Anaemia

Performing middle cerebral artery Doppler studies (Fig. 15-12) in cases of suspected fetal anaemia has revolutionised the management of this condition. Chronic fetal anaemia is usually secondary to a maternal infection such as parvovirus, or alloimmunisation. The physiological response to chronic anaemia is the development of a hyperdynamic fetal circulation. Raised peak velocities in the middle cerebral artery are linked to fetal anaemia[39,40] (Fig. 15-12C). Use of this technique accurately predicts anaemic fetuses, allowing the timing of any invasive testing to be at the point when fetal transfusions are clinically required. Middle cerebral artery Doppler peak velocities increase with gestational age.[40] In cases of acute fetal anaemia secondary to fetomaternal haemorrhage, Doppler studies are not helpful, and urgent delivery is indicated to allow neonatal resuscitation.

FETAL ABNORMALITY

Fetuses with autosomal trisomy may also have abnormal placentation with reduced tertiary villi formation.[41] An abnormal umbilical artery waveform should therefore prompt a detailed study of fetal structural anatomy and an assessment of amniotic fluid volume; karyotyping should also be considered.[34] This is particularly important in the presence of early-onset growth retardation (both symmetrical and asymmetrical), which has up to 20% association with abnormal karyotype.

Colour flow Doppler is of value in demonstrating abnormalities of the cord including true knots and a single umbilical artery (Fig. 15-13). Similarly, the use of colour Doppler will aid in the diagnosis of abdominal wall abnormalities such as omphaloceles and ectopia vesicae (Fig. 15-14).

The Fetal Circulation

The advent of colour and power Doppler has meant that it is now possible to visualise flow within many of the fetal vessels. These include the aorta, inferior vena cava, carotid, intracerebral and renal arteries. Furthermore, it is possible to study cardiac and cardiopulmonary haemodynamics. The detailed study of congenital cardiac abnormalities and the role of Doppler techniques are, however, beyond the scope of this chapter.

There is a redistribution of fetal blood flow in response to hypoxia with a selective increase in blood

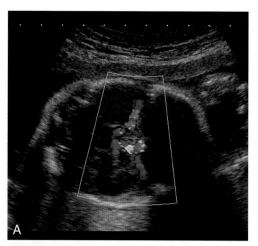

FIGURE 15-12 (A) Colour flow Doppler of the circle of Willis in the fetus. The middle cerebral arteries are demonstrated.

Continued

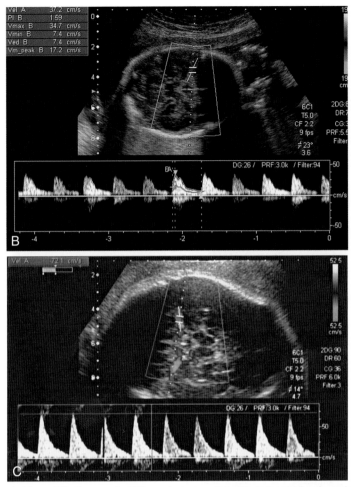

FIG.15-12—CONT'D (B) Spectral flow within the normal middle cerebral artery. Pulsatility index of 1.6 and a peak velocity of 37 cm/s. (C) Fetal anaemia increase in peak systolic flow velocity to 72 cm/s is demonstrated.

flow to the brain, heart and adrenal glands at the expense of the viscera. This redistribution reflects the morphological findings in IUGR, with the head continuing to grow at the expense of a relatively smaller abdomen. Similarly there is also reduced renal perfusion leading to reduced fetal urine production and hence reduction in amniotic fluid volume in the presence of chronic fetal compromise. Fetal outcome is thought to relate both to the severity and duration of hypoxia, as well as the gestational age at delivery.

THE FETAL CEREBRAL CIRCULATION

Whilst the fetal carotid artery can be examined, the middle cerebral artery is the most commonly interrogated of the intracerebral vessels. The skull is scanned as if to perform a biparietal diameter measurement. A colour Doppler examination is then performed in a plane slightly closer to the base of the skull, where the middle cerebral artery will be identified as a vessel coursing towards the probe from the circle of Willis in the Sylvian fissure (Fig. 15-12A).

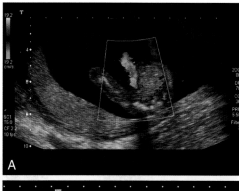

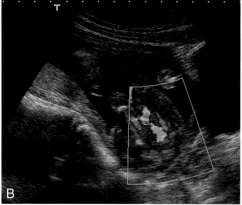

FIGURE 15-13 (A) Colour flow Doppler through the pelvis of a fetus with a single umbilical artery. (B) Single umbilical artery in the pelvis flanked by two femoral arteries.

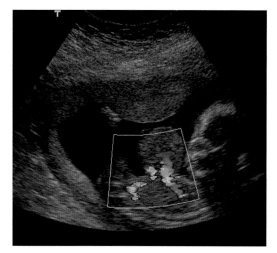

FIGURE 15-14 Omphalocele: colour flow Doppler demonstrates abnormal vessels within the anterior abdominal wall defect.

The middle cerebral artery pulsatility index rises until 32 weeks of gestation and then falls steeply (Fig. 15-7).[42]

Fetal haemodynamics suggest a brain-sparing effect in IUGR and evidence of cerebral redistribution by a decrease in the pulsatility index in the middle cerebral artery in the presence of established growth retardation is commonly considered an indicator for delivery[43,44] (Fig. 15-15). The presence of abnormal Doppler studies can also aid in the postnatal management of growth-restricted neonates who are at greater risk of ischaemic complications such as necrotising enterocolitis as a result of their intrauterine adaptations to a suboptimal environment.[45,46] Clinicians vary as to the stage in the progress of growth retardation at any given gestation when they will decide that the fetus should be delivered; there is no evidence that early intervention improves perinatal outcome.[47]

THE RENAL ARTERIES

Oligohydramnios consequent upon poor renal perfusion is a cardinal sign of IUGR. Although Doppler evaluation of the renal arteries is not used in clinical practice, colour Doppler of the renal vessels (Fig. 15-16) is useful to assess congenital renal abnormalities, such as renal agenesis, where the artery is also absent, although care should be taken as hypoplastic arteries may be difficult to demonstrate on ultrasound, and enlarged adrenal glands supplied by large adrenal vessels may be misidentified as kidney.

THE DUCTUS VENOSUS

The ductus venosus is an embryological channel which connects the fetal umbilical vein with the inferior vena cava and hence the right heart. In the fetus it carries most of the blood from the umbilical vein to the right atrium.

The ductus venosus is identified within the liver by following the umbilical vein in a sagittal plane into the fetal liver using colour Doppler. The ductus venosus arises at the junction of the umbilical vein and the left branch of the portal vein angling posteriorly and cephalad towards the inferior vena cava with which it makes an angle of 45 to 60°. Colour flow will demonstrate a high-velocity pattern with aliasing at low pulse repetition frequency (Fig. 15-17).

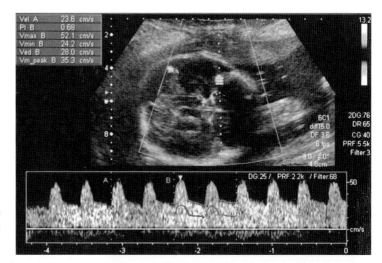

FIGURE 15-15 Middle cerebral artery flow in severe fetal compromise. There is a marked increase in diastolic flow as evidence of cerebral redistribution. The features imply ischaemic complication.

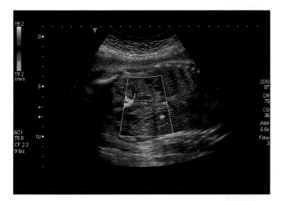

FIGURE 15-16 Coronal colour flow Doppler image of the fetus. There are two renal arteries, one of which arises from the iliac artery.

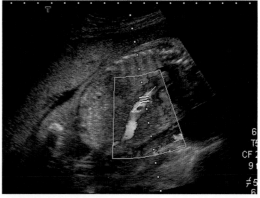

FIGURE 15-17 Oblique scan through the fetal abdomen with colour flow Doppler demonstrating the aliased flow within the ductus venosus. The Doppler sample volume is placed within the area of maximum aliasing.

Normal Doppler blood flow studies of the ductus venosus show a triphasic forward-flowing cycle reflecting ventricular systole, ventricular diastole and atrial systole (Fig. 15-18). Spectral analysis can therefore be used to reflect fetal ventricular function and cardiac afterload (Fig. 15-19). In the presence of end-stage hypoxaemia with hypoxic cardiomyopathy, there is a fall in cardiac function and hence rise in central venous pressure. This can be identified by absent end-diastolic, or reverse flow in the ductus venosus. The presence of reverse flow is associated with decreased fetal-maternal perfusion and fetal death.[48,49] In severely growth-restricted fetuses where the gestational age is close to viability, use of this

technique can help guide the clinician in deciding the exact moment at which delivery is required.

PLACENTAL ABNORMALITIES

The diagnosis of placenta praevia is largely performed by ultrasound imaging. Reporting of placental site at the routine second trimester transabdominal ultrasound has described incidences of low-lying placenta in excess of 40%,[50] so routine screening for placenta praevia in the second trimester is therefore not now widely used. By contrast, when there is antepartum haemorrhage, ultrasound is used to establish

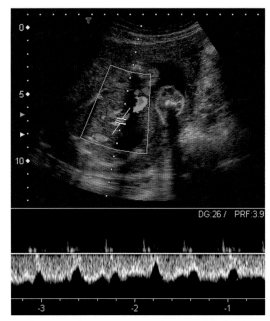

FIGURE 15-18 Normal spectral flow within the ductus venosus.

praevia. In this situation a vessel, or vessels, can be seen coursing from the margin of the placenta in close proximity to, or covering, the internal os. Similarly, other placental abnormalities can be documented: velamentous insertion of the cord can be identified with colour Doppler and chorioangioma can be differentiated from a placental haematoma by the demonstration of a rich vascular supply.[51]

Postpartum

A small amount of postpartum haemorrhage is a normal feature but when haemorrhage is prolonged, or heavy, the possibility of retained products of conception must be considered. Transvaginal ultrasound will frequently demonstrate abnormalities within the uterine cavity. As a general rule brightly reflective structures are taken to represent retained placental fragments and/or membrane; while echo-poor contents are thought to represent fresh or clotted blood. However, it is frequently difficult to differentiate between retained products of conception and uncomplicated blood clot.

the relationship of the placenta to the internal os. This is more commonly performed using transvaginal ultrasound. The addition of colour Doppler allows the demonstration of the rare but potentially serious vasa

There are changes in the blood flow characteristics of the uterine artery when there are retained products of conception: patients with residual trophoblast exhibit a resistance index in the myometrial vessels

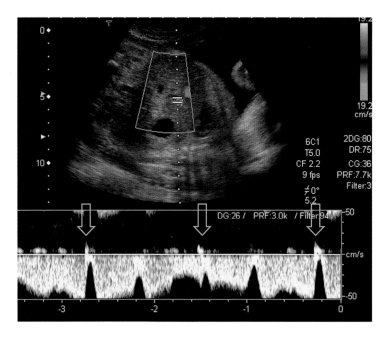

FIGURE 15-19 Intermittent flow reversal (arrows) within the ductus venosus in a cardiac dysrhythmia.

of 0.35±0.1; whereas those without residual tropho-blast have resistance indices in the myometrial vessels of 0.54±0.15. However, the combination of low-impedance flow and intrauterine material is common after abortion and does not necessarily imply retained products of conception. It may simply reflect physio-logical involution; the temporal course of return to non-pregnant flow characteristics in the uterine ves-sels has not been documented[52] (Fig. 15-20).

Trophoblastic Disease

Transvaginal ultrasound will demonstrate uterine abnormalities in persistent gestational trophoblastic tumour. However, the sensitivity of ultrasound imag-ing is only 70%, although abnormal uterine artery waveforms are seen in 90% of cases with persistent gestational trophoblastic tumour and raised uterine artery impedance may predict resistance to chemo-therapy.[53,54] However, magnetic resonance imaging (MRI) appears to be more sensitive in the detection of trophoblastic tumour, as it is more accurate at iden-tifying myometrial invasion and therefore establishing a diagnosis of choriocarcinoma.

Maternal Haemodynamics

Pregnancy is associated with marked changes in mater-nal haemodynamics. There is an increase in circulating blood volume with a corresponding increase in the cardiac output. This might be expected to have effects on blood flow to a number of the intra-abdominal organs, in addition to the effect that it has on uterine blood flow.

DOPPLER ULTRASOUND OF THE MATERNAL KIDNEY IN PREGNANCY

Doppler blood flow characteristics in the maternal kidney appear to alter little during pregnancy. Although certain authors report a slight reduction in the mean resistance index in renal artery examina-tions, this is not statistically significant. There is no doubt that volume flow is increased in pregnancy but this appears to be mediated largely by vasodilata-tion of the large supply vessels, although the absolute changes in flow velocity have not been investigated. There is no change in pulsatility or resistance indices in patients with essential hypertension.[55] There has been no documented change in these indices in pregnancy-induced hypertension. However, there is

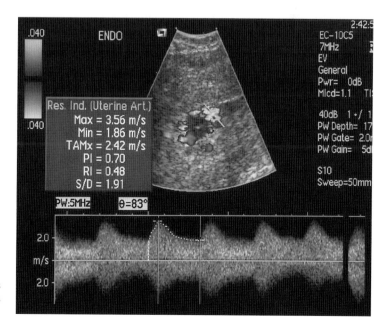

FIGURE 15-20 Spectral Doppler in retained products of conception. The resistance index of 0.48 implies residual trophoblast.

significant increase in acceleration time within the intrarenal vessels. This is suggestive of proximal vasospasm as being at least partly responsible for the pathogenesis of pregnancy-induced hypertension.[56,57]

There is no change in Doppler indices in patients presenting with progressive physiological dilatation of the collecting system of the kidneys during pregnancy. In the past this has been attributed to a combination of hormonal effects, together with a degree of mechanical obstruction of the ureter by the enlarging uterus. There is no correlation between the degree of dilatation of the collecting system and any change in the resistance index in uncomplicated cases, but it may be clinically useful in cases of suspected obstruction where Doppler ultrasound may show a significant difference between the affected and unaffected kidney. The obstructed kidney will usually show a resistance index differing by 0.04 or more than that in the unobstructed kidney. Resistance indices can be used as a discriminator in deciding which patients with loin pain in association with pregnancy should proceed to an intravenous urogram.[58]

Conclusions

The role of Doppler in obstetrics is an essential technology. The advent of colour Doppler has enabled more precise examination of the uteroplacental and fetoplacental circulations, together with more intricate examination of the fetal vasculature. However, fetomaternal haemodynamics are complex, showing variation in their response to many maternal and fetal physiological and pathological states. Currently Doppler methods appear capable only of detecting gross changes in placentation and gross changes of fetal well-being. For example, umbilical artery waveforms may be normal in a morphologically normal but small placenta. However, in experimentally induced acute hypoxia there is no alteration in fetomaternal flow as detected by Doppler techniques.[59]

In the same way, the role of uterine artery Doppler in the management of pregnancy is not clear cut. While apparently of value in patients with pre-existing maternal disease, its findings are not sufficiently sensitive or specific, nor does the use of screening Doppler affect perinatal morbidity and outcome.[60] Doppler ultrasound cannot be recommended as a screening procedure for the identification of pregnancy complications

in low-risk pregnancies. Doppler examination of the uterine and umbilical arteries between 18 and 26 weeks of gestation in high-risk pregnancies may be predictive of significant pregnancy complications, but at present there is insufficient evidence to suggest that the level of surveillance in the Doppler-negative group can be relaxed.

Doppler has most potential in the management of high-risk pregnancies such as those with pre-existing maternal disease, previously identified placental disease and those at high risk of fetal IUGR, or where IUGR is already established. Umbilical artery studies help identify fetuses at risk of hypoxia and acidaemia; when the results are applied clinically they contribute to reduced perinatal mortality rates. Doppler ultrasound of the fetal circulation may identify chronic hypoxia and there is evidence that documentation of redistribution of flow is important in the identification of fetal compromise (Tables 15-2 and 15-3). Doppler ultrasound has significantly impacted on the care of severe fetal anaemia.

It is likely that the future lies in comparative investigation of the uteroplacental, umbilical and one or more fetal vessels, together with the development of more sophisticated parameters of flow dynamics.

It is important, however, to stress that fetomaternal haemodynamics are not the only indicator of maternal or placental disease, or of fetal well-being. Doppler ultrasound may contribute to, but not replace, other methods of fetal and maternal surveillance.

REFERENCES

1. Pijnenborg R, Dixon G, Robertson WB, et al. Trophoblastic invasion of human decidua from 8 to 18 weeks of pregnancy. *Placenta* 1980;**1**:3–19.
2. Bewley S, Campbell S, Cooper D. Uteroplacental Doppler flow velocity waveforms in the second-trimester. A complex circulation. *Br J Obstet Gynaecol* 1989;**96**:1040–6.
3. Schulman H, Winter D, Farmakides G, et al. Doppler examinations of the umbilical and uterine arteries during pregnancy. *Clin Obstet Gynecol* 1989;**32**:738–45.
4. Bower S, Vyas S, Campbell S, et al. Colour Doppler imaging of the uterine artery in pregnancy: normal ranges of impedance to blood flow, mean velocity and volume flow. *Ultrasound Obstet Gynecol* 1992;**2**:261–5.
5. Schulman H, Fleischer A, Farmakides G, et al. Development of uterine artery compliance in pregnancy as detected by Doppler ultrasound. *Am J Obstet Gynecol* 1986;**155**:1031–6.
6. Fleischer A, Schulman H, Farmakides G, et al. Uterine artery Doppler velocimetry in pregnant women with hypertension. *Am J Obstet Gynecol* 1986;**154**:806–13.

7. Bower S, Schuchter K, Campbell S. Doppler ultrasound screening as part of routine antenatal screening: prediction of pre-eclampsia and growth retardation. *Br J Obstet Gynaecol* 1993;**100**:989–94.

8. Voigt HJ, Becker V. Doppler flow measurements and histomorphology of the placental bed in uteroplacental insufficiency. *J Perinat Med* 1992;**20**:139–47.

9. Kofinas AD, Espeland M, Swain M, et al. Correcting umbilical artery flow velocity waveforms for fetal heart rate is unnecessary. *Am J Obstet Gynecol* 1989;**160**:704–7.

10. Rightmire DA, Campbell S. Fetal and maternal Doppler blood flow parameters in postterm pregnancies. *Obstet Gynecol* 1987;**69**:891–4.

11. Bewley S, Cooper D, Campbell S. Doppler investigation of uteroplacental blood flow resistance in the second trimester: a screening study for pre-eclampsia and intrauterine growth retardation. *Br J Obstet Gynaecol* 1991;**98**:871–9.

12. Qu LR, Kan A, Masahiro N. Fetal circulation in relation to various maternal body positions. *Chung Hua Fu Chan Ko Tsa Chih* 1994;**29**:589–91.

13. Mulders LG, Jongsma HW, Wijn PF, et al. The uterine artery blood flow velocity waveform: reproducibility and results in normal pregnancy. *Early Hum Dev* 1988;**17**:55–70.

14. Morrow R, Ritchie K. Doppler ultrasound fetal velocimetry and its role in obstetrics. *Clin Perinatol* 1989;**16**:771–8.

15. Hastie SJ, Howie CA, Whittle MJ, et al. Daily variability of umbilical and lateral uterine wall artery blood velocity waveform measurements. *Br J Obstet Gynaecol* 1988;**95**:571–4.

16. Duggan PM, McCowan LM, Stewart AW. Antihypertensive drug effects on placental flow velocity wave forms in pregnant women with severe hypertension. *Aust N Z J Obstet Gynaecol* 1992;**32**:335–8.

17. Hirose S, Yamada A, Kasugai T, et al. The effect of nifedipine and dipyridamole on the Doppler blood flow waveforms of umbilical and uterine arteries in hypertensive pregnant women. *Asia Oceania J Obstet Gynaecol* 1992;**18**:187–93.

18. Castro LC, Allen R, Ogunyemi D, et al. Cigarette smoking during pregnancy: acute effects on uterine flow velocity waveform. *Obstet Gynecol* 1993;**81**:551–5.

19. Morrow RJ, Ritchie JW, Bull SB. Maternal cigarette smoking: the effects on umbilical and uterine blood flow velocity. *Am J Obstet Gynecol* 1998;**159**:1069–71.

20. North RA, Ferrier C, Long D, et al. Uterine artery flow velocity waveforms in the second trimester for the prediction of pre-eclampsia and fetal growth retardation. *Obstet Gynecol* 1994;**83**:378–86.

21. NICE Clinical Guideline 62, Antenatal Care. www.nice.org.uk/CG062fullguideline; March 2008.

22. Ferrier C, North RA, Becker G, et al. Uterine artery waveform as a predictor of pregnancy outcome in women with underlying renal disease. *Clin Nephrol* 1994;**42**:362–8.

23. Johnstone FD, Steel JM, Haddad NG, et al. Doppler umbilical artery flow velocity waveforms in diabetic pregnancy. *Br J Obstet Gynaecol* 1992;**99**:135–40.

24. Ben-Ami M, Battino S, Geslevich Y, et al. A random single Doppler study of the umbilical artery in the evaluation of pregnancies complicated by diabetes. *Am J Perinatol* 1995;**12**:437–8.

25. Kofinas AD, Penry M, Simon NV, et al. Interrelationship and clinical significance of increased resistance in the uterine arteries in patients with hypertension or pre-eclampsia or both. *Am J Obstet Gynecol* 1992;**166**:601–6.

26. Giles WB, Trudinger BJ, Baird PJ. Fetal umbilical artery flow velocity waveforms and placental resistance: pathological correlation. *Br J Obstet Gynaecol* 1985;**92**:31–8.

27. Mires G, Dempster J, Patel NB, et al. The effect of fetal heart rate on umbilical artery flow velocity waveforms. *Br J Obstet Gynaecol* 1987;**94**:665–9.

28. Gill RW, Trudinger BJ, Garrett WJ, et al. Fetal umbilical venous flow measured in utero by pulsed Doppler and B-mode ultrasound. *Am J Obstet Gynecol* 1980;**139**:720–5.

29. Kofinas AD, Penry M, Swain M, et al. The effect of placental laterality on uterine artery resistance and development of pre-eclampsia and intrauterine growth retardation. *Am J Obstet Gynecol* 1989;**161**:1536–9.

30. Erskine RLA, Ritchie JWK. Umbilical artery blood flow characteristics in normal and growth-retarded fetuses. *Br J Obstet Gynaecol* 1985;**92**:605–10.

31. McParland P. Modern approach to the poorly grown fetus. *Ir Med J* 1992;**85**:88–9.

32. Trudinger BJ, Cook CM, Giles WB, et al. Fetal umbilical artery velocity waveforms and subsequent neonatal outcome. *Br J Obstet Gynaecol* 1991;**98**:378–84.

33. Neilson JP. Doppler ultrasound in high-risk pregnancies. In: Enkin MW, Keirse MJNC, Renfrew MJ, et al., editors. *Pregnancy and childbirth module. Cochrane Database of Systematic Reviews,* No. 03889. London: BMJ Publishing; 1993.

34. Poulain P, Palaric JC, Paris-Liado J, et al. Fetal umbilical Doppler in a population of 541 high-risk pregnancies: prediction of perinatal mortality and morbidity. Doppler Study Group. *Eur J Obstet Gynecol Reprod Biol* 1994;**54**:191–6.

35. Cruz-Martinez R, Figueras F, Oros D, et al. Cerebral blood perfusion and neurobehavioral performance in full term small-for-gestational-age. *Am J Obstet Gynecol* 2009;**201**:474e1–7.

36. Zimmermann P, Alback T, Koskinen J, et al. Doppler flow velocimetry of the umbilical artery, uteroplacental arteries and fetal middle cerebral artery in prolonged pregnancy. *Ultrasound Obstet Gynecol* 1995;**5**:189–97.

37. Faber R, Viehweg B, Burkhardt U. Predictive value of Doppler ultrasound findings in twin pregnancies. *Zentralbl Gynäkol* 1995;**117**:353–7.

38. Giles WB, Trudinger BJ, Cook CM, et al. Umbilical artery flow velocity waveforms and twin pregnancy outcome. *Obstet Gynecol* 1988;**72**:894–7.

39. Vyas S, Nicolaides KH, Campbell S. Doppler examination of the middle cerebral artery in anaemic fetuses. *Am J Obstet Gynecol* 1990;**162**:1066–8.

40. Mari G. Noninvasive diagnosis by Doppler ultrasonography of fetal anemia due to maternal red-cell alloimmunization. *N Engl J Med* 2000;**342**:9–14.

41. Rochelson B, Kaplan C, Guzman E, et al. A quantitative analysis of placental vasculature in the third-trimester fetus with autosomal trisomy. *Obstet Gynecol* 1990;**75**:59–63.

42. Vyas S, Nicolaides KH, Bower S, et al. Middle cerebral artery flow velocity waveforms in fetal hypoxaemia. *Br J Obstet Gynaecol* 1990;**97**:797–803.

43. Rowlands DJ, Vyas SK. Longitudinal study of fetal middle cerebral artery flow velocity waveforms preceding fetal death. [Comment in *Br J Obstet Gynaecol* 103(8):852]. *Br J Obstet Gynaecol* 1995;**102**:888–90.

44. Society for Maternal-Fetal Medicine Publications Committee, Berkley E, Chauhan SP, Abuhamad A. Doppler assessment of the fetus with intrauterine growth restriction. *Am J Obstet Gynecol.* 2012;**206**:300–8.

45. Hackett GA, Campbell S, Gamsu H, et al. Doppler studies in the growth-retarded fetus and prediction of neonatal necrotising enterocolitis, haemorrhage, and neonatal morbidity. *Br Med J* 1987;**294**:13–16.

46. Laurin J, Marsal K, Persson PH, et al. Ultrasound measurements of fetal blood flow in predicting fetal outcome. *Br J Obstet Gynaecol* 1987;**94**:940–8.

47. The GRIT Trial Study Group. Infant wellbeing at 2 years of age in Growth Restriction Intervention Trial (GRIT): multicentred randomized controlled trail. *Lancet* 2004;**364**:513–20.

48. Gudmunsson S, Tulzer G, Huhta JC, et al. Venous Doppler velocimetry in fetuses with absent end-diastolic blood velocity in the umbilical artery. *J Matern Fetal Invest* 1993;**3**:196.

49. Baschat AA, Gembruch U. Triphasic umbilical venous blood flow with prolonged intrauterine survival in intrauterine growth retardation. *Ultrasound Obstet Gynecol* 1996;**8**:201–5.

50. Ott W. Placenta praevia. *Ultrasound Obstet Gynecol* 1993;**139**:1493–4.

51. Heinonen S, Ryynanen M, Kirkinen P, et al. Perinatal diagnostic evaluation of velamentous umbilical cord insertion: clinical, Doppler, and ultrasonic findings. *Obstet Gynecol* 1996;**87**:112–17.

52. Dillon EH, Case CQ, Ramos IM, et al. Endovaginal ultrasound and Doppler findings after first-trimester abortion. *Radiology* 1993;**186**:87–91.

53. Dobkin GR, Berkowitz RS, Goldstein DP, et al. Duplex ultrasonography for persistent gestational trophoblastic tumor. *J Reprod Med* 1991;**36**:14–16.

54. Long MG, Boultbee JE, Langley R, et al. Doppler assessment of the uterine circulation and the clinical behaviour of gestational trophoblastic tumours requiring chemotherapy. *Br J Cancer* 1992;**66**:883–7.

55. Zeeman GG, McIntire DD, Twickler DM. Maternal and fetal artery Doppler findings in women with chronic hypertension who subsequently developed superimposed pre-eclampsia. *J Matern Fetal Neonatal Med* 2003;**14**(5):318–23.

56. Myake H, Nakai A, Kshino T, et al. Doppler velocimetry of maternal renal circulation in pregnancy induced hypertension. *J Clin Ultrasound* 2001;**29**(8):449–55.

57. Nakai A, Asakura H, Oya A, et al. Pulsed Doppler US findings of renal interlobar arteries in pregnancy induced hypertension. *Radiology* 1999;**213**(2):423–8.

58. Weston MJ, Dubbins PA. The diagnosis of obstruction: colour Doppler ultrasonography of renal blood flow and ureteric jets. *Curr Opin Urol* 1994;**4**:69–74.

59. Trudinger BJ, Giles WB, Cook CM. Flow velocity waveforms in the maternal uteroplacental and fetal umbilical placental circulations. *Am J Obstet Gynecol* 1985;**152**:155–63.

60. Newnham JP, O'Dea MR, Reid KP, et al. Doppler flow velocity waveform analysis in high-risk pregnancies: a randomised control trial. *Br J Obstet Gynaecol* 1991;**98**:956–63.

Chapter 16

Interventional and Intraoperative Doppler

Michael T. Corwin and John P. McGahan

Introduction

Ultrasound is the preferred modality for performing imaging-guided interventional procedures. Advantages over other modalities such as CT include real-time guidance allowing precise needle placement, portability, relatively low cost, and lack of ionising radiation.[1,2] The addition of colour Doppler has been shown to be of great utility during interventional procedures. The primary benefit is the enhanced ability to visualise blood vessels during needle placement. Other advantages include improved needle visualisation and timely identification of procedural complications (Box 16-1). Specific Doppler applications can be divided into pre-procedure planning, intra-procedural guidance, and post-procedure monitoring.

Pre-Procedure Planning

AVOIDANCE OF BLOOD VESSELS

The most important use of colour Doppler ultrasound in interventional procedures is visualisation of blood vessels along the needle trajectory. This allows the vessels to be avoided as the needle is advanced, thereby minimising the risk of bleeding.[3] Alternatively, in some situations such as arteriography or venography, colour may be useful to localise vessels for puncture. The focus of this chapter will be the use of colour Doppler for non-vascular interventional procedures.

The addition of colour Doppler to imaging guidance has been shown to reduce the risk of bleeding in both percutaneous liver and kidney biopsies.[4–6] Good guidance technique routinely incorporates colour Doppler imaging immediately prior to needle placement anywhere in the body. Specific vessels (Table 16-1) should be identified during certain common interventional procedures (Fig. 16-1).

In fine needle aspiration of thyroid nodules and lymph nodes, colour Doppler is used to avoid the internal jugular veins and carotid arteries and their major branches (Fig. 16-2). In the chest, colour Doppler ultrasound has been shown to improve vessel visualisation during transthoracic needle aspiration biopsies.[7,8] During mediastinal biopsy, not only should the great vessels be visualised, but a specific search for the internal mammary arteries and veins must be performed. Intercostal vessels can be avoided by advancing the needle directly over ribs, as the vessels run along the inferior margin of the ribs. However, a search for intercostal vessels with colour Doppler is warranted, especially if the needle must be directed close to the inferior margin of the rib in order to target the lesion.

Ultrasound-guided percutaneous liver biopsy can be performed using a sub-xiphoid approach to access the left lobe, or an intercostal approach into the right lobe. Although both techniques are acceptable, some authors favour a sub-xiphoid approach to avoid damage to intercostal structures and avoid traversing the pleura.[9] However, a recent study reported a 0.8% (6/776) rate of significant bleeding complications from percutaneous US-guided liver biopsy, all from the left lobe approach.[10] Four of the six cases were attributed to superior epigastric artery injury. These vessels lie approximately 4 cm from midline at the level of the xiphoid process. Therefore the superior epigastric arteries must be identified and avoided during left lobe biopsies or any other procedure in the epigastric region. If they cannot be visualised, a midline approach is preferred in order to avoid these vessels. Likewise, the inferior epigastric arteries should be identified during any puncture in the lower abdomen or pelvis, such as

BOX 16-1 APPLICATIONS OF DOPPLER IN INTERVENTIONAL ULTRASOUND

USES OF COLOUR DOPPLER IN INTERVENTIONAL ULTRASOUND

Avoidance of blood vessels

Identification of vascular lesions (pseudoaneuryms/AV fistulas)

Targeting vascularised tissue for biopsy

Needle localisation

Monitoring aspiration or injections

Catheter placement and patency

Identifying post-procedure bleeding

TABLE 16-1 Specific Vasculature Structures That Doppler US can Identify and Help Avoid When Performing Biopsies, Aspirations, or Drainages in Various Body Regions	
Procedure site	**Vessels to identify**
Neck/thyroid	Carotid arteries/jugular veins
Mediastinum	Internal mammary artery
Chest/upper abdomen	Intercostal vessels
Left liver/epigastric region	Superior epigastric artery
Abdomen/pelvis	Inferior epigastric artery and abdominal wall varices

paracentesis (Fig. 16-3). Additionally, as paracentesis is often performed in cirrhotic patients with portal hypertension, colour Doppler should be also used to identify enlarged abdominal wall varices.

During liver biopsy colour Doppler can decrease bleeding risk by visualisation and avoidance of major intrahepatic vasculature. Fine needle aspiration biopsy under US guidance is an established technique for distinguishing between bland and malignant portal vein thrombus. Colour Doppler improves visualisation of the thrombus by identifying flow surrounding it or within it, and can guide needle placement directly into the thrombus without traversing patent portions of the portal vein and helping avoid the adjacent hepatic artery.[11] Colour Doppler is useful to distinguish hepatic vessels from bile ducts when

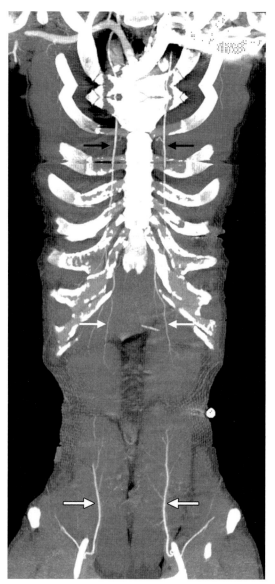

FIGURE 16-1 Thick slab coronal MIP image from a CTA shows the positions of the internal mammary (black arrows), superior epigastric (white arrows), and inferior epigastric (block arrows) arteries. These must be identified and avoided during procedures involving an anterior approach.

performing transhepatic cholangiography. Colour and spectral Doppler US can identify tumour neovascularity. It is important to avoid such vessels as they lack a normal coagulation response and have a higher propensity for bleeding (Fig. 16-4). Puncture of these vessels can result in aspiration of a large amount of

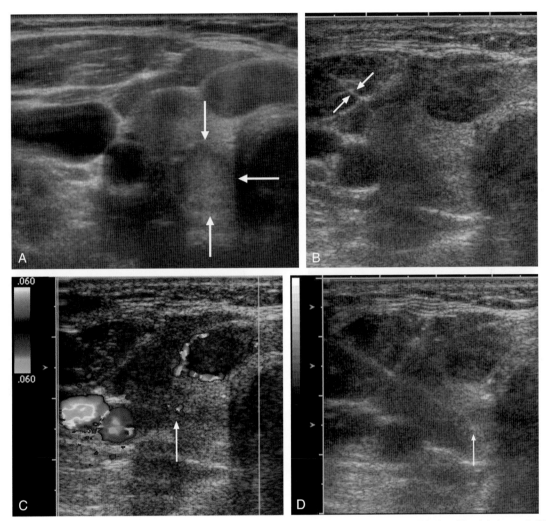

FIGURE 16-2 Thyroid fine needle aspiration biopsy. (A) Grey scale US image shows an isoechoic posterior right thyroid nodule (arrows). (B) The proximal needle (arrows) is visualised within hypoechoic muscle but the tip is difficult to identify as it enters more echogenic tissue. (C) Colour Doppler image shows colour flow at the tip of the needle (arrow) as it is gently jiggled back and forth, as well as demonstrating the internal jugular vein and carotid artery. (D) After the needle tip and vessels are identified, colour Doppler is turned off and the needle tip (arrow) is seen in the nodule while avoiding the vessels.

blood during FNA which will degrade the specimen and reduce diagnostic yield.

IDENTIFICATION OF VASCULAR LESIONS

A less common but highly important use of colour Doppler ultrasound is the identification of vascular lesions such as pseudoaneurysms and arteriovenous fistulas (AVFs) prior to performing an intervention. On grey scale US, a pseudoaneurysm can appear to be a cystic lesion or fluid collection and aspiration or drainage may be requested. Puncture of such a lesion could result in a life-threatening haemorrhage. This scenario may be encountered in the setting of acute pancreatitis, where pseudocysts are common. However, splenic (or any branch of the celiac axis) artery pseudoaneurysm can mimic a pseudocyst and must be excluded before performing an intervention. Colour Doppler US can easily identify the vascular nature of these lesions by demonstrating the characteristic swirling blood in a 'yin-yang' pattern (Fig. 16-5).

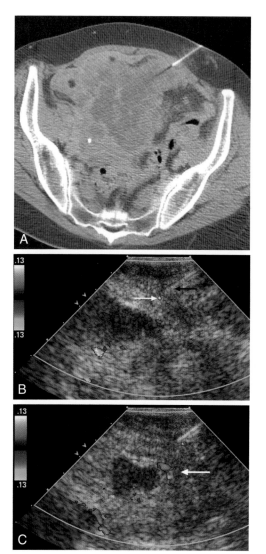

FIGURE 16-3 CT- and US-guided pelvic mass biopsy. (A) CT was used for initial superficial needle placement during percutaneous biopsy of a large heterogeneous pelvic mass. (B) Colour Doppler was then utilised and revealed the needle trajectory (black arrow) was directed towards the inferior epigastric artery (white arrow). Slight repositioning allowed for the needle to be advanced avoiding the artery as shown in (C). Also note the tumour vessel (arrow) that was identified and avoided.

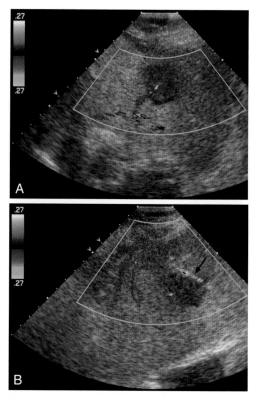

FIGURE 16-4 Hypoechoic liver lesion biopsy in a patient with metastatic breast cancer. (A) Colour Doppler image shows a tumour vessel along the posterior aspect of the liver mass. (B) Colour Doppler image showing the biopsy trajectory (arrow) in the anterior portion of the mass in order to avoid this vessel.

The use of colour Doppler in the treatment of pseudoaneurysms is discussed elsewhere in this book.

Arteriovenous fistulas have been reported as a complication of renal biopsies in 3–18%.[12] Although often asymptomatic, they are of particular importance in renal transplant recipients who often undergo

multiple biopsies. These lesions must be identified and avoided prior to repeat biopsy in order to minimise the risk of serious bleeding. Arteriovenous fistulas are rarely seen on grey scale US but can be easily identified on colour Doppler. Tissues surrounding the fistula vibrate due to the high-velocity blood flow and may show a flash of colour noise – the equivalent of a palpable thrill or audible bruit. The feeding artery will demonstrate aliasing unless the pulse repetition frequency is increased. Spectral Doppler tracings show high-velocity, low-resistance waveform in the feeding artery, and high-velocity, arterialised flow in the draining vein (see Chapter 10, Fig. 10-19).

EVALUATING TISSUE PERFUSION

While it is important to avoid macroscopic blood vessels when performing an interventional procedure to

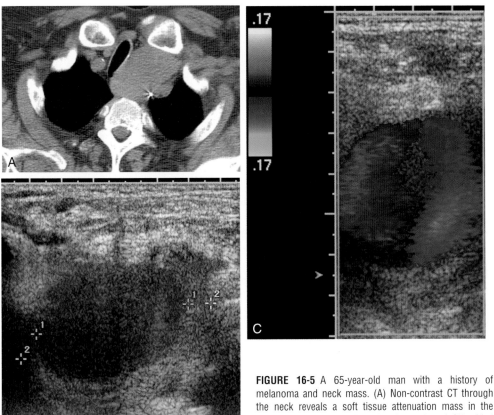

FIGURE 16-5 A 65-year-old man with a history of melanoma and neck mass. (A) Non-contrast CT through the neck reveals a soft tissue attenuation mass in the superior mediastinum displacing the trachea. A CT-guided biopsy was requested, however, the lesion was first studied with US. (B) Grey scale US reveals a hypoechoic mass, however colour Doppler (C) shows the classic 'yin-yang' pattern of a pseudoaneurysm and biopsy was deferred.

minimise bleeding risk, it can be beneficial to identify perfusion within lesions in order to target these areas for biopsy. A common pitfall in image-guided percutaneous biopsy is the sampling of non-viable or necrotic tissue leading to non-diagnostic results. Colour Doppler US can be used to direct biopsy towards vascularised portions of lesions in order to increase diagnostic yield. Additionally, if a target lesion is difficult to visualise on grey scale ultrasound, colour Doppler US can identify neovascularity which may help localise the lesion. This is especially useful in hypervascular tumours such as hepatocellular carcinoma, and in cases of local recurrence after tumour resection or radiofrequency ablation as it may be difficult to distinguish post-surgical or post-RFA changes from recurrent tumour.

Intra-Procedural Applications

IMPROVED NEEDLE VISUALISATION

Real time visualisation of the needle tip is an advantage of US-guided intervention. Generally, the needle should only be advanced when the tip can be seen in order to ensure successful access to the target lesion and to avoid inadvertent puncture of adjacent structures. Unfortunately, it can be difficult to clearly delineate the needle tip and that is a common source of frustration when performing US guided interventions. Visualisation of the needle is particularly difficult when it traverses tissues that have high echogenicity similar to that of the needle (fatty livers), when the needle is advanced parallel to the insonating beam, and with small-gauge needles. Many techniques have been described to improve needle tip visualisation, such as roughening the surface of the needle tip, Teflon coating, and the so-called 'pump manoeuvre' where the needle stylet is gently moved back and forth within the needle. The addition of colour Doppler US is a useful adjunct to improve needle visualisation.[11,13] Colour Doppler detects motion of any kind and therefore the movement of the needle or inner stylet is more easily detected and the needle localised (Fig. 16-2).

As mentioned above, needle visualisation can be particularly difficult when the needle is advanced parallel to the insonating beam because the low angle of insonation causes the US waves to be reflected away from the transducer. Needle visualisation is best when it is as close to perpendicular as possible (90° to the US beam) on grey scale imaging. Conversely, the Doppler shift is greatest when the moving structure is parallel (0°) to the US beam. Therefore, colour Doppler US is of particular benefit when parallel needle trajectory is required.

If needle placement is performed using real-time colour Doppler, it is important to properly adjust the colour Doppler sensitivity in order to avoid a 'snowstorm' of colour signal with minor movement of the adjacent tissue or patient. Additionally, the temporal resolution (frame rate) will be decreased when colour Doppler is on and therefore should be turned off once blood vessels are identified and needle position is confirmed.

MONITORING ASPIRATION, INJECTION, AND CATHETER PLACEMENT

One of the main interventional applications of US is guidance for fluid collection aspiration or drainage. Examples include renal or liver cyst aspiration, pancreatic pseudocyst aspiration or drainage, and abscess drainage throughout the abdomen and pelvis. Additionally, US-guided percutaneous cyst sclerosis is a useful technique for treatment of symptomatic benign cysts. A wide variety of agents have been used for sclerosis including alcohol and doxycycline, and cyst sclerosis has been described in practically every organ in the body. Colour Doppler US can help visualise the moving fluid during aspiration or injection and can assist in determining catheter position and patency.

During aspiration of fluid collections, the moving fluid through the needle will produce a line of colour on colour Doppler which can aid in needle localisation. Likewise a line of colour will be seen with injection of fluid during cyst sclerotherapy. Colour Doppler has also been shown to be useful in evaluating drainage catheter position and patency after placement.[14] Pigtail catheters can be surprisingly difficult to visualise with grey scale US. Improved detection can be obtained by aspirating the catheter or injecting sterile saline, both of which will lead to colour signal with Doppler imaging (Fig. 16-6). Visualising colour signal at the side ports when injecting saline or aspirating will also confirm catheter patency. Saline should be injected slowly to avoid the snowstorm pattern which will obscure the catheter.

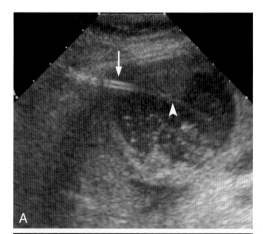
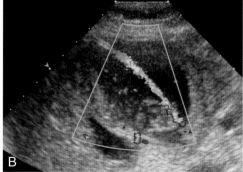

FIGURE 16-6 Percutaneous cholecystostomy. (A) Grey scale image shows inner stylet within the catheter (arrow) and the catheter (arrowhead) advancing over the stylet into the gallbladder though the tip is difficult to see within the sludge and stones. (B) Colour Doppler image obtained while gently aspirating the catheter clearly delineates the course of the catheter within the gallbladder.

Post-Procedure Monitoring

POST-PROCEDURE BLEEDING

US-guided percutaneous liver and renal biopsies are widely established techniques for diagnosing both diffuse parenchymal disease and focal lesions. The rate of serious bleeding complications has been reported at 0.5% for liver biopsies and 0.7% for kidney biopsies.[15] However, the risk may be increased in patients with abnormal coagulation parameters such as low platelets, prolonged bleeding time, or elevated INR. In fact, many patients referred for these procedures have such coagulopathies due to their underlying hepatic or renal disease. Although appropriate correction of such deficiencies will reduce the risk: when it occurs, bleeding from these procedures can be life-threatening. Therefore prompt detection of post-biopsy bleeding is of paramount importance.

Recently colour Doppler US has been shown to be useful in identifying bleeding after both US-guided liver biopsy and RFA. After needle withdrawal, colour Doppler evaluation of the needle tract can reveal a line of colour signal ('patent track' or 'colour line sign'), indicating bleeding through the needle track[16,17] (Figs 16-7–16-9). This sign has been shown to indicate

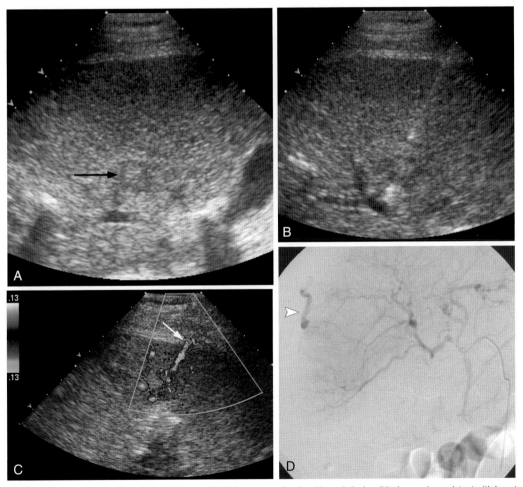

FIGURE 16-7 'Colour line sign' after liver RFA. (A) Grey scale US image reveals a focal hepatic lesion (black arrow) consistent with hepatocellular carcinoma in this cirrhotic patient. (B) US-guided RFA was performed. (C) Colour Doppler image following probe removal reveals a 'colour line' along the track (white arrow) consistent with the 'colour line sign.' This persisted for 15 minutes and therefore the patient was referred for angiography (D) which revealed active arterial extravasation at the ablation site (white arrowhead). This was successfully coil embolised.

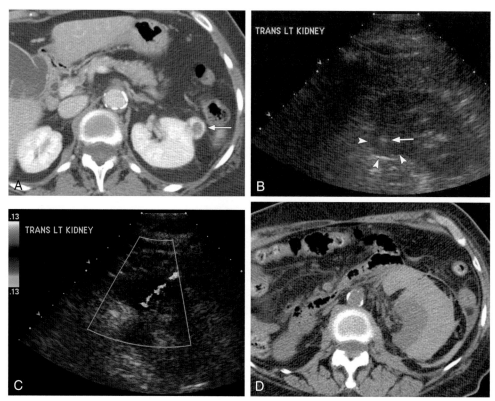

FIGURE 16-8 'Colour line sign' after renal RFA. (A) Contrast-enhanced CT reveals a peripherally enhancing solid left renal mass (arrow). (B) Grey-scale US image shows the needle tip (white arrow) within the mass (arrowheads). (C) Colour Doppler image following ablation reveals the 'colour line sign' which persisted for greater than 5 minutes. (D) Non-contrast CT following the procedure reveals large left subcapsular haematoma.

a significantly higher risk of clinically important post-procedure bleeding when it persists for five minutes after needle withdrawal following liver biopsy. The absence of this finding was predictive of a lack of significant bleeding with a negative predictive value of 99%.[17] As this technique can be performed quickly and easily, we recommend using colour Doppler after all percutaneous biopsies of solid organs to assess for the line sign. If present, immediate pressure can be applied to the biopsy site to help tamponade the bleeding. The patient can be positioned with the biopsy site down forcing apposition of the biopsied organ against the body wall for five minutes. US can then be used to re-check for the absence or persistence of the line sign and further management decisions can be made at that point.

VASCULAR COMPLICATIONS

Arteriovenous fistulas are a known complication of percutaneous renal biopsy. The true incidence is unknown, with estimates ranging from 3–18%.[12] Although most are asymptomatic, some may cause complications such as hypertension or haematuria. Although these lesions are occult on grey scale imaging, colour Doppler US will easily identify these lesions as described above. One study found small localised flow disturbances consistent with AVFs in 12 of 77 patients using colour Doppler US immediately after renal biopsy.[12] Importantly, most of these lesions resolved by 24 hours and none were symptomatic, therefore routine treatment is not indicated. However knowledge of their presence is important in the rare patient that does become symptomatic.

Intraoperative Colour Doppler Procedures

EQUIPMENT

While standard ultrasound probes are ideal for daily use in the ultrasound department, they are usually not suitable for intraoperative use. Specific probes are designed for both laparoscopic and intraoperative applications. These probes are typically small and are designed to gain access into tight anatomical regions during surgery. They are configured as end-fire or side-fire probes which are usually multi-frequency (ranging from 5–9 MHz depending on their particular use and manufacturer). The intraoperative abdomen transducers are usually small linear array probes, some with novel designs, including those that can be placed on the end of the user's finger. These probes may have higher frequencies for increased resolution. However, for other surgical procedures including guidance of intraoperative spinal cord and/or the brain surgery, transducer frequencies usually range from 7–12 MHz. Laparoscopic ultrasound probes are designed to fit through different-size laparoscopic ports usually in the range of 1 cm in diameter. Also the shaft of laparoscopic probes is fairly long (usually 25–30 cm) so they can reach from the laparoscopic port to the target organ such as the liver.

Probe sterilisation for intraoperative use includes placing a sterile covering over the transducer and cable. Maintaining meticulous sterile technique is mandatory in the operating suite. Probes are usually soaked in sterilising solution before intraoperative use to minimise significant contamination if there is a break in the sterile covering.

Intraoperative ultrasound provides increased resolution compared to transcutaneous sonography as the signal degradation from overlying fat, muscle and bone is eliminated. For instance, with the increased resolution of intraoperative liver ultrasound additional small solid nodules which are not detected on transcutaneous ultrasound are often identified. It has been estimated that intraoperative ultrasound detects more focal liver lesions compared to preoperative ultrasound, CT or even MRI.[18]

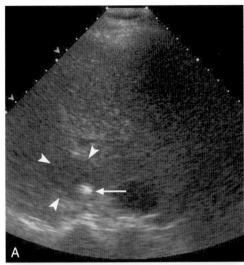
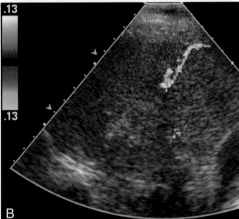
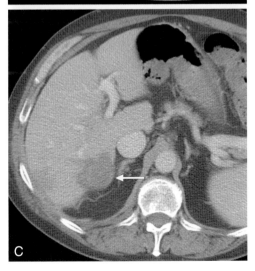

FIGURE 16-9 'Colour line sign' after liver RFA without significant bleeding. (A) Grey scale US image reveals RFA probe (arrow) within the focal liver lesion (arrowheads). (B) Colour Doppler image following RFA shows the 'colour line sign'. However, this persisted for less than 5 minutes and contrast-enhanced CT (C) following the procedure shows the ablation zone (arrow) but no significant haemorrhage.

USES OF INTRAOPERATIVE COLOUR DOPPLER ULTRASOUND

While this discussion will not go into great detail about specific parameters utilised for Doppler sonography in a target area, it will give an overview of intraoperative colour and/or Doppler ultrasound. For the exact parameters, such as predicting stenosis with Doppler in specific target areas, please consult other relevant chapters. The use of colour Doppler during surgical procedures can be classified into five different applications. These include the following:

    (a) Planning of surgery.
    (b) Utilisation of colour Doppler during surgery.
    (c) Predicting intraoperative outcome.
    (d) Confirming the success of surgery.
    (e) Identifying any potential surgical complications.
Many times intraoperative Doppler is utilised more than once during the course of a surgical procedure.

PLANNING SURGERY

Intraoperative Doppler ultrasound is very helpful in planning surgery. Within the abdomen either laparoscopic or open ultrasound imaging and Doppler can be utilised for surgical planning of the liver, pancreas and kidney. Ultrasound is used for defining tissue planes, identifying anomalous vessels or demonstrating tumour invasion.[19,20] For instance, in surgical resection of the liver, identification of lobar and segmental anatomy is aided by the use of colour Doppler. Colour Doppler ultrasound is important to help define a plane for resection. Thus, colour Doppler may demonstrate major vessels to allow dissection in the most avascular plane in the liver or kidney. The middle hepatic vein is a critical landmark demarcating the plane between the right and left lobe of the liver (Fig. 16-10). Anomalous vasculature is readily identified by colour Doppler sonography. For instance, accessory arterial supply is frequently identified in the liver such as either a replaced right hepatic artery originating from the SMA or a replaced left hepatic artery from the left gastric artery. Intraoperative colour Doppler is also extremely helpful in predicting the extent of disease. For instance, while preoperative ultrasound or CT may not demonstrate vascular invasion by tumour, it can be precisely localised with colour Doppler ultrasound during surgery. Further research has shown added value of the use of contrast-enhanced intraoperative ultrasound in detecting increased number of colorectal liver metastases, as compared to preoperative imaging or intraoperative ultrasound.[21]

Colour Doppler ultrasound has utility in numerous other surgical applications. For instance, intraoperative Doppler can be used to precisely localise arterial venous malformation of the brain, identifying the least disruptive surgical approach. Doppler has now replaced intraoperative angiography for confirmation of successful resection by not only demonstrating absence of colour flow of the AVM after resection; but also by identifying normalisation of resistance index in the feeding arteries[22] (Fig. 16-11). Likewise, neurosurgical resection of large intracavernous paraclinoid aneurysms can be evaluated to assess blood flow of the parent and branch vessel with microvascular Doppler sonography.[23] Colour Doppler ultrasound can be used in both preoperative and intraoperative planning and decision making in head and neck surgery.[24]

USE OF ULTRASOUND DURING SURGERY

Intraoperative Doppler ultrasound is very helpful to demonstrate success of surgery by re-evaluating vessel patency during difficult surgical dissection (Fig. 16-10). Also intraoperative blood flow to solid organs can be evaluated with intraoperative sonography.[25,26] It can demonstrate ancillary findings,

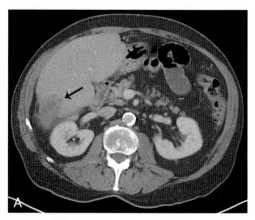

FIGURE 16-10 Metastatic colon cancer, right lobe of the liver with right hepatectomy and use of intraoperative ultrasound. (A) CT scan demonstrating one of the multiple hepatic metastases (arrow) noted within the right lobe of the liver.

Continued

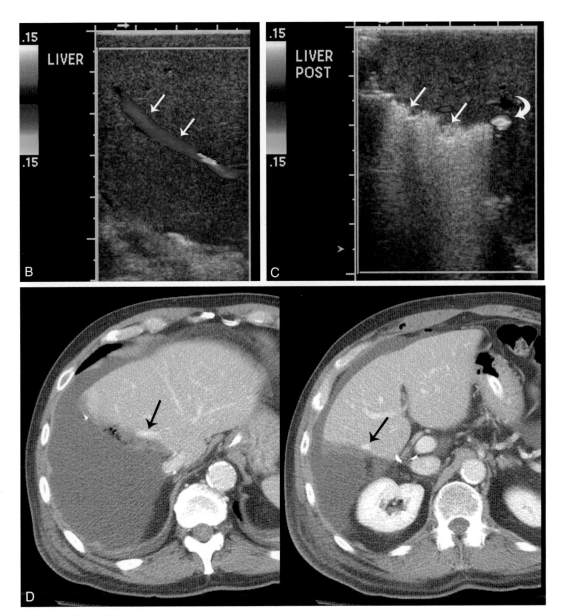

FIGURE 16-10—CONT'D (B) Intraoperative ultrasound demonstrates the middle hepatic vein (arrows) used to define the plane between the right and left lobe of the liver. There was no tumour invasion into the middle hepatic vein. (C) During surgery, there was acoustic shadowing at the resection margin (arrow), but patency of the middle hepatic vein (curved arrow). (D) Postoperative CT demonstrates right hepatectomy with preservation of the middle hepatic vein (arrow) seen on two different regions within the liver.

including critical vessel stenosis during surgery (Fig. 16-12).

PREDICTING OUTCOMES

Microemboli can be a potential problem with any vascular surgical procedure. For example, small deposits of debris can develop at the surgical site during carotid endarterectomy or thoracic endovascular aortic repair (TEVAR) and may embolise to the brain. Intraoperative detection of these microemboli is critically important to the surgical outcome since microembolism during surgery increases the risk of perioperative

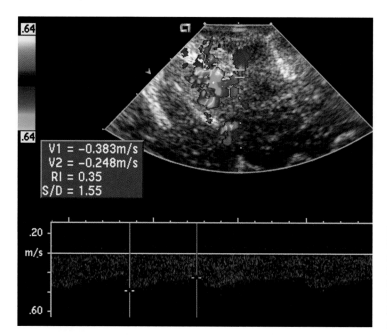

V1 = −0.383m/s
V2 = −0.248m/s
RI = 0.35
S/D = 1.55

FIGURE 16-11 Doppler US to guide AVM resection. Colour and spectral Doppler evaluation identifies the arteriovenous malformation (AVM) nidus and its feeding artery. The direction of flow in the feeding artery is away from the transducer. A spectral Doppler tracing obtained over this artery shows low-resistance flow (RI 0.35) as would be expected with an AVM.

stroke. Intraoperative Doppler ultrasound is used to monitor the signal from within the middle cerebral artery during the vascular surgery. A transcranial Doppler probe is placed on the thinnest portion of calvarium in the region of the temporal bone. The identification of increased spectral reflection from the microemboli, mimicking turbulence, guides intraoperative decision making, specifically increasing the use of platelet antagonists or anticoagulation.[27–29]

CONFIRMING SUCCESS OF SURGERY

Intraoperative Doppler sonography may be used in a number of different circumstances to confirm an appropriate surgical outcome. For instance, after clipping of cerebral aneurysm, evaluation of the aneurysm and associated vessel after clip positioning is enabled by Doppler sonography. Doppler sonography, however, is limited in some cases especially when multiple clips are placed due to acoustic shadowing from them.[30] Intraoperative Doppler sonography has been applied for surgical treatment of the median arcuate ligament syndrome. It can be utilised to demonstrate stenosis of celiac artery and post-stenotic dilatation before the release of the median arcuate ligament; and, afterwards, it can be used to confirm decompression of the celiac artery.[31] It is used to predict success of vascular surgery, such as bypass

grafts that may connect to vessels beyond an area of stenosis. Intraoperative confirmation of appropriate flow profiles and lack of flow restriction in the bypass graft is critical to successful surgery (Fig. 16-13).

IDENTIFYING COMPLICATIONS OF SURGERY

Probably the most important role of intraoperative colour Doppler is the timely identification of potential complications or inadequate outcomes. Identification of a critical arterial stenosis, an internal flap or a continued area of narrowing, allowing immediate surgical correction, is important to the success of carotid endarterectomy (Fig. 16-14). It obviates the need for reoperation. In one series 11% of cases of carotid endarterectomy were immediately revised because of persistent stenosis demonstrated with intraoperative duplex sonography.[32]

Another major role for intraoperative Doppler sonography is identifying either arterial or venous thrombosis immediately before operative closure. This is especially important in the area of transplantation. For instance, intraoperative Doppler ultrasound can detect hepatic artery thrombosis allowing immediate revision of the anastomosis.[33] Likewise, in renal transplantation, intraoperative colour duplex scanning can detect vascular complications such as renal vein thrombosis, arterial dissection, vasospasm, or arterial occlusion[34,35] (Fig. 16-15).

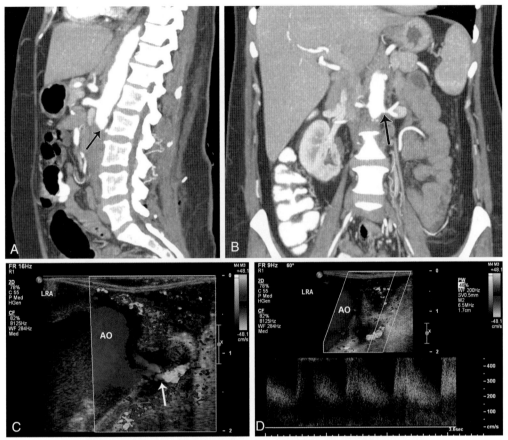

FIGURE 16-12 Intraoperative ultrasound of left renal artery stenosis and aortic occlusion. (A) Sagittal CT image of the abdomen demonstrates complete aortic occlusion (arrow). (B) Coronal CT image demonstrates narrowing of the left renal artery (arrow). (C) After aortic thrombectomy, intraoperative colour Doppler ultrasound confirms aortic patency, but identifies turbulence in the left renal artery (arrow). (D) Intraoperative spectral Doppler demonstrated peak systolic velocity in the left renal artery of greater than 600 cm per second, indicative of persistent high-grade left renal artery stenosis which became manifest after thrombectomy reestablished flow. (AO = aorta).

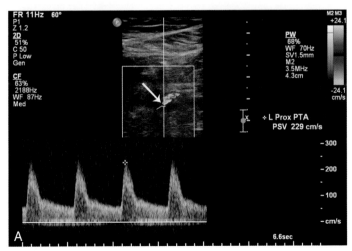

FIGURE 16-13 Superficial femoral artery (SFA) to posterior tibial artery (PTA) bypass graft, intraoperative evaluation. (A) Preoperative Doppler US examination demonstrates Doppler cursor placed on proximal posterior tibial artery (arrow) with peak systolic velocity of 229 cm per second. Proximal to this, velocity was in the range of 80–90 cm per second.

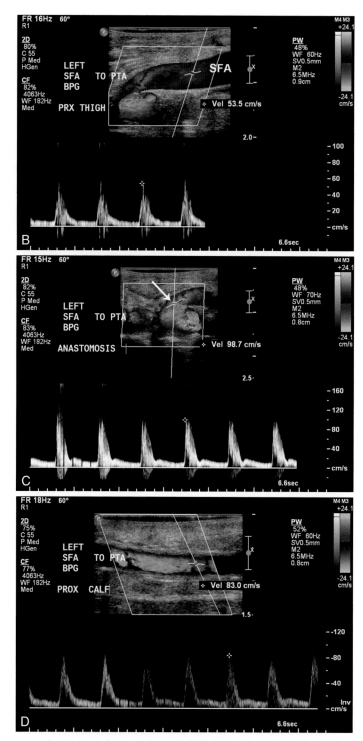

FIGURE 16-13—CONT'D (B) After surgical anastomosis of the SFA to the PTA, colour Doppler evaluation of the superficial femoral artery (SFA) demonstrates velocity in the range of 53 cm per second. (C) At the site of anastomosis (arrow) of the superficial femoral artery to the posterior tibial artery, velocities are 98 cm per second. (D) Downstream within the posterior tibial artery, velocity is 83 cm per second. Intraoperative ultrasound therefore confirmed successful anastomosis without stenosis.

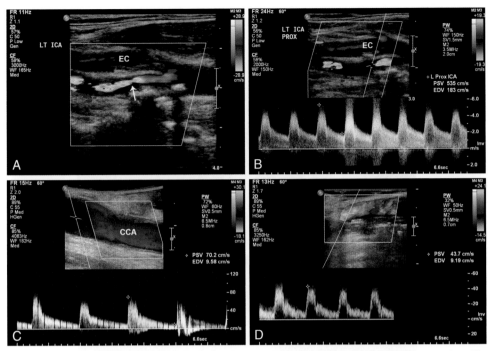

FIGURE 16-14 Intraoperative ultrasound to evaluate successful internal carotid endarterectomy. (A) Preoperative colour US examination demonstrates focal internal carotid artery stenosis (arrow). (B) Spectral Doppler confirms high-grade stenosis with peak systolic velocity of 535 cm per second and end diastolic velocity of 183 cm per second. (C) Intraoperative post-endarterectomy evaluation of the internal carotid artery along the previously stenotic area demonstrates a good surgical outcome with peak systolic velocity of 45 cm per second and without residual stenosis or flap.

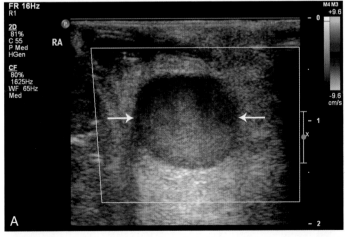

FIGURE 16-15 Intraoperative evaluation of occluded renal artery to transplanted kidney. (A) Intraoperative Doppler ultrasound of the main renal artery to renal transplant demonstrates no flow (arrows). The occluded artery was immediately opened and the thrombus removed.

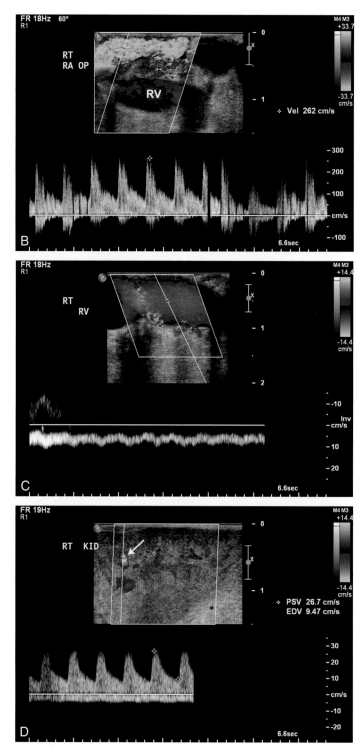

FIGURE 16-15—CONT'D (B) Afterwards, the renal artery is patent with good Doppler flow but with elevation of the peak systolic velocity. (RV = renal vein). (C) Intraoperative Doppler of the main renal vein demonstrates normal venous flow. (D) Intraoperative Doppler cursor (arrow) placed on an inter-lobar artery of the transplanted kidney demonstrates good systolic and diastolic flow with appropriate resistance. Note brisk up-stroke during systole. This patient had a normal postoperative course.

Conclusions

Colour Doppler US is a valuable tool when performing US-guided interventions. Its use can minimise the risk of complications such as bleeding by improving blood vessel visualisation, identifying vascular lesions such as pseudoaneurysms, improving needle visualisation, and allowing for rapid assessment of post-procedural bleeding. Intraoperative Doppler sonography is helpful in planning surgery and confirming success or identifying suboptimal results that can be revised before closure.

REFERENCES

1. McGahan J. Invasive Ultrasound Priciples (Biopsy, Aspiration, and Drainage). In: McGahan J, Goldberg BB, editors. *Diagnostic Ultrasound*, vol. 1, 2nd ed. New York, NY: Informa Healthcare USA, Inc.; 2008.
2. Matalon TA, Silver B. US guidance of interventional procedures. *Radiology* 1990;**174**(1):43–7.
3. Rubens DJ, Gottlieb RH, Fultz PL. Role of colour Doppler imaging in interventional sonography. *J Clin Ultrasound* 1999;**27**(5):259–71.
4. Lencioni R, Caramella D, Bartolozzi C. Percutaneous biopsy of liver tumors with colour Doppler US guidance. *Abdom Imaging* 1995;**20**(3):206–8.
5. Polakow J, Ladny JR, Dzieciol J, et al. Ultrasound guided percutaneous fine-needle biopsy of the liver: efficacy of colour Doppler sonography. *Hepatogastroenterology* 1998;**45**(23):1829–30.
6. Granata A, Floccari F, Ferrantelli A, et al. Does systematic preliminar colour Doppler study reduce kidney biopsy complication incidence? *Internat J Nephrol* 2011;**2011**:419093.
7. Gorguner M, Misirlioglu F, Polat P, et al. Colour Doppler sonographically guided transthoracic needle aspiration of lung and mediastinal masses. *J Ultrasound Med* 2003;**22**(7):703–8.
8. Yang PC. Ultrasound-guided transthoracic biopsy of the chest. *Radiol Clin North Am* 2000;**38**(2):323–43.
9. Nazarian LN, Feld RI, Herrine SK, et al. Safety and efficacy of sonographically guided random core biopsy for diffuse liver disease. *J Ultrasound Med* 2000;**19**(8):537–41.
10. Vijayaraghavan G, Sheehan D, Zheng L, et al. Unusual complication after left-lobe liver biopsy for diffuse liver disease: severe bleeding from the superior epigastric artery. *AJR Am J Roentgenol* 2011;**197**(6):W1135–9.
11. Longo JM, Bilbao JI, Barettino MD, et al. Percutaneous vascular and nonvascular puncture under US guidance: role of colour Doppler imaging. *Radiographics* 1994;**14**(5):959–72.
12. Werner M, Osadchy A, Plotkin E, et al. Increased detection of early vascular abnormalities after renal biopsies by colour Doppler sonography. *J Ultrasound Med* 2007;**26**(9):1221–6.
13. Hamper UM, Savader BL, Sheth S. Improved needle-tip visualisation by colour Doppler sonography. *AJR Am J Roentgenol* 1991;**156**(2):401–2.
14. Gerscovich EO, Budenz RW, Lengle SJ. Assessment of catheter placement and patency by colour Doppler ultrasonography. *J Ultrasound Med* 1994;**13**(5):367–70.

15. Atwell TD, Smith RL, Hesley GK, et al. Incidence of bleeding after 15,181 percutaneous biopsies and the role of aspirin. *AJR Am J Roentgenol* 2010;**194**(3):784–9.
16. McGahan JP, Wright L, Brock J. Occurrence and value of the colour Doppler 'line sign' after radiofrequency ablation of solid abdominal organs. *J Ultrasound Med* 2011;**30**(11):1491–7.
17. Kim KW, Kim MJ, Kim HC, et al. Value of 'patent track' sign on Doppler sonography after percutaneous liver biopsy in detection of postbiopsy bleeding: A prospective study in 352 patients. *AJR Am J Roentgenol* 2007;**189**(1):109–16.
18. Sahani DV, Kalva SP, Tanabe KK, et al. Intraoperative US in patients undergoing surgery for liver neoplasms: comparison with MR imaging. *Radiology* 2004;**232**(3):810–14.
19. Torzilli G, Botea F, Donadon M, et al. Minimesohepatectomy for colorectal liver metastasis invading the middle hepatic vein at the hepatocaval confluence. *Ann Surg Oncol* 2010;**17**(2):483.
20. Sethi AS, Regan SM, Sundaram CP. The use of a Doppler ultrasound probe during vascular dissection in laparoscopic renal surgery. *J Endourol* 2009;**23**(9):1377–82.
21. Ruzzenente A, Conci S, Iacono C, et al. Usefulness of Contrast-Enhanced Intraoperative Ultrasonography (CE-IOUS) in patients with colorectal liver metastases after preoperative chemotherapy. *J Ultrasound Med* Oct 11 2012;**17**(2):281–7.
22. Dempsey RJ, Moftakhar R, Pozniak M. Intraoperative Doppler to measure cerebrovascular resistance as a guide to complete resection of arteriovenous malformations. *Neurosurgery* 2004;**55**(1):155–60; discussion 160–151.
23. Xu BN, Sun ZH, Jiang JL, et al. Surgical management of large and giant intracavernous and paraclinoid aneurysms. *Chin Med J* 2008;**121**(12):1061–4.
24. Gravvanis A, Tsoutsos D, Delikonstantinou I, et al. Impact of portable duplex ultrasonography in head and neck reconstruction. *J Craniofac Surg* 2012;**23**(1):140–4.
25. Mues AC, Okhunov Z, Badani K, et al. Intraoperative evaluation of renal blood flow during laparoscopic partial nephrectomy with a novel Doppler system. *J Endourol* 2010;**24**(12):1953–6.
26. Ou HY, Huang TL, Chen TY, et al. Early modulation of portal graft inflow in adult living donor liver transplant recipients with high portal inflow detected by intraoperative colour Doppler ultrasound. *Transplant Proc* 2010;**42**(3):876–8.
27. Brosig T, Hoinkes A, Seitz RJ, et al. Ultrasound turbulence index during thromboendarterectomy predicts postoperative cerebral microembolism. *Cerebrovasc Dis* 2008;**26**(1):87–92.
28. Bismuth J, Garami Z, Anaya-Ayala JE, et al. Transcranial Doppler findings during thoracic endovascular aortic repair. *J Vasc Surg* 2011;**54**(2):364–9.
29. Ogasawara K, Suga Y, Sasaki M, et al. Intraoperative microemboli and low middle cerebral artery blood flow velocity are additive in predicting development of cerebral ischemic events after carotid endarterectomy. *Stroke* 2008;**39**(11):3088–91.
30. Heiroth HJ, Etminan N, Steiger HJ, et al. Intraoperative Doppler and Duplex sonography in cerebral aneurysm surgery. *Br J Neurosurg* 2011;**25**(5):586–90.
31. Tsujimoto H, Hiraki S, Sakamoto N, et al. Laparoscopic treatment for median arcuate ligament syndrome: the usefulness of intraoperative Doppler ultrasound to confirm the decompression of the celiac artery. *Surg Laparosc Endosc Percutan Tech* 2012;**22**(2):e71–5.
32. Ott C, Heller G, Odermatt M, et al. Intraoperative duplex ultrasonography in carotid endarterectomy: the impact on indication

for immediate revision and intermediate-term outcome. *Vasa* 2008;**37**(2):151–6.

33. Gu LH, Fang H, Li FH, et al. Prediction of early hepatic artery thrombosis by intraoperative colour Doppler ultrasound in pediatric segmental liver transplantation. *Clin Transplant* Feb 13 2012;**26**(4):571–6.

34. Sadej P, Feld RI, Frank A. Transplant renal vein thrombosis: role of preoperative and intraoperative Doppler sonography. *Am J Kidney Dis* 2009;**54**(6):1167–70.

35. Thalhammer C, Aschwanden M, Bilecen D, et al. Intraoperative colour duplex ultrasound during renal transplantation. *Ultraschall Med* 2008;**29**(6):652–6.

Chapter 17

Microbubble Ultrasound Contrast Agents

Jonathan D. Berry, Peter N. Burns and Paul S. Sidhu

Background

In the past 15–20 years, the practice of contrast-enhanced ultrasound (CEUS) has moved from a technique used in a few centres to a widely employed imaging modality that is used worldwide. This change in practice has been facilitated by an appreciation of the importance of the technique in day-to-day ultrasound practice, together with the development and increased availability of both CEUS-capable equipment and the contrast agents themselves.

The principle of ultrasound microbubble contrast agents is based on the peculiar augmentation of echo strength by small bubbles of gas. Unlike other imaging modalities, the majority of which have benefited from contrast-enhancing agents for many years, contrast enhancement in ultrasound was developed relatively recently. The phenomenon of gas-induced ultrasound contrast was first observed when during echocardiography an injection of indocyanine green through a catheter resulted in transient echo enhancement in the region of the catheter tip.[1] This observed enhancement was the result of small air bubbles forming in the catheter tip and strongly scattering ultrasound energy back towards the transducer. Following this there has been progress in understanding the physics of ultrasound contrast enhancement and applying it to the development of encapsulated microbubble agents and imaging technologies for clinical use.

Characteristics of Microbubble Ultrasound Contrast

Ultrasound contrast agents in current use are typically small (3–5 μm diameter) gas-filled bubbles, which are slightly smaller than an erythrocyte (Fig. 17-1). Microbubble contrast agents are physiologically inert, non-toxic and pass through the pulmonary circulation following intravenous injection. The microbubbles contain either air or an inert gas, encapsulated either by a thin shell composed of a biocompatible material such as a lipid, protein or more recently, synthetic polymer.

The intense echo enhancement observed with microbubbles is a result of the high compressibility of the gas they contain. A microbubble undergoes volumetric oscillation while being insonated, to a greater degree than a rigid sphere of similar size, and consequently scatters more energy. In addition there is a fortuitous relationship between the size of microbubble that is able to pass through a capillary and that which will resonate at the frequencies typically used in general ultrasound imaging (3–5 MHz).[2] As such, at the resonant frequency, the returning echoes from a microbubble are maximised in such an effective manner that these microbubbles behave as though they are many orders of magnitude larger than their actual physical size.

When microbubbles are forced by the ultrasound imaging beam into resonant oscillation, they exhibit nonlinear motion, much as does the string of a musical instrument when plucked or struck. This results in the generation of harmonics in the ultrasound echoes, analogous to the overtones produced by a musical instrument. Just as these give the instrument its particular recognizable timbre when playing the same note, so the harmonic echoes from bubbles contain a characteristic pattern of frequencies that allows them to be distinguished from those of tissue, even though they arise from the same ultrasound beam. Ultimately, as acoustic power is increased physical disruption of the microbubbles begins to occur, producing

351

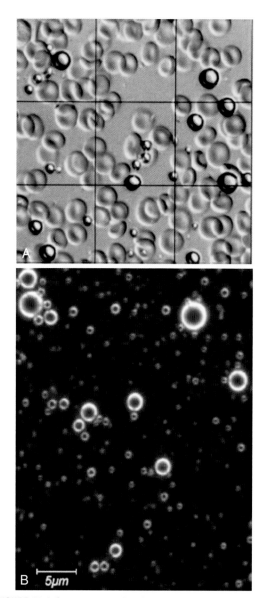

FIGURE 17-1 Contrast agents for ultrasound. (A) Perfluoropropane bubbles with a protein shell (Optison™), seen here against a background of red blood cells. (B) Lipid-coated microbubbles of perfluoropropane gas (Definity™) are seen under a dark field microscope.

Safety of Microbubble Contrast

Concern over potential bio-effects associated with the use of ultrasound contrast agents has led to many experimental studies assessing whether the presence of microbubbles can act as cavitation seeds, thereby potentiating bio-effects. This has been reviewed by ter Haar[4] and by the World Federation for Ultrasound in Medicine and Biology.[5,6] Although it has been shown that adding contrast agents to blood decreases the threshold for cavitation and related bio-effects (e.g., haemolysis, platelet destruction), no significant effects have been reported in circumstances that are comparable to the bubble concentrations and ultrasound exposure used in a low Mechanical Index (MI) diagnostic clinical examination. Nonetheless, it remains prudent to apply the ALARA (*As Low As Reasonably Achievable*) exposure principle to contrast ultrasound examinations by using the lowest MI, the shortest acoustic exposure time, the lowest contrast agent dose and the highest ultrasound frequency that is consistent with obtaining adequate diagnostic information.

At least 5 million injections of microbubble contrast for clinical diagnosis have been performed worldwide. These injections are very well tolerated and have an excellent safety record, with post-market surveillance suggesting that the predominant cause of severe adverse events is an anaphylactoid reaction, with an estimated rate of 1 in 7000 for both the perflutren microspheres approved for cardiac indications in the United States[6] and the sulphur hexafluoride microspheres approved in Europe.[7] This level of adverse events is comparable to that of most analgesics and antibiotics and lower than that for other imaging contrast agents, such as those used in CT imaging.[8] A study by the Italian Society for Ultrasound in Medicine and Biology of more than 23 000 injections of a sulphur hexafluoride microsphere showed no deaths and two serious adverse events, giving a serious adverse event rate of less than 1:10 000.[7]

Although there is currently no Food and Drug Administration (FDA)-approved radiologic indication in the United States, there is extensive experience with ultrasound contrast in echo-cardiology. A review of more than 18 671 hospitalised patients undergoing echocardiography in an acute setting in a single centre

echoes at fractions of harmonic intervals which can also be identified by the receiving instrument. The disruption of bubbles may be used to therapeutic advantage, such as drug delivery and cell membrane poration.[3]

reported no effect on mortality from using contrast in this group.[9] Furthermore, an analysis of registry data from 4 300 966 consecutive patients who underwent transthoracic echocardiography at rest during hospitalisation showed that 58 254 of these patients were given the contrast agent Definity™.[10] Acute, crude mortality was no different between groups, but closer analysis revealed that in patients undergoing echocardiography, those receiving the contrast agent were 24% less likely to die within 1 day compared with patients not receiving contrast. Nonetheless, after four deaths of acutely ill cardiac patients, North American labelling currently advises caution when using microbubble agents in patients with severe cardiopulmonary compromise.[11] At least one contrast agent is currently undergoing clinical development in the United States and seeking the first FDA approval for a radiologic indication in the USA.

Commercially Available Contrast Agents

(See Table 17-1.)

The need to form biologically and physically stable microbubbles in commercial quantities in a simple, cost-effective fashion has led to the development of a variety of microbubble technologies. At the time of writing, commercially available contrast agents approved for intravenous administration include the agents listed in Table 17-1, the majority of experience and data are derived from studies employing Sonovue™ in Europe and Asia, Definity™ in North America and Sonazoid™ in Japan.

Optison™ uses perfluoropropane gas which has slow diffusion into and low solubility in blood, extending the life of the agent. Excretion of the gas is ultimately through the lungs. Albumin provides the soft shell of the microbubble for which the only licensed clinical indication is cardiac imaging.

SonoVue™ consists of sulphur hexafluoride encased by a phospholipid. The microbubbles are prepared by mixing the provided carrier fluid and freeze dried powder. Once prepared, the bubbles remain stable in the vial for several hours. The stability of this formulation in vivo allows real time imaging to occur for several minutes following administration. Licensed clinical indications for use of this agent include cardiac, macrovascular, liver and breast applications.

Definity™ is licensed in the United States for cardiac use and comprises lipid-stabilised octafluoropropane gas. The indications include opacification of the cardiac chambers and improved delineation of the endocardial borders; in Canada, Definity™ is additionally approved for radiological applications in the abdomen and pelvis.

Sonazoid™ is a lipid-stabilised perfluorobutane microbubble that allows both continuous vascular and late-phase Kupffer cell imaging.[12] First licensed for use in Japan, it is envisaged that Sonazoid™ will be increasingly employed in the field of focal hepatic lesion detection and follow up post hepatic radio-frequency ablation.

TABLE 17-1	Characteristics of Some Commercially Available Ultrasound Contrast Agents			
Brand name	**Producer**	**Gas**	**Stabilisation**	**Approved Applications**
Sonazoid™	GE Healthcare	Perfluorobutane	Hydrogenated egg phosphatidyl serine	Abdominal
Optison™	GE Healthcare	Perfluoropropane	Albumin	Cardiac
SonoVue™	Bracco	Sulphur hexafluoride	Phospholipid	Cardiac Vascular Hepatic Breast
Definity™	Lantheus Medical Imaging	Octafluoropropane	Phospholipid	Cardiac Abdomen Pelvis

Ultrasound Technologies Used in Contrast Imaging

The physical characteristics of microbubbles have allowed the development of a variety of contrast-specific imaging techniques. Equipment manufacturers attach a variety of proprietary names to the techniques employed; many of these share the same principles of operation and the majority of high-specification ultrasound machines have contrast-specific modes available.

HARMONIC IMAGING

One simple method to distinguish bubbles from tissue is to excite the bubbles so as to produce harmonics and then detect these in preference to the fundamental frequency echo from tissue (Fig. 17-2A). Key factors in the harmonic response of an agent are the incident pressure of the ultrasound field, the frequency, the size distribution of the bubbles, and the mechanical properties of the bubble capsule – a stiff capsule will dampen oscillations and attenuate the nonlinear response. Although simple and effective, this method halves the bandwidth of the image, reducing its resolution and can be confounded by the propagation of a second 'tissue' harmonic echo which results from non-linear propagation of ultrasound by non-bubble bearing structures, so reducing the image contrast. It is rarely used in modern systems.

PHASE INVERSION IMAGING

Phase or pulse inversion imaging (PII) achieves a better differentiation between bubbles and tissue without loss of resolution.[13] PII involves transmission of an initial imaging pulse followed by a second pulse which is an inverted version of the first. The two resulting echoes are then summed: if they are scattered from a linear target, this sum is zero. However, because microbubbles produce non-linear scatter, the sum of the two signals from a microbubble will not be zero (Fig. 17-2B). In addition to allowing a wider bandwidth to be used than in harmonic imaging, PII also allows relatively low insonation pressures (low MI) which reduces the risk of microbubble disruption. This technique allows for continuous real time imaging during vascular phases, allowing detection of vascular patterns peculiar to different liver tumours. Inclusion of a third pulse of lower amplitude than the other two pulses allows detection of nonlinear echoes at the fundamental frequency,

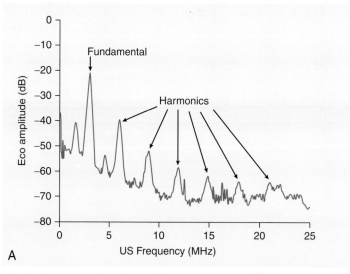

FIGURE 17-2 (A) Harmonic emission from microbubbles. Microbubbles are insonated at 3 MHz and the echo analysed for its frequency content. The largest peak of the energy in the echo is at the 3 MHz fundamental, but that there are clear secondary peaks in the spectrum at 6, 9, 12, 15 and 18 MHz, as well as peaks between these harmonics ('ultra-harmonics') and below the fundamental (the 'sub-harmonic'). Harmonic imaging and Doppler aim to separate and process the second harmonic echo only, which is about 18 dB less than that of the fundamental echo signal.

Continued

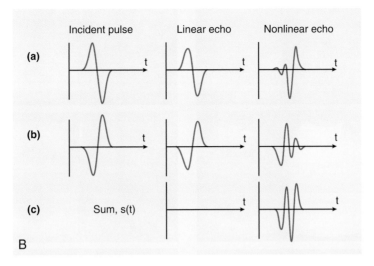

FIGURE 17-2—CONT'D (B) Principle of Pulse Inversion Imaging. A pulse of sound (a) is transmitted into the body and echoes are received from agent and tissue. A second pulse (b), which is an inverted copy of the first, is then transmitted in the same direction and the two resulting echoes summed. Linear echoes from tissue are inverted copies of each other and cancel to zero (c, middle). Microbubble echoes are distorted copies of each other, so that the even nonlinear components of these echoes reinforce each other when summed, producing a strong harmonic signal (c, right side).

which improves penetration of the contrast image. This method is sometimes called 'power modulation pulse inversion' (PMPI) or 'contrast pulse sequence' (CPS).[14]

QUANTIFICATION TECHNIQUES

Quantification of microbubbles is complicated by the fact that there is no simple unit of quantification of the contrast echo which can be measured reliably and reproducibly. Furthermore, contrast imaging using the multi-pulse sequences such as PMPI and CPS described above are subject to multiple artifacts including motion artifact from patient or operator movement which can be difficult to avoid in long examinations. Initial work in the field of quantification of microbubbles focused on assessment of a number of variables including time to arrival, wash-in/wash-out characteristics, time to peak and the area under the curve (Fig. 17-3). With advances in technology, quantification techniques have progressed to allow microbubbles to be used for true, functional imaging in the form of dynamic contrast-enhanced ultrasound (DCE-US). Unlike other functional imaging techniques, DCE-US avoids the need for ionising radiation and so may be used repeatedly to monitor, for example, tumour response to treatment.[15]

Artifacts

Artifacts occur predominantly with the older high MI imaging techniques.[16] One of the most commonly seen artifacts when using microbubbles to enhance conventional Doppler studies is that of 'blooming' in which colour pixels appear to extend beyond the bounds of the vessel (Fig. 17-4). This phenomenon may prove problematic when objective computer analysis of contrast enhancement is required. While the problem arises partly from multiple re-reflections between adjacent microbubbles, it is also in part due to limitations of the hardware analysis of the Doppler signal.

A further artifact resulting from limitations in the ultrasound hardware is the apparent reversal of Doppler flow following administration of contrast. This effect represents overloading of the Doppler circuitry and once appreciated is easily recognised.

Intravascular contrast may make high-velocity shifts detectable, which pre-contrast were not detectable. Whilst this may initially appear to be a desirable effect, it can be problematic when absolute angle-corrected values are required for clinical decision making, for example in assessment of internal carotid artery stenosis.

Sharp spikes of Doppler 'noise' may occasionally be seen, which may arise from collapse of the microbubbles.

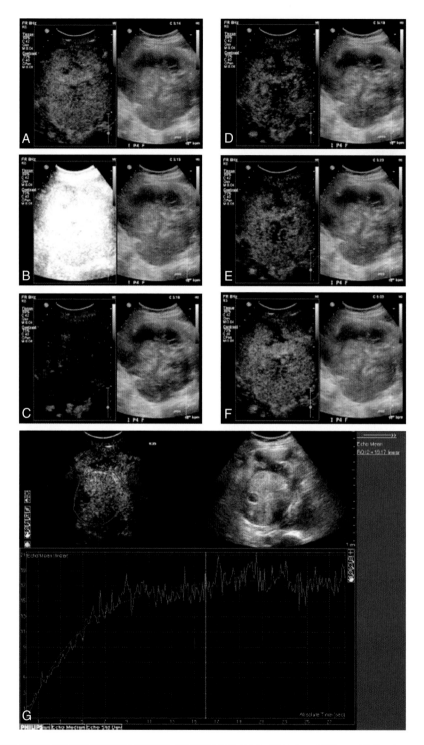

FIGURE 17-3 Dynamic contrast-enhanced ultrasound (DCE-US). Disruption-replenishment imaging used to quantify flow in a renal cell carcinoma in a patient undergoing anti-angiogenic treatment. A sequence of side-by-side contrast images (conventional on right, simultaneous CEUS on left) of a large renal cell carcinoma is made during a steady intravenous infusion of the agent Definity™. (A) $t = -1$ sec, the tumour is enhanced. (B) $t = 0$ sec, a brief, high MI 'flash' disrupts bubbles within the scan plane. (C) $t = 1$ sec, new bubbles begin to wash in to the scan plane. (D-F) $t = 4$ sec, 8 sec and 18 sec after flash, the scan plane is fully replenished. (G) Off-line analysis software measures wash-in for a region-of-interest from the cine-loop record in a similar case. The steeper the slope, the greater the flow rate; the higher the plateau, the greater the vascular volume. Disruption-replenishment imaging thus allows quantitation of tumour flow and total vascular volume.

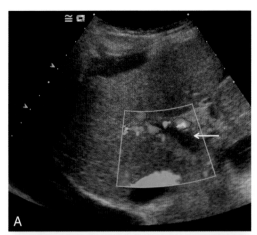
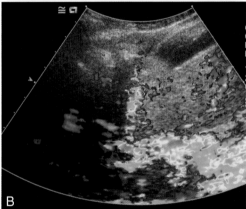

FIGURE 17-4 A commonly seen artifact when using microbubbles is 'blooming' in which colour pixels appear to extend beyond the bounds of the vessel. (A) Baseline colour Doppler image at the level of the porta hepatis demonstrating absence of colour signal in the portal vein (arrow) but colour is present in the overlying hepatic artery. (B) Following the administration of SonoVue™ 'blooming' from the hepatic artery obscures the portal vein.

'Pseudo-enhancement' may arise from echogenic structures which are non-perfused but lie distal to a body of bubbles. This artefact is commonly seen after radio-frequency ablation of liver lesions where it can be misinterpreted as an incomplete ablation.

Clinical Applications of Microbubble Contrast

CARDIAC

Cardiology represents the single greatest area of use of microbubble contrast agents with several established and evolving applications.

Echocardiography

Patient factors including obesity and lung disease render a significant number of echocardiograms non-diagnostic, particularly in the case of stress echocardiography. Microbubble contrast agents allow improved delineation of the endocardial border and detection of wall motion abnormalities, as a result, up to 74% of otherwise non-diagnostic studies may be 'rescued'.[17] Use of microbubbles allows additional information regarding regional and global left ventricular function to be acquired during a stress echocardiography examination. Furthermore, valvular disease may be more accurately assessed by contrast-enhanced Doppler.

Myocardial Perfusion

Assessment of myocardial perfusion offers potential for the diagnosis of acute myocardial infarction, as well as assessing perfusion during stress testing. The combination of the more robust microbubbles with low MI techniques allows a more comprehensive myocardial assessment. Furthermore, the application of intermittent high-power pulses to destroy the microbubbles allows assessment of the rate of refilling of the myocardial micro-circulation, so providing a measure of micro-circulation perfusion. Studies indicate contrast echocardiography to be highly sensitive for the detection of acute coronary syndrome offering the hope of rapid bedside diagnosis and treatment for this life-threatening condition.[18]

Coronary Arteries

Localisation and quantification of the degree of coronary artery stenosis may be performed using intermittent harmonic imaging techniques. Analogous to the assessment of micro-circulation described above, coronary artery flow rate may be calculated by intermittent destruction of microbubbles and measurement of time taken for microbubbles to reaccumulate. Motion of the cardiac wall is a major problem that has yet to be satisfactorily resolved with respect to this assessment.

LIVER

Unenhanced ultrasound is the first-line investigation of liver disease but continues to be perceived as less accurate in terms of detection and staging of focal lesions when compared to contrast-enhanced CT or

MR imaging. Nearly all the ultrasound contrast agents available have been used to study liver lesions, consequently much of our understanding regarding in vivo behaviour has been gained from studies of liver abnormalities.[19]

Focal Liver Lesions

For focal liver lesions, the important aspects of the examination are the detection and then characterisation of lesions into benign and malignant abnormalities. Real-time low MI microbubble imaging is analogous to the phases seen with contrast-enhanced CT, except imaging with microbubbles is in real-time and repeatable. Microbubble ultrasound contrast displays an early (arterial) phase at around 10 to 35 seconds post intravenous administration, followed by a portal venous phase at approximately 30 to 120 seconds (Fig. 17-5). Depending on the formulation of the microbubble contrast agent there may then be a liver-specific phase as the microbubbles are taken up within the Kupffer cells.[20]

Initial studies employing the high mechanical index imaging technique of stimulated acoustic emission (SAE) showed the potential of microbubbles to improve the detection of liver lesions but this has now been superseded by nonlinear techniques with low MI.[21] Imaging of a focal liver lesion during different vascular phases provides clues to the identity of the lesion with good correlation between the findings on microbubble contrast-enhanced ultrasound and CT or MR imaging.[22]

Current practice when characterising hepatic lesions is as follows: the liver lesion is identified with B-mode imaging then, with the transducer held stationary over the lesion, continuous imaging is performed for 180 seconds after injection of a bolus of microbubble contrast (followed by a saline flush) via a peripheral vein. Using this technique nearly all benign focal hepatic lesions can be confidently characterised, thus negating the need for the patient to proceed to more expensive, time-consuming and potentially harmful investigations.[23] There is a growing body of evidence to assist the practitioner when performing such liver lesion characterisation, with pathways firmly established.[23,24]

Haemangiomas typically display progressive enhancement from the periphery of the lesion, mirroring that seen on CT and MR imaging (Fig. 17-6).

Focal fatty sparing, focal fatty change and regenerative nodules may have alarming appearances with contrast-enhanced CT and MR imaging but reassuringly display iso-enhancement compared to surrounding liver parenchyma following microbubble contrast administration.

Focal nodular hyperplasia, a benign vascular anomaly, tends to enhance strongly with microbubble contrast, demonstrating a characteristic central hyperenhancing 'star', often with a non-enhancing central scar (Fig. 17-7).

Hepatic adenomas, which on occasion may be very large and associated with haemorrhage, generally show increased enhancement in the arterial and porto-venous phases, becoming iso-enhancing with surrounding parenchyma on delayed imaging.

Simple liver abscesses are readily diagnosed on B-mode imaging but if there is diagnostic uncertainty, administration of microbubble contrast shows a rim of increased enhancement with a poorly reflective

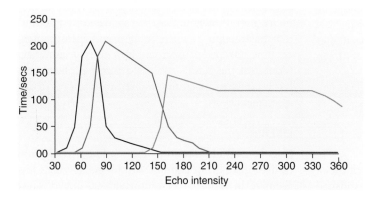

FIGURE 17-5 Characterisation of focal liver lesions is based on the dual blood supply of hepatic artery and the portal vein, with three overlapping vascular phases defined: arterial phase 10–35 seconds (blue line, lesion vascularity), portal-venous phase 30–120 seconds (red line, information on wash-out) and late phase >120 seconds (green line, sinusoid pooling or cell uptake). Microbubbles disappear 240–360 seconds after injection.

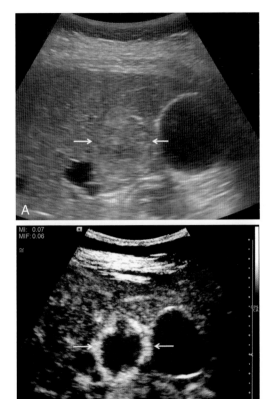

FIGURE 17-6 A haemangioma shows progressive enhancement from the periphery of the lesion. (A) Baseline image of an atypical focal liver lesion (arrows). (B) Microbubble-enhanced image in the late phase demonstrates 'creeping' enhancement from the periphery (arrows) typical of a haemangioma.

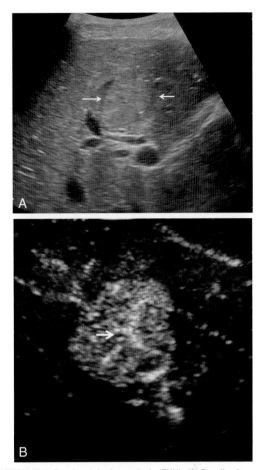

FIGURE 17-7 Focal nodular hyperplasia (FNH). (A) Baseline image of an iso-reflective focal liver lesion (arrows). (B) Microbubble-enhanced image in the arterial phase demonstrates a 'spoke-wheel' pattern of rapid enhancement (arrow) typical of an FNH.

central area. Occasionally enhancing septa may be seen within the abscess and the surrounding liver segment may show increased enhancement secondary to hyperaemia (Fig. 17-8).

Differentiating benign from malignant lesions is generally dependent on the 'wash-out' of enhancement leaving a 'black-hole' in the liver relative to surrounding tissue. As with other imaging modalities the ultrasound characteristics of liver metastases depend on the source of the primary. In general metastases are poorly enhancing in portal-venous and late phases (Fig. 17-9). The early arterial phase may demonstrate either hypervascularity or hypovascularity, but there is still discussion about these features,[25] as it is possible that all metastases may demonstrate brief hypervascularity. However, metastases universally 'wash-out'.[26]

Hepato-cellular carcinomas (HCC) can be extremely difficult to identify within a cirrhotic liver on B-mode imaging, thus limiting the effectiveness of surveillance ultrasound imaging in this group of high-risk patients. CEUS may assist in the detection of these tumours although there are no recommendations on guidance for the routine use of CEUS in surveillance ultrasound imaging. With microbubble contrast, HCC tend to be strongly enhancing in the arterial phase (Fig. 17-10), although this is short-lived and imaging of the entire liver in the narrow time

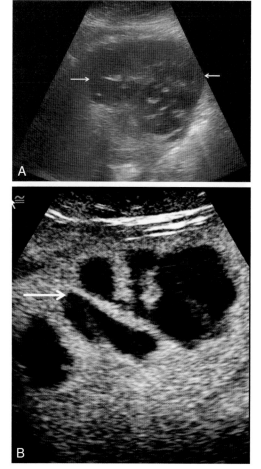

FIGURE 17-8 Liver abscess. (A) Baseline image of a mixed reflective focal liver lesion (arrows). (B) Microbubble-enhanced image in the portal venous phase demonstrates a low reflective 'liquid' abscess with septations (arrow) visible.

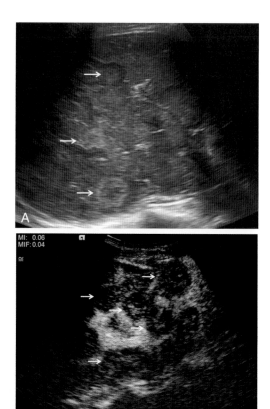

FIGURE 17-9 Malignant lesions washout in the late portal-venous phase to demonstrate the 'black-holes' of liver metastases. (A) Baseline image of multiple breast cancer metastases in the right lobe of the liver (arrows). (B) Following administration of microbubble contrast, there is washout at 2 min 32 sec of contrast from the multiple liver lesions (arrows).

window can be difficult. HCC are iso- or hypo-enhancing in the porto-venous phase and hypo-enhancing on delayed imaging.[27] An HCC may show some late phase enhancement, depending on the degree of differentiation of the tumour, with the wash-out prolonged and incomplete.[28]

Liver Transplantation and Liver Vasculature

Microbubble contrast agents are a useful diagnostic tool for ultrasound imaging in liver transplantation.[29]

Pre-transplant assessment of the native liver paren-chyma and hepatic vasculature is essential but with a cirrhotic, highly attenuating liver, visualisation of the vessels may be problematic. Demonstration of portal vein patency is improved with the use of microbubble contrast ('Doppler rescue')[30] (Fig. 17-11). If a trans-jugular intra-hepatic portal-systemic shunt (TIPSS) is present and possible occlusion is suspected, the administration of microbubbles will demonstrate low flow that may not be evident on the normal colour Doppler study of the TIPSS.

In the post-transplant liver, documentation of the patency of the hepatic artery is paramount since com-promise of this vessel may result in bile duct ischae-mia, necrosis and bile duct leaks, leading to eventual

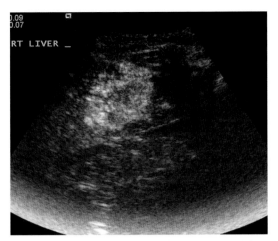

FIGURE 17-10 Hepatocellular carcinoma showing strong enhancement shortly after injection of microbubble contrast agent.

re-transplantation. If a hepatic artery spectral Doppler trace is not demonstrated using standard Doppler, using microbubble contrast may negate the need for arteriography or CT angiography.[31]

SPLEEN

The spleen is often a technically difficult organ to visualise adequately on B-mode ultrasound, several conditions within and around the spleen may cause diagnostic confusion. Aside from the assessment of splenic injury, the use of microbubble contrast will enhance the operator's confidence when assessing focal splenic lesions.[32] Splenunculi occur in up to 30% of the population, they may be multiple and can be found at locations remote from the spleen, when they may be mistaken for enlarged lymph nodes,

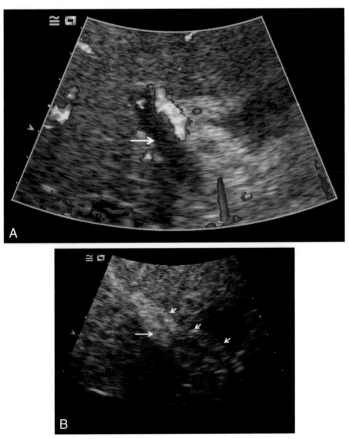

FIGURE 17-11 Confirmation of portal vein patency. (A) No colour flow signal is seen in the portal vein (arrow) despite optimisation of the Doppler parameters. (B) Following CEUS the portal vein is confirmed to be patent (long arrow) with visualisation of a long length of the main hepatic artery (short arrows).

particularly when multiple. Microbubble contrast will accurately demonstrate that the parenchymal enhancement of the splenunculi matches the main spleen and shows a clear vascular hilum.

Focal Splenic Lesions

In a patient with no known primary malignancy an incidentally discovered focal splenic lesion will usually be benign. Cavernous haemangiomas are the most common benign solid splenic lesion; usually small and solitary, they may occasionally be multiple and >2 cm in diameter. With large haemangiomas, microbubble contrast demonstrates a centripetal enhancement pattern, analogous to that seen in liver haemangiomas. Other benign solid lesions in the spleen are rare but include lymphangioma and hamartoma, both of which show varying degrees of enhancement after microbubble administration.

Simple splenic cysts, either congenital or acquired, rarely cause diagnostic uncertainty. Abscesses in the spleen may have ultrasound appearances ranging from cystic to solid and generally appear avascular on both Doppler ultrasound and microbubble-enhanced ultrasound. Splenic infarction typically occurs in patients with infective endocarditis or myeloproliferative disorders and is often difficult to visualise on initial B-mode ultrasound but may show lack of vascular perfusion on colour Doppler ultrasound and improved conspicuity with the use of CEUS.[33]

Primary malignant tumours of the spleen, such as lymphoma and angiosarcoma, do occur but they are both rare.[34] More common, although still unusual, are metastatic deposits in the spleen. Evidence suggests that malignant splenic disease tends to enhance in the arterial phase, then shows rapid wash out in the delayed phase when compared to adjacent normal spleen.[35] The majority of malignant deposits are serosal (causing scalloping of the spleen surface) as opposed to parenchymal, the primary neoplasm is most commonly in the ovary. In cases of known malignant disease within the spleen CEUS may be used to monitor disease response to treatment.

PANCREAS

Whilst CT is the imaging modality for the detection of focal pancreatic lesions, CEUS may be utilised to characterise lesions detected at CT. Adenocarcinoma is the most common primary malignancy of the pancreas and this tends to be hypo-enhancing in all phases when compared to adjacent normal parenchyma.[36] In contrast, the highly vascular neuroendocrine tumours tend to hyper-enhance in the arterial phase.[37] Cystic pancreatic lesions can present a particular diagnostic challenge with differentiation between mucin-producing tumours, serous cystadenomas and benign or post-inflammatory cysts occasionally being difficult. Improved characterisation of pancreatic lesions has been achieved by combining the high spatial resolution of endoscopic ultrasound with the advantages of CEUS in the form of contrast enhanced endoscopic ultrasound (CE-EUS).[38]

Patients with pancreatitis frequently need repeat imaging to assess for complications such as pancreatic necrosis, splenic vein occlusion and pseudo-cyst formation. CEUS may be employed in this setting to avoid the need for multiple CT scan.

GASTROINTESTINAL TRACT

The primary use of CEUS in the field of gastroenterology is in the assessment of inflammatory bowel disease, particularly Crohn's disease. Measurement of bowel wall thickening, luminal narrowing and wall vascularity can diagnose and potentially quantify disease activity, together with the extent of any chronic strictures.[39] In addition, some of the complications associated with Crohn's disease may be assessed with CEUS, including abscess formation and fistula tracks.

RENAL

The main objectives of renal ultrasound are assessment of size, vascular interrogation and exclusion of pelvi-calyceal dilatation. Assessment of renal masses often requires further imaging with CT or MRI. Microbubble contrast administration results in rapid, avid enhancement of the renal cortex within a few seconds, followed by the outer medulla and then gradual filling in of the pyramids. The kidneys of patients with chronic renal impairment generally enhance less avidly and for a shorter period than those with normal renal function.[40]

Focal Renal Lesions

There is now evidence that CEUS is more sensitive than CT in detecting vascularity in hypovascular

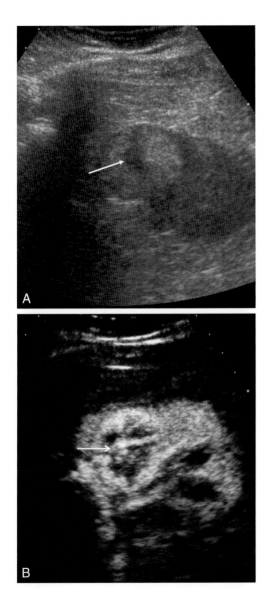

FIGURE 17-12 A renal carcinoma. (A) On the baseline image a complex mass is present at the upper aspect of the left kidney (arrow). (B) Following CEUS abnormal vessels are demonstrated within the tumour (arrow) confirming the malignant nature of the lesion.

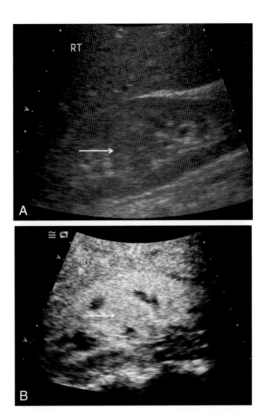

FIGURE 17-13 Column of Bertin. (A) On the baseline image a possible mass is present at the mid aspect of the right kidney (arrow). (B) Following CEUS normal vascularity and perfusion identical to the renal cortex is demonstrated within the mass (arrow), in keeping with a column of Bertin.

renal lesions and is as accurate as CT at characterising complex cystic lesions as benign or malignant[41] (Fig. 17-12). Renal 'pseudo-tumours', such as a prominent column of Bertin, can be difficult to differentiate from real renal masses. CEUS may be of assistance in such cases by confirming or excluding the presence of abnormal vessels and the patency of the renal vein (Fig. 17-13).

Following percutaneous ablation of a focal renal lesion, CEUS assists in both visualisation of the lesion and whether it remains vascularised and therefore viable.

Renal Vasculature

Although Doppler ultrasound of the renal arteries is an accepted screening examination for renal artery stenosis, this technique is technically challenging. Problems arise in visualising the entire renal artery, identifying accessory arteries and obtaining accurate spectra due to patient factors and being unable to access a suitable angle on the artery. Microbubble contrast enhancement may overcome some of these problems and increase the success rate of the examination.[42] Microbubble contrast is useful in the visualisation of the vessels after renal transplantation. Viability of the transplant is dependent on patency of both the renal artery and vein; microbubble contrast can aid in the diagnosis of renal artery stenosis or renal vein thrombosis, as well as assess the overall perfusion of the transplant and identification of areas of reduced or absent flow[43] (Fig. 17-14).

ABDOMINAL TRAUMA

CT remains the modality of choice in poly-trauma but in patients who suffer a site-specific low-energy injury, the radiation burden of a whole-body CT may be difficult to justify and it is often only one or two organs in which injury is suspected, for example the spleen and left kidney with left-flank blunt trauma. CEUS may be used as an adjunct to Focused Assessment with Sonography in Trauma (FAST) to assess the organs in question with studies indicating it to be more sensitive than standard ultrasound in the detection of solid organ injury and almost as sensitive as CT.[44] Active hepatic haemorrhage is best visualised in the arterial phase of CEUS imaging, whilst lacerations and haematomas are best seen in the delayed phase, when their lack of enhancement is emphasised by adjacent enhancing parenchyma (Fig. 17-15). The splenic parenchyma generally displays prolonged enhancement which is initially patchy and is then more homogeneous by approximately 40–60 seconds after bolus injection. As in the liver, lacerations of the spleen reveal themselves as linear branching non-enhancing structures

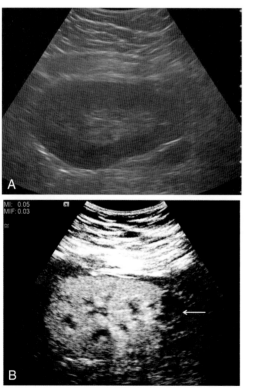

FIGURE 17-14 Segmental infarction in a transplant kidney. (A) On the B-mode image the transplant kidney appears normal. (B) Following CEUS there is an area of non-perfusion (arrow) at the lower aspect of the transplant kidney consistent with an infarction (biopsy proven).

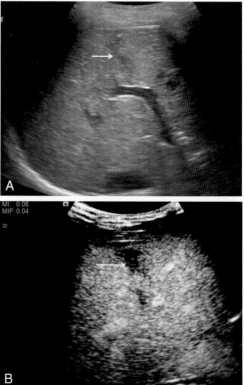

FIGURE 17-15 The subtle abnormality on the B-mode image is seen to be a laceration on the contrast image. (A) An area of reflective inconsistency is seen in the right lobe of the liver (arrow). (B) Following CEUS there is no perfusion of the liver at this site (arrow) demonstrating the presence of a liver laceration.

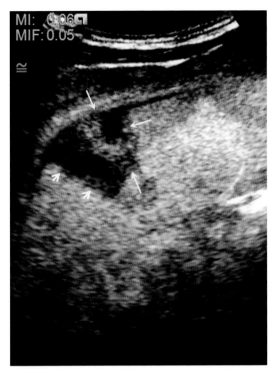

FIGURE 17-16 Splenic laceration: Microbubble contrast enhancement shows no perfusion of the spleen at the site of a laceration (short arrows), with an adjacent area of contusion and haematoma (long arrows) and a thin layer of fluid around the spleen.

whilst sub-capsular haematoma tends to be a curvilinear non-enhancing structure (Fig. 17-16).

Both spleen and kidney enhance avidly with microbubble contrast and therefore the dose used tends to be less than that for liver imaging. The kidneys tend to enhance for a shorter time (approximately 2 minutes) than the spleen.[45] As with the spleen and liver, lacerations of the kidneys are generally linear non-enhancing structures whilst complete avulsion of the kidney results in diffusely poorly or non-enhancing renal parenchyma.

Vesico-Ureteric Reflux (VUR)

The standard methods for the investigation of VUR involved ionising radiation. Since the majority of patients are children; this is undesirable and therefore the option of using intra-vesical administration of microbubble contrast is appealing. Early attempts realised the potential for this technique but recognised some of the practical difficulties in the implementation of the method. More recently studies have indicated that the use of microbubbles for the investigation of VUR is a sensitive test and this has now become standard practice in many departments.[46]

Hystero Contrast Salpingography (HyCoSy)

In the investigation of sub-fertility, Fallopian tube patency has traditionally been established by hysterosalpingography (HSG), a technique requiring both iodinated contrast and irradiation of the pelvic organs. The use of HyCoSy avoids these risks. Instillation of microbubble contrast into the uterine cavity is performed using trans-vaginal ultrasound, the passage of contrast through the Fallopian tubes and spillage into the pelvis may be followed in real time.[47] Currently, this may be used as a screening test for tubal patency but it cannot yet provide detailed anatomical delineation of tubal pathology and its positive predictive value for the detection of occluded Fallopian tube remains low.[48] Consequently, some would argue that the high negative predictive value of conventional HSG means that this should remain the investigation of choice. Furthermore whilst both HSG and HyCoSy can result in significant patient discomfort some studies have suggested that pain is more common with HyCoSy.[49]

SCROTUM

Ultrasound is the imaging choice for the testis and is usually sufficient for diagnostic purposes. Occasionally, findings may be equivocal and in such cases CEUS may be of assistance. With small testicular tumours it may be difficult to demonstrate internal vascularity and therefore the lesion could be misinterpreted as benign. CEUS provides operator confidence regarding the true nature of such lesions.[50,51] Segmental testicular infarction, trauma to the testis and inflammation may all be demonstrated more effectively through the use of CEUS (Fig. 17-17).[52,53]

PROSTATE

Whilst trans-rectal ultrasound is routinely used for targeted biopsy of the prostate gland, real time and Doppler US are of limited value in the assessment of prostate tumours with both poor sensitivity and specificity. Low MI endocavity CEUS raises the possibility of

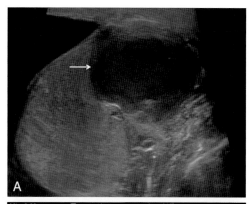

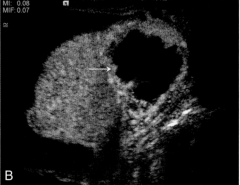

FIGURE 17-17 Testicular abscess. (A) There is a low reflective rounded abnormality in the lower pole of the testis (arrow) in a patient with severe epididymo-orchitis. (B) Following CEUS the rounded lesion is seen to be an abscess with a liquid centre and irregular wall (arrow).

improved tumour site detection. Initial data indicate that the technique is of assistance in directing targeted biopsies towards the site of primary tumour but specificity remains a problem; areas of benign hyperplasia may masquerade as malignancy.[54]

BREAST

Although the superficial nature of breast tissue and the angiogenesis often associated with malignancy should mean that breast tumours would be a suitable subject for interrogation with CEUS, several studies have failed to demonstrate any convincing patterns of enhancement that can reliably differentiate malignant from benign breast lesions.[55] Whilst CEUS may not be of benefit in the detection of the primary breast tumour there are hopes that CEUS quantification

techniques may assist in assessment of tumour response to treatment. In addition, microbubbles are an effective method for the detection of sentinel lymph nodes prior to surgery.[56]

Lungs and Pleura

This limited application of CEUS is confined to the assessment of peripheral regions of consolidated or collapsed lung and thickened pleural membranes. Avascular areas of pulmonary infarction resulting from an embolic event may be differentiated from pneumonia and simple collapse.[57] In addition, CEUS may be employed when performing targeted biopsy of peripheral lung lesions to distinguish necrotic (and therefore probably non-diagnostic) tissue from vascularised regions of the tumour.

VASCULAR
Trans-Cranial Ultrasound

Assessment of intra-cranial vessels using standard Doppler ultrasound is limited by the severe attenuation of the signal due to the poor temporal bone window (see Chapter 3). Microbubble contrast agents can overcome this problem and allow improved visualisation of these vessels. In one study, CEUS technically improved the images in 77% of patients,[58] with the basal arteries of the circle of Willis being adequately depicted in up to 85% of patients.[59] Through the use of CEUS and imaging via the foramen magnum, the intra-cranial vertebral arteries, the basilar artery and some of the cerebellar vessels can be imaged more easily.[60]

Carotid Artery

Microbubble contrast use in the assessment of carotid arteries is focused on three areas. The first is to accurately visualise flow within the carotid artery, a task that is frequently complicated by overlying calcified plaque and vessel tortuosity. In one study, on baseline colour Doppler imaging 21% of vessel stenoses were not identified, compared with only 6% after microbubble contrast.[61] The second area is differentiation between vessel occlusion and a high-grade stenosis, a distinction which can be difficult to make with standard colour Doppler but using microbubbles decreases the false-negative rate from 30% to 17%.[62]

Finally, when MR imaging is contraindicated, CEUS may be employed in the assessment of carotid artery dissection.[63] There has also been some interest in the imaging of angiogenesis within plaque with CEUS as a measure of plaque vulnerability.[64]

Aorta

Patient factors frequently render US imaging of the aorta sub-optimal. CEUS may assist in such situations by improving delineation of the lumen of the aorta, as well as assessment of potential leakage and dissection.[65] Endovascular aneurysm repair (EVAR) is now an established technique, although the potential long-term complications remain unknown. Long-term surveillance of these devices with CT imaging carries a significant cumulative radiation dose, therefore the concept of surveillance with CEUS is appealing. Evidence suggests that CEUS surveillance is both safe and effective and in some cases, superior to CT imaging[66] (Fig. 17-18).

MUSCULO-SKELETAL

Microbubble contrast is finding applications in the study of articular inflammatory disease. Several studies have shown synovial enhancement in patients with synovial inflammation confirmed with MR imaging.[67] Furthermore, CEUS may assist in differentiation

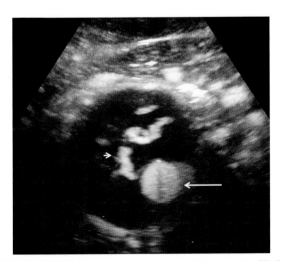

FIGURE 17-18 On this transverse image through the aorta, the CEUS image demonstrates a leak (short arrow) from the main body of the EVAR (long arrow).

between active synovitis and other causes of peri-articular swelling, such as fibrotic pannus and fluid collections, which can be of prognostic value. Adjacent bursae and tendons may also be elegantly demonstrated.[68] Microbubbles therefore have a role not only in diagnosis but also in monitoring disease progression and response to therapy.

THERAPY

The currently available microbubbles consist of gas contained within a shell. Potential exists to attach a 'cargo' and effectively use the microbubble as a vehicle to transport a therapeutic agent to a specified site. Ultimately this may prove to be a more important application of microbubbles than any of those discussed above. Perhaps the most interesting use would be in the area of gene therapy where the initial hopes of effective treatments have often been limited by lack of suitable delivery mechanisms. Sonoporation, the mechanism by which cell membranes are rendered porous to large molecules by ultrasound, is enhanced in the presence of microbubbles. It has been shown in animal models that this process can deliver gene therapy agents.[69] In addition to gene therapy, there are also possibilities for other therapeutic initiatives, including delivery of chemo-therapeutic agents, with the site of delivery being defined by selective microbubble disruption. Evidence suggests this technique could prove particularly effective.[70]

REFERENCES

1. Gramiak R, Shah PM. Echocardiography of the aortic root. *Invest Radiol* 1968;**3**:356–66.
2. Stride E, Saffari N. Microbubble ultrasound contrast agents: a review. *Proc Inst Mech Eng [H]* 2003;**217**:429–47.
3. Porter TR, Xie F, Li S, et al. Increased ultrasound contrast and decreased microbubble destruction rates with triggered ultrasound imaging. *J Am Soc Echocardiogr* 1996;**9**:599–605.
4. ter Haar G. Ultrasonic contrast agents: safety considerations reviewed. *Eur J Radiol* 2002;**41**:217–21.
5. Barnett SB, ter Haar G, Ziskin MC, et al. International recommendations and guidelines for the safe use of diagnostic ultrasound in medicine. *Ultrasound Med Biol* 2000;**26**:355–66.
6. Bouakaz A, de Jong N. WFUMB Safety Symposium on Echo-Contrast Agents: nature and types of ultrasound contrast agents. *Ultrasound Med Biol* 2007;**33**:187–96.
7. Piscaglia F, Bolondi L. The safety of SonoVue in abdominal applications: retrospective analysis of 23188 investigations. *Ultrasound Med Biol* 2006;**32**:1369–75.
8. International Collaborative Study of Severe Anaphylaxis . Risk of anaphylaxis in a hospital population in relation to the use

of various drugs: an international study. *Pharmacoepidemiol Drug Saf* 2003;**12**:195–202.

9. Kusnetzky LL, Khalid A, Khumri TM, et al. Acute mortality in hospitalized patients undergoing echocardiography with and without an ultrasound contrast agent. Results in 18,671 consecutive studies. *J Am Coll Cardiol* 2008;**51**:1704–6.

10. Main ML, Ryan RC, Davis TE, et al. Acute mortality in hospitalized patients undergoing echocardiography with and without an ultrasound contrast agent: multicentre registry results in 4,300,966 consecutive patients. *Am J Cardiol* 2008; **102**:1742–6.

11. Main ML. Ultrasound contrast agent safety: from anecdote to evidence. *JACC Cardiovasc Imaging* 2009;**2**:1057–9.

12. Edey AJ, Ryan SM, Beese RC, et al. Ultrasound imaging of liver metastases in the delayed parenchymal phase following administration of Sonazoid™ using a destructive mode technique (Agent Detection Imaging™). *Clin Radiol* 2008;**63**:1112–20.

13. Tiemann K, Lohmeier S, Kuntz S, et al. Real-time contrast echo assessment of myocardial perfusion at low emission power: first experimental and clinical results using power pulse inversion imaging. *Echocardiography* 1999;**16**:799–809.

14. Eckersley RJ, Chin CT, Burns PN. Optimising phase and amplitude modulation schemes for imaging microbubble contrast agents at low acoustic power. *Ultrasound Med Biol* 2005;**31**:213–19.

15. Leen E, Averkiou M, Arditi M, et al. Dynamic contrast enhanced ultrasound assessment of the vascular effects of novel therapeutics in early stage trials. *Eur Radiol* 2012;**1**:10–12.

16. Forsberg F, Liu JB, Burns PN, et al. Artifact in ultrasonic contrast agents studies. *J Ultrasound Med* 1994;**13**:357–65.

17. Nihoyannopoulos P. Contrast echocardiography. *Clin Radiol* 1996;**51**:28–30.

18. Senior R, Becher H, Monaghan MJ, et al. Contrast echocardiography: evidence-based recommendations by European Association of Echocardiography. *Eur J Echocardiogr* 2009;**10**:194–212.

19. Wilson SR, Burns PN. Microbubble-enhanced US in body imaging: What role? *Radiology* 2010;**257**:24–39.

20. Forsberg F, Goldberg BB, Liu JB, et al. Tissue-specific US contrast agent for evaluation of hepatic and splenic parenchyma. *Radiology* 1999;**210**:125–32.

21. Blomley MJK, Albrecht T, Wilson SR, et al. Improved detection of metastatic liver lesions using pulse inversion harmonic imaging with Levovist: a multicentre study. *Radiology* 1999;**213**:491.

22. Burns PN, Wilson SR. Focal liver masses: enhancement patterns on contrast-enhanced images–concordance of US scans with CT scans and MR images. *Radiology* 2007;**242**:162–74.

23. Wilson SR, Burns PN. An algorithm for the diagnosis of focal liver masses using microbubble contrast enhanced pulse inversion sonography. *AJR Am J Roentgenol* 2006;**186**:1401–12.

24. Claudon M, Cosgrove D, Albrecht T, et al. Guidelines and good clinical practice recommendations for contrast enhanced ultrasound (CEUS) – update 2008. *Ultraschall Med* 2008;**29**:28–44.

25. Murphy-Lavallee J, Jang HJ, Kim TK, et al. Are metastases really hypovascular in the arterial phase? The perspective based on contrast-enhanced ultrasonography. *J Ultrasound Med* 2007;**26**:1545–56.

26. Bhayana D, Kim TK, Jang HJ, et al. Hypervascular liver masses on contrast-enhanced ultrasound: the importance of washout. *AJR Am J Roentgenol* 2010;**194**:977–83.

27. Nicolau C, Vilana R, Bru C. The use of contrast-enhanced ultrasound in the management of the cirrhotic patient and for the detection of HCC. *Eur Radiol* 2004;**14**:P63–P71.

28. Claudon M, Cosgrove D, Albrecht T, et al. Guidelines and Good Clinical Practice Recommendations for Contrast Enhanced Ultrasound (CEUS) – Update 2008. *Ultraschall Med* 2008;**29**:28–44.

29. Berry JD, Sidhu PS. Microbubble contrast-enhanced ultrasound in liver transplantation. *Eur Radiol* 2004;**14**:P96–P103.

30. Marshall MM, Beese RC, Muiesan P, et al. Assessment of portal venous patency in the liver transplant candidate: a prospective study comparing ultrasound, microbubble-enhanced colour Doppler ultrasound with arteriography and surgery. *Clin Radiol* 2002;**57**:377–83.

31. Sidhu PS, Shaw AS, Ellis SM, et al. Microbubble ultrasound contrast in the assessment of hepatic artery patency following liver transplantation: role in reducing frequency of hepatic artery arteriography. *Eur Radiol* 2004;**14**:21–30.

32. Peddu P, Shah M, Sidhu PS. Splenic abnormalities: a comparative review of ultrasound, microbubble enhanced ultrasound and computed tomography. *Clin Radiol* 2004;**59**:777–92.

33. Gorg C, Bert T. Contrast enhanced sonography of focal splenic lesions with a second generation contrast agent. *Ultraschall Med* 2005;**26**:470–7.

34. von Herbay A, Barreiros AP, Ignee A, et al. Contrast-enhanced ultrasonography with SonoVue: differentiation between benign and malignant lesions of the spleen. *J Ultrasound Med* 2009;**28**:421–34.

35. Yu X, Yu J, Liang P, et al. Real-time contrast-enhanced ultrasound in diagnosing of focal spleen lesion. *Eur J Radiol* 2012;**81**:430–6.

36. Numata K, Ozawa Y, Kobayashi N, et al. Contrast-enhanced sonography of pancreatic carcinoma: correlations with pathological findings. *J Gastroenterol* 2005;**40**:631–40.

37. Dietrich CF, Braden B, Hocke M, et al. Improved characterisation of solitary pancreatic tumours using contrast enhanced transabdominal ultrasound. *J Cancer Res Clin Oncol* 2008;**134**:635–43.

38. Dietrich CF. Contrast-enhanced low mechanical index endoscopic ultrasound (CELMI-EUS). *Endoscopy* 2009;**41**: E43–5.

39. Ripolles T, Martinez MJ, Paredes JM, et al. Crohn disease: correlation of findings at contrast-enhanced US with severity at endoscopy. *Radiology* 2009;**253**:241–8.

40. Correas JM, Claudon M, Tranquart F, et al. The kidney: imaging with microbubble contrast agents. *Ultrasound Q* 2006;**22**:53–66.

41. Quaia E, Bertolotto M, Cioffi V, et al. Comparison of contrast-enhanced sonography with unenhanced sonography and contrast-enhanced CT in the diagnosis of malignancy in complex cystic renal masses. *AJR Am J Roentgenol* 2008;**191**:1239–49.

42. Claudon M, Plouin PF, Baxter GM, et al. Renal arteries in patients at risk of renal arterial stenosis: multicentre evaluation of the Echo-enhancer SH U 508A at color and spectral Doppler US. *Radiology* 2000;**214**:737–46.

43. Harvey CJ, Sidhu PS. Ultrasound contrast agents in genitourinary imaging. *Ultrasound Clin North Am* 2011;**5**:489–506.

44. Catalano O, Aiani L, Barozzi L, et al. CEUS in abdominal trauma: multi-centre study. *Abdom Imaging* 2009;**34**:225–34.

45. Piscaglia F, Nolsøe C, Dietrich C, et al. The EFSUMB Guidelines and Recommendations on the Clinical Practice of Contrast Enhanced Ultrasound (CEUS). Update 2011 on non-hepatic applications. *Ultraschall Med* 2012;**32**:33-59.

46. Darge K. Voiding urosonography with US contrast agents for the diagnosis of vesicureteric reflux in children. II.

Comparison with radiological examinations. *Pediatr Radiol* 2008;**38**:54–63.

47. Ayida G, Harris P, Kennedy S, et al. Hysterosalpingo-contrast sonography (HyCoSy) using Echovist-200 in the outpatient investigation of infertility patients. *Br J Radiol* 1996;**69**:910–13.

48. Lanzani C, Savasi V, Leone FP, et al. Two-dimensional HyCoSy with contrast tuned imaging technology and a second generation contrast media for the assessment of tubal patency in an infertility program. *Fertil-Steril* 2009;**92**:1158–61.

49. Stacey C, Brown C, Manhire A, et al. HyCoSy – as good as claimed? *Br J Radiol* 2000;**73**:133–6.

50. Lock G, Schmidt C, Helmich F, et al. Early experience with contrast enhanced ultrasound in the diagnosis of testicular masses; a feasibility study. *Urology* 2011;**77**:1049–53.

51. Patel K, Sellars ME, Clarke JL, et al. Features of testicular epidermoid cysts on contrast enhanced ultrasound and real time elastography. *J Ultrasound Med* 2012;**31**:1115–22.

52. Bertolotto M, Derchi LE, Sidhu PS, et al. Acute segmental testicular infarction at contrast-enhanced ultrasound: early features and changes during follow-up. *AJR Am J Roentgenol* 2011;**196**:834–41.

53. Lung PF, Jaffer OS, Sellars ME, et al. Contrast enhanced ultrasound (CEUS) in the evaluation of focal testicular complications secondary to epidiymitis. *AJR Am J Roentgenol* 2012;**199**:W345–54.

54. Strazdina A, Krumina G, Sperga M. The value and limitations of contrast-enhanced ultrasound in detection of prostate cancer. *Anticancer Res* 2011;**31**:1421–6.

55. Sorelli PG, Cosgrove DO, Svensson WE, et al. Can contrast-enhanced sonography distingush benign from malignant breast masses. *J Clin Ultrasound* 2010;**38**:177–81.

56. Sever AR, Mills P, Jones SE, et al. Preoperative sentinel node identification with ultrasound using microbubbles in patients with breast cancer. *AJR Am J Roentgenol* 2011;**196**:251–6.

57. Gorg C. Transcutaneous contrast-enhanced sonography of pleural-based pulmonary lesions. *Eur J Radiol* 2007;**64**:213–21.

58. Otis SM, Rush M, Boyajian R. Contrast-enhanced transcranial imaging. Results of an American phase-two study. *Stroke* 1995;**26**:203–9.

59. Postert T, Braun B, Meves S, et al. Contrast-enhanced transcranial color-coded sonography in acute hemispheric brain infarction. *Stroke* 1999;**30**:1819–26.

60. Seidel G, Kaps M. Harmonic imaging of the vertebrobasilar system. *Stroke* 1997;**28**:1610–13.

61. Sitzer M, Rose G, Furst G, et al. Characteristics and clinical value of an intravenous echo-enhancement agent in evaluation of high-grade internal carotid stenosis. *J Neuroimaging* 1997;**7**:S22–5.

62. Furst G, Saleh A, Wenserski F, et al. Reliability and validity of non-invasive imaging of internal carotid artery pseudo-occlusion. *Stroke* 1999;**30**:1444–9.

63. Clevert DA, Sommer WH, Zengel P, et al. Imaging of carotid arterial diseases with contrast-enhanced ultrasound (CEUS). *Eur J Radiol* 2011;**80**:68–76.

64. Shalhoub J, Owen DRJ, Gauthier T, et al. The use of contrast enhanced ultrasound in carotid arterial disease. *Eur J Vasc Endovasc Surg* 2010;**39**:381–7.

65. Clevert DA, Stickel M, Johnson T, et al. Imaging of aortic abnormalities with contrast-enhanced ultrasound. A pictorial comparison with CT. *Eur Radiol* 2007;**17**:2991–3000.

66. Clevert DA, Sommer WH, Meimerakis G, et al. Contrast-enhanced ultrasound compared with multislice computed tomography for endovascular aneurysm repair surveillance. *Ultrasound* 2011;**19**:11–19.

67. Carotti M, Salaffi F, Manganelli P, et al. Power Doppler sonography in the assessment of synovial tissue of the knee joint in rheumatoid arthritis: a preliminary experience. *Ann Rheum Dis* 2002;**61**:877–82.

68. Klauser AS, Franz M, Arora R, et al. Detection of vascularity in wrist tenosynovitis: power Doppler ultrasound compared with contrast-enhanced grey-scale ultrasound. *Arthritis Res Ther* 2010;**12**:R209.

69. Price RJ, Skyba DM, Kaul S, et al. Delivery of colloidal particles and red blood cells to tissue through microvessel ruptures created by targeted microbubble destruction with ultrasound. *Circulation* 1998;**98**:1264–7.

70. Lentacker I, Geers B, Demeester J, et al. Design and evaluation of doxorubicin-containing microbubbles for ultrasound triggered doxorubicin delivery: cytotoxicity and mechanisms involved. *Mol Ther* 2010;**18**:101–8.

Appendix: System Controls and Their Uses

Paul L. Allan

In addition to the basic choice of transducer type and frequency for the examination in hand, there are many other factors on a Doppler ultrasound system which need to be adjusted. Despite the efforts of the manufacturers to automate and simplify things, it is still necessary to adjust continually many of the scan and Doppler parameters during the course of an examination. Is the vessel superficial or deep? Is flow fast or slow, high volume or low volume? Most systems now come with a variety of preset programs for different situations: peripheral arteries, veins, cerebrovascular, etc.; together with automatic image and spectral display optimisation. Many also have the facility to allow users to save their own program preferences, which is a convenient option to store preferred settings once a satisfactory set up has been achieved for a particular type of examination. Whilst the manufacturer's presets allow the basic appropriate settings to be employed at the start of an examination, fine adjustments will still be required during the course of the examination to make the most of the available information. Familiarity with the ultrasound system, together with experience, enable skilled operators to set up their system appropriately for the examination being performed. Different manufacturers sometimes use different names for the same controls or functions; it is not possible to give an exhaustive list of all the possible options on the range of modern equipment now available but the following notes describe the basic controls, or parameters on most systems that can be adjusted during the course of an examination to improve and maximise the information that is obtained from the examination.

General Principles

TRANSDUCER FREQUENCY

The highest frequency which will achieve the highest resolution consistent with adequate penetration for imaging is normally chosen. The Doppler frequency used by any transducer is often 1–2 MHz below the imaging frequency, although modern equipment has a wide range of receive frequencies such as 5–14 MHz. In addition to the basic imaging requirements, it should be remembered that the deeper a vessel lies, the longer it takes a sound pulse to travel there and back, so that the Nyquist limit becomes very relevant (Chapter 1), limits the Doppler frequencies that can be used and therefore the frequency shifts/velocities that can be recorded accurately.

B-MODE IMAGE

For colour Doppler examinations this should be set up with relatively low overall gain, so that the image is a little on the dark side as the software tends to allocate colour to darker areas, rather than to areas which contain echoes. See 'Colour write priority' below.

TRANSMIT POWER

The transmit power of the system should be set at the lowest level consistent with an adequate examination, especially during obstetric and gynaecological examinations. It is better to start at a medium level and increase the power only after other measures to improve system sensitivity have been tried, such as adjusting colour gate size, removing filters, adjusting the scale/pulse repetition rate. For low mechanical index (MI) contrast studies (see Chapter 17) the transmit power should be set as low as possible and the MI reading ideally should be less than 0.4. Modern systems often have contrast-agent-specific programs already installed, or the relevant settings can be obtained from the supplier of the contrast agent.

UPDATE/DUPLEX/TRIPLEX

In duplex ultrasound there is the ability to acquire and display both real time imaging and spectral Doppler information either simultaneously, or alternately. Simultaneous display results in degradation of both the image and the spectral display as the computer has to process data from both sources. The update facility allows the operator to set the system to handle either imaging data, or Doppler data. This results in a higher quality of display for the selected mode and it is usually used for acquisition of the best-quality spectral display for analysis. Simultaneous duplex scanning is of some value in the initial stages of an examination in order to position the sample volume in a specific area of interest. Triplex mode refers to the simultaneous acquisition, processing and display of colour Doppler, spectral display and imaging information. As with duplex scanning, this requires significant division of processing power and consequent compromise in the quality of the display. Newer systems with more powerful computers are less prone to these problems but there is still a division of processing power and experienced operators will still tend to switch between imaging and spectral Doppler for optimal results.

AUTOMATIC IMAGE OPTIMISATION

Many systems now have automatic image optimisation controls which adjust factors such as time gain compensation, receiver gain and colour Doppler gain to improve the image. In some cases this facility can also be applied to the spectral display. These can be useful in getting a reasonable initial display but should not be relied upon entirely and the operator needs to make the final adjustments to obtain the best images.

Colour Doppler Controls

COLOUR BOX

This defines the area of the image over which colour Doppler data are acquired. It can be adjusted for size, position and direction/angulation. It is better to keep the box as small and as superficial as practical because larger areas take more processing power and time. Larger sizes and greater angulations may therefore reduce frame rates. Greater angulation also reduces sensitivity, which can therefore be improved by reducing the degree of angulation of the colour box, for instance when examining deeper segments of the femoral vein in larger legs. Deeper boxes need slower pulse repetition frequencies, therefore limiting the size of shift that can be measured without aliasing.

COLOUR MAP

Choose a colour map that has good contrast for the identification of aliasing. Maps which grade to white at each end, or to very pale colours, do not give as much information about aliasing as those which have significantly different colours, such as pale green and pale orange. Variance maps were said to register the amount of spectral broadening in the colour map, although this is not easy to appreciate and may, in fact, not be true as this 'variance' seems to reflect the velocity, rather than spectral broadening. Variance maps are most frequently used in cardiological examinations. In addition, colour tags can be put into the scale so that velocities above or below the chosen range can be identified.

COLOUR GAIN

The colour gain is set to the optimal level. This can be identified by turning up the gain until noise/colour speckle is seen in the colour box and then backing off slightly on the overall colour gain. It should also be adjusted to remove any spill of the colour map over the boundaries of the vessel seen on the B-mode images; this is sometimes called colour bleeding. Colour gain often needs to be increased if the colour box is moved to a deeper location.

COLOUR SCALE

The colour scale should be set to levels appropriate for the range of velocities under investigation. It should be remembered that colour Doppler only gives information on the mean Doppler shift in a pixel; the mean velocity in a pixel is only calculated when an angle correction for that pixel is performed. The colour scale is closely related to the pulse repetition frequency, or sampling rate; this has to be above the Nyquist limit for the frequency shift being measured.

If it is set too low then aliasing will occur; this can be rectified by increasing the colour scale range, also known as the pulse repetition frequency. If it is set too high then there will be poor colour sensitivity for slower velocities, resulting in inadequate colour fill-in across the vessel.

COLOUR INVERSION

This changes the colour map display for mapping the direction of blood flow in relation to the transducer, e.g. red for flow towards the transducer and blue for away from the transducer, or vice versa.

COLOUR GATE

This relates to the size of the colour pixels, a smaller size gives better spatial resolution, whereas a larger size provides better sensitivity at the expense of spatial and sometimes temporal resolution.

COLOUR BASELINE

The colour baseline can be adjusted to provide a wider range of shifts on one side or the other, depending on the characteristics of the blood flow in the vessel being examined and particularly if the flow is in only one direction.

COLOUR FILTERS

These help remove low-frequency noise and clutter from the image. It is best to set filters at the lowest level compatible with an acceptable image as they also remove low-frequency shift information from the image.

COLOUR WRITE PRIORITY

A pixel in the image can display either B-mode imaging information, or colour Doppler information. The colour write priority facility allows the relative priorities for these two types of information to be defined. High colour priority results in colour information being displayed in areas which might contain low-intensity imaging information, for instance at the margins of vessels. Alternatively, high imaging priority results in grey scale information displacing colour information, such as might occur with reverberation artefacts appearing within the vessel lumen amongst the colour Doppler information.

COLOUR PERSISTENCE

This reflects the amount of frame-averaging which occurs. A low level of persistence results in an image which has a fast temporal response but may have a poor signal-to-noise ratio. A high level of persistence improves the signal-to-noise ratio by summating data from several frames, but this results in an impaired temporal response, so that pulsatile flow information is dampened.

Power Doppler Controls

Although the power mode is intrinsically simpler than velocity mode, there are still several controls and options which influence the power image.

POWER MAPS

Most systems offer a variety of colour maps from which the operator can select according to personal preference, usually a yellow- or magenta-based scale is used for display of power Doppler information. The threshold or sensitivity can be varied; this results in changes in the transparency of the power box. When the power map background is opaque the sensitivity is maximal. Various degrees of increasing translucency are available so that sensitivity can be traded for imaging and anatomical information.

POWER GAIN

This is similar to colour gain and amplifies the received Doppler signal. Excessive gain will result in unnecessary noise and artefact in the image.

SCALE

The energy scale affects the sensitivity of the system for signal intensities of varying strengths: lower scales are more sensitive to lower-intensity signals, which will also increase flash artefact. On some systems the power Doppler scale is linked to the filter settings.

DYNAMIC RANGE

As in spectral Doppler, this affects the range of signal intensities over which the available colour scale is spread and the appearance of the Doppler information on the screen: increasing the dynamic range will tend to increase the amount of colour on the screen.

POWER BOX STEERING ANGLE

As with the colour box, the power box can be adjusted for size, position and direction/angulation. Although the power display is much less dependent on angle than the velocity display, there may still be loss of the power signal at 90° because these low Doppler frequencies fall below the motion discrimination filter cut-off level. In most situations, steering the power Doppler box does not have much effect on the display; however, the loss of signal at 90° may be overcome by having a degree of angulation of the transducer.

POWER/COLOUR HYBRID IMAGES

Many systems now allow a hybrid image containing both power Doppler and colour Doppler data to be displayed. This aims to combine the sensitivity of power Doppler with the directional and velocity information from colour Doppler. On some systems, the relative contributions from the two sources can be adjusted.

FILTERS

Motion discrimination filters in power Doppler are used to filter out excessive signal noise from structures, other than blood, which are moving in the Doppler box. Low filter settings provide more sensitivity but are more prone to flash artefacts, whereas higher filter settings reduce flash artefacts but will also filter out some blood flow information.

Spectral Controls

SPECTRAL GAIN

This affects the receiver gain for the spectral display. As in B-mode imaging, the level should be adjusted in order to give a balanced distribution of grey shades across the displayed spectra. Excessive or inadequate levels of gain will produce erroneous estimates of Doppler shift/velocity.

SPECTRAL DYNAMIC RANGE

This can be varied to optimise the display of particular frequency shifts. A narrow dynamic range results in the loss of low-intensity shifts above and below the main shift frequencies. Conversely a wide dynamic range, particularly if associated with a high level of

spectral receiver gain, can result in artefactual broadening of the spectra displayed. Further manipulation of the spectral display can be performed by altering the postprocessing algorithms on some systems in order to emphasise, or suppress, particular frequency shifts. In normal practice a simple linear allocation is most convenient.

SPECTRAL SCALE

Altering the scale affects the pulse repetition frequency and thus the range of shifts which can be registered without aliasing. In practice the scale is adjusted so that the Doppler waveform is displayed without wrap-around, which indicates aliasing. The scale may be displayed as either a KHz scale for frequency shift, or a velocity scale. The use of velocity, rather than frequency shift, allows some comparison of different examinations, performed with different transducer frequencies and with different angles of insonation.

SPECTRAL INVERSION

This allows the operator to change the orientation of the display. Many operators prefer to display both arterial and venous waveforms above the baseline, even if flow is away from the transducer. However, care is therefore required when assessing the vertebral arteries for reverse flow, or the leg veins for reflux, as errors may occur if spectral inversion is not recognised. Some centres do not allow spectral inversion because of the potential for misinterpretation, particularly in relation to examinations for venous insufficiency.

SPECTRAL SWEEP SPEED

A medium speed is adequate for most arterial work, with a slower speed better for venous flow. A fast sweep speed is useful for acceleration time measurement and waveform analysis, particularly if there is tachycardia.

ANGLE CORRECTION

The measurement of the angle of insonation relative to the direction of flow is required in spectral Doppler in order to convert frequency shift information into velocity information and also in colour Doppler to convert mean pixel shifts into mean velocities. The main direction of flow may not necessarily be parallel to the vessel wall and colour Doppler is useful in precise positioning of the angle-correction cursor along the line of the jet. The angle of insonation should be less than 60° or the errors in velocity calculation become significant.

GATE SIZE

This defines the range of depths from which Doppler data are collected. The gate should be positioned across the lumen of the vessel but clear of the walls in order to reduce wall thump artefact. The position of the gate which corresponds to the maximum Doppler shift is located using a combination of the colour map for initial positioning and then refining this using the operator's ears, which are the most sensitive and efficient spectral analyser available; with experience, your ears will register when the peak frequency shift is obtained. If an assessment of volume flow is being made, the gate should be wide enough to encompass the entire vessel width so that all the flow contributes to the signal and the time-averaged mean velocity will be most representative. Smaller gates give a cleaner signal, especially with laminar flow, but at the expense of a reduction in sensitivity.

FILTERS

Removal of low-frequency noise and clutter arising from the vessel wall and surrounding tissues contributes to a cleaner signal, but filters should be set as low as is practical, otherwise low-frequency shifts from slow blood flow will be filtered out, which could result in the mistaken impression of absent diastolic flow in arteries, or occlusion in veins. In practice it is best to keep the filters set at the lowest setting and only increase filtration as required during an examination.

Conclusions

Modern systems allow the operator to preset many of these parameters and create different personal profiles/setups for different types of examination such as veins, carotids, renal, etc. However, it should be remembered that ultrasound is a dynamic examination and, even with modern equipment, the best results will be obtained if the system controls are adjusted to optimum settings for the task in hand, rather than relying on the preset profiles alone.

Index